The Voice
and Voice Therapy

FIFTH EDITION

Daniel R. Boone
University of Arizona

Stephen C. McFarlane
University of Nevada Medical School

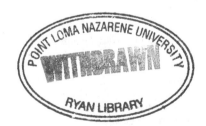

PRENTICE HALL, Englewood Cliffs, New Jersey 07632

Library of Congress Cataloging-in-Publication Data

BOONE, DANIEL R.
    The voice and voice therapy/Daniel R. Boone, Stephen C.
  McFarlane—5th ed.
      p.   cm.
    Includes bibliographical references and index.
    ISBN 0-13-030677-0
    1. Voice disorders. 2. Larynx—Diseases. I. McFarlane, Stephen
  C. II. Title.
      [DNLM: 1. Voice—physiology. 2. Voice Disorders—etiology.
  3. Voice Disorders—therapy. 4. Voice Disorders—diagnosis.
  5. Speech, Alaryngeal. 6. Voice Training   WV 500 B724v   1993]
  RF540.B66   1993
  616.85'5—dc20
  DNLM/DLC   93-32168
  for Library of Congress   CIP

Editorial/production supervision,
    interior design, and electronic page makeup: Kari Callaghan Mazzola
Acquisitions editor: Charlyce Jones Owen
Cover design: DeLuca Design
Production coordinator: Mary Ann Gloriande

© 1994, 1988, 1983, 1977, 1971 by Prentice-Hall, Inc.
A Paramount Communications Company
Englewood Cliffs, New Jersey 07632

Printed in the United States of America
10 9 8 7 6 5 4 3 2 1

ISBN 0-13-030677-0

PRENTICE-HALL INTERNATIONAL (UK) LIMITED, *London*
PRENTICE-HALL OF AUSTRALIA PTY. LIMITED, *Sydney*
PRENTICE-HALL CANADA INC., *Toronto*
PRENTICE-HALL HISPANOAMERICANA, S.A., *Mexico*
PRENTICE-HALL OF INDIA PRIVATE LIMITED, *New Delhi*
PRENTICE-HALL OF JAPAN, INC., *Tokyo*
SIMON & SCHUSTER ASIA PTE. LTD., *Singapore*
EDITORA PRENTICE-HALL DO BRASIL, LTDA., *Rio de Janeiro*

Contents

Chapter 6 *Voice Therapy for Special Problems*   210

Chapter 7 *Therapy for Resonance Disorders*   244

Chapter 8 *Evaluation and Voice Therapy in Various Settings*   272

Preface

The writing of the first edition of *The Voice and Voice Therapy* began about twenty-five years ago. Although a number of voice improvement books or voice science books were available at the time, each with its own distinctive following, clinical voice textbooks were few in number. The European influence on voice rehabilitation was seen in the early writings of Emil Froeschels, Godfrey Arnold, Muriel Morley, Margaret Greene, Deso Weiss, and Friedrich Brodnitz. Among the prominent American clinical voice writers up to twenty-five years ago were Virgil Anderson, G. Oscar Russell, Robert West, Georgianna Peacher, Harlan Bloomer, Paul Moore, Jon Eisenson, and John Irwin. When *The Voice and Voice Therapy* was first published in 1971, the three principal clinical voice textbooks used in some American universities were Greene's *The Voice and Its Disorders*, Van Riper and Irwin's *Voice and Articulation*, and Brodnitz's *Vocal Rehabilitation*.

Voice evaluation and therapy have improved immeasurably during the life span of this book. Twenty-five years ago, because of lack of computer-based instrumentation, voice measurement was more primitive, focusing more on static measurement (such as voice pitch) than on dynamic aspects of voicing (such as mucosal wave movement). Likewise, lacking good instrumental feedback to the patient, voice therapy had to rely more on the patient's ear (and the clinician's) than on visual confirmation of various vocal achievements. Clinician–patient caring and effective clinical interaction between clinician and patient were primary factors in bringing about clinical change (better-sounding voices, smaller nodules, etc.). These factors still play an important role.

The fifth edition of this book reflects continuous changes in vocal rehabilitation. We have attempted to integrate much of the mushrooming clinical voice research into these pages, so that particular research findings might have clinical utilization in the various clinical settings in which voice clinicians work.

We would like to thank the following reviewers: Charles L. Wilhelm, *Fort Hays State University*; Richard Ham, *Florida State University*; Joseph S. Attanasio, *Montclair State College*; Colette L. Coleman, *California State University–Sacramento*. We have complied with our readers' and reviewers' requests that we keep the basic eight-chapter format used in the four previous editions. In Chapter 1, we take a look at how the voice is influenced by the larynx in its ever-changing biological, emotional, and linguistic roles. In Chapter 2, we attempt to integrate new knowledge specific to laryngeal physiology as we review vocal tract structure and voice function. The voice disorders seen in our present clinics are described in Chapter 3. Significant textual changes can be found in Chapter 4, in which we present the latest diagnostic-evaluative procedures that are used in many clinics. Our Chapter 5 continues to be one of the most valuable chapters in the book (according to our clinical readers) with its procedural presentations of twenty-five voice therapy approaches. Chapter 6 becomes a bit longer in each successive edition, looking at voice therapy for special problems ranging from spasmodic dysphonia to laryngectomy. In Chapter 7, we look at resonance problems, their evaluation, and their management. Chapter 8 is a totally new chapter that looks at the practice of voice evaluation/therapy in various settings, such as schools, hospitals, clinics, and private practice.

Since our fourth edition, there has been a marked increase in the study of voice disorders, their evaluation, and their management. Since 1987, we have the new *Journal of Voice*, published by the Voice Foundation. This new quarterly journal has proved to be an important source for increasing the literature on voice, combining the perspectives of the physician, the singing and voice coach, the voice scientist, and the speech-language pathologist. Also, within the American Speech-Language-Hearing Association is a special interest group for members who are interested in the voice and its disorders. There also appear to be more courses related to voice pathology in graduate training programs.

There is dynamic world interest in the voice and voice disorders. Worldwide conferences and symposia and a burgeoning world literature are all contributing to our understanding of voice disorders and their treatment. This new edition of *The Voice and Voice Therapy* comes out at an exciting time in the evolution of the study of voice disorders and their treatment. We hope we have portrayed that excitement here.

Daniel R. Boone, Ph.D.
Stephen C. McFarlane, Ph.D.

Chapter 1

The Voice and Voice Therapy

This book focuses on voice disorders, voice evaluation, and voice therapy. A voice disorder is often a symptom of laryngeal dysfunction and is sometimes a symptom of serious laryngeal disease. Although we consider in this chapter the important biological role the larynx plays in human survival, we center on the many facets of voice from the simple expressions of emotion to our most complex spoken communication. We see how voice disorders can seriously interfere with effective communication. We look at specific voice disorders, some the result of a faulty laryngeal mechanism (such as vocal cord paralysis) and some the result of using the vocal mechanisms incorrectly (such as the hoarseness heard in functional dysphonia).

In the ensuing chapters of the book, we look closely at the vocal tract and how it works, with attention given to understanding particular voice disorders and their evaluation, followed by methods of case management and voice therapy.

THE BIOLOGICAL FUNCTION OF THE LARYNX

In Chapter 2, the total structures of the airway are introduced. Names and function are given to the various components of the vocal tract, beginning with the structures and mechanics of respiration, followed by voice function (phonation), and ending with a look at the structures and mechanisms that contribute to vocal resonance.

A description of the biological aspects of laryngeal function provides us an early hint of how the biological demands of the airway and the larynx will always take precedence over artistic or communicative vocal production. When the brain signals the body's need for renewal of oxygen in the breath cycle, we automatically take in a breath. Oxygen-ladened air flows through the passages of the upper airway into the lungs, followed by the outgoing carbon-dioxide-loaded air flowing out of the body through the airway. This transportation of air into and out of the lungs is the primary function of the airway. Protecting the airway for an unobstructed passage of the air supply is the larynx. The primary biological function of the larynx is to keep fluids and foods from going into the airway (aspiration).

The larynx sits in a vital site at the front, bottom of the throat (pharynx) and at the top of the windpipe (trachea). As fluids and chewed food (bolus) come down the posterior throat, they are diverted from the lower throat (hypopharynx) into the open esophagus, where they continue their journey through the esophagus down into the stomach. As part of the swallowing act, the laryngeal mechanism rises high (elevating the esophagus and trachea with it) in the neck. As the swallow progresses, the tongue comes back, pushing against the epiglottis cartilage of the larynx, which from this pushing action closes over the open larynx.

Whenever the larynx plays this sphincteral role of closing off the airway to permit the posterior passage of liquids or food, the entire laryngeal body rises. Also, in fear situations, the larynx may reflexively elevate as part of its primary role in protecting the airway. Some voice patients, sometimes those with excessive fears, will attempt voice with the larynx in its elevated "protector" posture. Such excessive laryngeal elevation is not a good posture for producing a normal voice.

Besides the elevating capability of the larynx, which helps prevent aspiration, airway closure is aided by three laryngeal muscle valves, described in Chapter 2 as the aryepiglottic folds, the ventricular folds (false folds), and the thyroarytenoid muscles (the true vocal cords, or vocal folds). The most vertical of these valve pairs in the larynx are the aryepiglottic folds, which are considered part of the supralarynx. Under vigorous valving conditions, such as severe coughing, they begin to approximate (adduct) each other. Below them are the ventricular folds; only during vigorous adductory activities, like the cough, do they approach each other. The lowest and more medial of the three laryngeal valves are the thyroarytenoid muscles, the true vocal folds (cords). During swallow, they always adduct to prevent possible aspiration. Also, the individual has fine control of the true folds with some capability of altering their shape, length, and tension, producing various voicing changes.

When an individual breathes naturally, all three valve sites are open.

The vocal folds are open in a paramedian position (halfway between open and closed); on inspiration, the vocal folds separate a bit more (abduct) and on expiration, they move slightly toward (adduct) each other. If the individual were to cough, all three valve sites would adduct medially, closing off the airway. In Chapter 2, we discover that normal voice (phonation) is achieved by the true vocal folds adducting with the outgoing airstream passing between them, setting them into vibration. The vertical changes of laryngeal height and the degree of adductory or abductory positioning can have a profound influence on the sound of the voice. We will see in Chapter 3 that inadequate adduction can lead to no voice (aphonia); excessive vocal fold adduction produces an extremely tight-sounding voice (spasmodic dysphonia).

THE EMOTIONAL FUNCTION OF THE LARYNX

As early as 3 months old, the infant seems to express emotions by making laryngeal sounds. Certainly, the care giver can soon detect differences in the emotional state of the baby by changes in the sound of the baby's vocalizations: A cry from hunger may sound different from a cry of discomfort or the vocalization of anger. Contentment (after a full stomach or being held) can be heard in the cooing responses of the baby. From early infancy throughout the life span, the sound of one's vocalization often mirrors one's internal emotional state.

Our voice can sound happy or sad, contented or angry, secure or unsafe, placid or passionate. How one feels affectively may be heard in the sound of the voice as well as in changes of the prosodic rhythm patterns of vocalization. Our emotional status plays a primary role in the control of respiration; for example, nervousness can be heard in one's shortness of breath. Our emotional state seems to dictate the vertical positioning of the larynx, the relative relaxation of the vocal folds, the posturing and relaxation of the muscles of the pharynx and tongue.

One's emotionality can be heard in the voice, a fact that can be threatening to the professional singer, or harmful to sales for the nervous salesperson, or embarrassing to someone who sounds like he or she is crying when actually happy. Our mood state can be harmful to voice. Many voice disorders are the result of various affective excesses; for example, a young professional woman attempts to use normal conversational voice when her larynx is postured in a high, sphincterally closed position, resulting in a tight, tense voice. Her problem may be more related to unchecked and unrealistic fear than it is to faulty use of the vocal mechanisms per se.

Because emotionality and vocal function are so closely entwined, effective voice therapy often requires the treatment of the total person and not just fixating on the remediation of voice symptoms. Therefore, as we will see in ensuing chapters, getting to know the patient is an important prerequisite to taking a case history or making an instrumental-perceptual voice evaluation. Voice clinicians have long recognized that the patient in the office may not resemble the same person in play settings; the patient's voice will change according to his or her mood state. To assess voice realistically, we have to observe and listen to the patient in various life settings.

THE LINGUISTIC FUNCTION OF THE VOICE

Voice seems to hold spoken language together. From the primitive emotional vocalization that may color what we say to the skilled use of voice stress to emphasize a particular utterance, the voicing component of spoken language plays a primary role. It is not always what we say that carries the message, but how we say it.

New interest in infant vocalization is producing a fascinating literature. By the time typical 1-year old babies utter their first word, they have already used their voice in highly elaborate jargon communication. While human babies all seem to babble about the same way from 4 to 6 months of age, babbling becomes more language differentiated beyond that age. That is, babies no longer sound alike after 6 months; rather, they begin to sound like the primary language they have been hearing. The melody of the parent language, or its prosody, begins to color the vocalizations of the baby. The jargon of Chinese babies begins to sound like the sweeping tonal patterns of the Chinese language; the guttural sounds of an Arab language begin to be heard in the jargon of Arab babies.

These prosodic vocal patterns exist far beyond the individual word or segment. In fact, such voicing is known as suprasegmental phonation. In young babies, suprasegmental vocalization far exceeds the voicing of actual word segments. As babies acquire new words, they often place them in the proper place of their ongoing voicing rhythm. If they want to say "milk," rather than say the word in isolation, they are far more likely to say the word at the end of a jargon phrase, such as "gawa na ta milk." The jargon leading up to the word is suprasegmental voicing. The jargon voice carries an uncoded message with no specific meaning but seems to convey some general meaning by the overall sound of it. The mood and need state of the baby influence the sound of the vocalization. And it appears that the sound of our voice colors the meaning of what we say for a lifetime.

Although jargon speech appears to diminish after the first 18 months of life, we continue to use suprasegmental vocalization in all aspects of spoken communication. We add vocal stress patterns to augment the meaning of what we say. The actual words we say are only part of the communication. The "how we say it" is conveyed by various vocal stress strategies, such as changing loudness, grouping words together on one breath, changing pitch level, changing vocal quality and resonance to match our mood. These stress changes of the suprasegmentals of what we say can be produced with or without intent. That is, if it serves our purpose, we can sound angry by talking louder, or we may sound angry despite our best efforts to hide our anger from our listener. Once again, the voice carries much of the message. The same words spoken or written may convey different messages (as any lawyer taking depositions will tell you) depending on the stress patterns given the words by the speaker, with or without intent.

Considering the role of the voice in both emotional and linguistic expression, it is no wonder that people with voice disorders may find themselves handicapped in their communication. A young girl with vocal nodules, for example, may have developed them in part from excessive emotional vocalization (such as constantly yelling). Once the nodules were developed, however, she may be unable to use the vocal suprasegmentals and stress patterns she had previously used in communication. As anyone knows who has ever suffered a complete loss of voice from severe laryngitis, the lack of voice prevents you from being you. Somehow whisper and gesture do not carry the communication effectiveness that normal voice allows you to add to the words you say.

While a primary role of the human larynx appears to be biological (guarding the airway), laryngeal voicing plays a vital role in the expression of both emotional and linguistic communication. When we add the voicing dimensions of acting and singing as laryngeal functions, we can truly appreciate the amazing artistic capabilities of the vocal tract (that a few people are fortunate to have and sometimes use). The role of the human larynx is obviously more complex and more subtle than the way the larynx functions as an airway protector in most other mammals.

Physical disorders of the airway, larynx, and resonating cavities can affect all of these functions: biological, emotional, linguistic, and artistic. We will look at various physically caused voice disorders in Chapter 3, such as a disorder of vocal cord paralysis. With unilateral paralysis, typically the patient cannot bring his or her vocal folds together adequately, preventing the production of normal voice.

VOICE DISORDERS RELATED TO ORGANIC PROBLEMS

While the majority of voice problems may well be functional in origin, some of them are physically caused by various airway disorders. We classify these physical problems as organic voice disorders.

Any voice problem that lasts more than a week should be medically investigated for possible physical causation. Sometimes the required treatment will be medical-surgical, and voice therapy will only help to find and maintain the best possible voice. Some organic voice problems are static, relatively fixed, and not responsive to medical treatment; for these problems, voice therapy becomes the only remediation possible. Although specific disorders of voice related to organic problems and their management will be presented in Chapter 6, let us consider a voice problem related to a physical cause:

> Charles, a 58-year-old chef, began to experience a shortness of breath that allowed him to say only about five words per breath. Physical examination indicated that he had severe pulmonary emphysema, probably directly related to his smoking about three packs of cigarettes daily. In fact, he reported to his doctor that in his 20s and 30s, he had smoked four packs a day, but he had cut back because the continuous smoking interfered with his preparing meals in his restaurant. Extensive pulmonary and respiratory testing revealed that Charles had lost most of his lung elasticity, which was confirmed by his inability to empty his lungs quickly on various tests. When asked to count as far as he could on one breath, he could count only to five; he could prolong a vowel for only 8 seconds. Endoscopic examination showed that Charles had additive growth along the glottal margin of the vocal folds, a condition diagnosed as leukoplakia. Although no medical treatment was recommended for Charles's pulmonary emphysema, much of the leukoplakia was removed surgically. In voice therapy, Charles practiced extending his expirations. With practice, he could count to 15 on one breath, extend vowels for over 15 seconds, and say 8 to 10 words on one expiration. Functionally, despite the irreversible lung disease, Charles was able to increase his ability to say more words with less shortness of breath. Following the surgery on his vocal folds, he received some voice therapy to help establish a voice pitch level he found acceptable.

The case of Charles illustrates a speech-voice problem caused by two organic diseases, pulmonary emphysema and laryngeal leukoplakia. Voice therapy helped the patient learn to breathe more efficiently for speech; in effect, Charles learned to say more words per expiration. Surgical removal of the laryngeal lesions followed by voice therapy helped to reestablish an acceptable voice. As illustrated here, voice therapy can often be effective in helping voice patients with various organic voice problems develop the best voice possible.

Impairment in Respiration

The respiratory system functions as the activator of voice. The expiratory airflow pressures and volumes passing between the approximated vocal folds set the folds into vibration, which produces voice. Therefore, any compromise of respiratory function can have a direct effect on speech (number of words said) and voice (loudness, pitch, quality). Lung volume may be reduced by space-occupying lesions in the lungs, such as various forms of cancer or fluids in the lung; a reduction in air volume will reduce the amount of air the speaker can use for voice. Diseases of the airway, such as bronchitis or emphysema, can decrease lung elasticity and make it more difficult for the patient to sustain airflow and voicing. Although organic disease of the respiratory system may require medical treatment, voice therapy can often help patients develop the best respiratory control possible for speech and voice. Like Charles, most voice patients can improve their functional respiratory expiration by working on it directly.

Impairment in the Movement of the Folds

There are several physical ways that the movement of the vocal folds may be impaired. The vocal folds normally move toward one another (adduct) for phonation by the active contraction of the intrinsic laryngeal muscles. The folds are held together by active muscle contraction during phonation, working against the tendency to be blown apart by the airflow beneath and between them. The adduction of the folds is sometimes compromised by destruction of the nerves that innervate these laryngeal muscles, as described in Chapter 3. This produces weakness or paralysis of the laryngeal muscles, resulting in vocal fold paralysis.

Other neuromuscular problems may prevent normal vocal fold approximation as a result of some kind of destruction within the cerebrum, perhaps as a result of a stroke or some form of degenerative disease. When phonation is impaired because of a problem in the central nervous system (CNS), the problem is usually part of a *dysarthria* (speech-voice-fluency impairment secondary to CNS involvement). We discuss dysarthria and its voice symptoms in greater detail in Chapter 6. Overall management of voice problems related to neural innervation requires medical care as well as the short-range and long-range participation of a speech-language pathologist.

Sometimes, the movement of the vocal folds may be inhibited by a laryngeal web growing between the glottal margin of each fold. If such a web is identified, it is usually removed surgically, followed by intensive voice therapy, which is necessary for reestablishing voice.

Mass-Size Changes in the Vocal Folds

A severe cold accompanied by laryngitis is a good example of a voice problem related to a mass-size change of the vocal folds. In laryngitis, for example, the patient experiences severe swelling and redness of the membrane that covers the vocal folds; this irregular thickening along the total anterior to posterior border of the folds contributes to the lowering of pitch and the hoarseness we commonly hear in laryngitis.

A common additive mass to the vocal folds is either vocal nodules or vocal polyps, usually the result of continuous vocal abuse and misuse. Most of the mass-size changes that lead to dysphonia are clearly observable growths, such as the wartlike papilloma seen in the larynges of children or the leukoplakia-type lesion described in the case illustration of Charles. The mass added to the vocal fold will drastically change the vibratory characteristic of that fold and will usually result in a lowering of fundamental frequency. The added mass is often on the margin of the vocal fold, and so it prevents the two folds from optimally approximating each other.

Occasionally, a patient may demonstrate some kind of endocrine or metabolic disorder that changes the mass of the vocal folds and results in voice changes that are difficult for the patient to tolerate. Most additive lesions to the vocal folds, unilateral or bilateral, can change the sound of the voice by lowering pitch, decreasing loudness, and increasing breathiness.

Resonance Changes

The majority of resonance problems are related to excessive nasality (*hypernasality*) or insufficient nasality (*hyponasality* or *denasality*). Although some people are hypernasal for wholly functional reasons (their natural voice is always nasal sounding), the majority of people with hypernasality speak that way for physical reasons. Obvious effects, like an unrepaired cleft palate or a short soft palate, will allow excessive coupling between the oral and nasal cavities, which results in an escape of air and sound waves through the nose. Some patients with hypernasality have difficulty moving the muscles of the throat and soft palate because of weakness or paralysis of the muscles. This form of hypernasality, perhaps the result of a stroke or a symptom of a progressive neurological disease, is classified as a dysarthria. Some speech and voice therapies provided for patients with dysarthria are presented in Chapter 6. Management of patients with excessive nasal resonance is detailed in Chapter 7.

The opposite problem, insufficient nasal resonance, or denasality, is usually caused by some kind of obstruction in the nasopharyngeal and nasal cavities. Allergies, enlarged adenoidal tissue, and severe head colds are typical physical problems that may cause denasality. The primary treatment and management of patients with denasality is medical-surgical; voice therapy for denasality is rarely helpful.

FUNCTIONAL VOICE DISORDERS

Most voice disorders do not appear to have an organic or physical cause but are related to misusing the vocal mechanisms, known as functional dysphonia. People with functional voice problems produce their faulty voices in different ways. Some do not coordinate their respiratory functions with what they want to say. They may not take big enough breaths for the length of the planned utterances, which could require them to take "catch-up breaths" in the middle of vocal passages. They may also expire too much air before they begin to speak. Such lack of coordination between respiratory control and phonation demand is a typical functional voice problem. Often some therapy in developing a quick and adequate inspiration, followed by some practice in extending the length of the expiration, can correct this problem.

Another functional voice problem is a person speaking at too low or too high a pitch level, having a voice that always appears inappropriately loud or hoarse (despite the normal appearance of the vocal folds). Occasionally, patients with severe voice symptoms seem to shut down the entire airway, not only shutting the vocal folds and the laryngeal structures above them, but retracting the tongue and contracting the muscles of the throat. Such patients require voice therapy directed at creating an open airway, as observed when they yawn and then sigh. Functional abuse (such as excessive throat clearing) and vocal misuse (such as yelling) can eventually lead to actual tissue changes of the vocal folds (such as nodules or polyps), which contribute further to what sounds like a faulty voice.

The following description of a young boy with vocal nodules illustrates a functional voice disorder that is frequently observed in a young primary school population:

Eli, age 7, was described by his parents as a boy "who was always talking, yelling, and letting the family know that he was around." For the past year Eli often demonstrated a low-pitched, hoarse voice, particularly toward the end of the day, after many hours of noisy play. His hoarseness was noticed by his pediatrician, who subsequently referred him to an ear-nose-throat specialist, an otolaryngologist. Initial attempts by the otolaryngologist at indirect laryngoscopy were unsuccessful because of the boy's intolerance for the laryngeal mirror. After a second visit, however, the physician was able to see Eli's vocal folds, and he found small bilateral vocal nodules. Eli was then referred to the speech-language pathologist in the same hospital, who took a thorough case history from both the parents and the boy. A number of abusive noises the boy produced were heard, and a gross determination was made of how often these abuses occurred. The speech-language pathologist saw Eli for several sessions, during which he provided graphic materials that showed Eli in language he could understand how abusing his voice had produced the "little bumps he now had on his vocal folds." The counseling was coupled with requests that Eli make serious attempts to curb his yelling and funny noises. Each time he found himself making a noise, he was asked to chart it on a time graph the clinician gave him to take home. After several weeks of monitoring his yelling behavior with the help of his parents, Eli returned for another visit with the otolaryngologist. This time laryngoscopy showed that Eli's nodules were much smaller. It appeared that curbing his vocal abuses lessened the laryngeal strain he was experiencing, which reduced the size of his vocal nodules.

The management of Eli's voice problem required a few sessions of counseling specific to his vocal abuses. If he had needed voice therapy over a longer period of time, the focus of his therapy would have been to discover what kind of abuse or misuse was present and then to design a program to reduce that abuse. We would also have searched with him for the best voice he could produce.

The voice clinician must continually search for the patient's best and most appropriate voice production. This searching is necessary because so much vocal behavior is highly automatic, particularly the dimensions of pitch and quality. The patient cannot deliberately break down vocalization into various components and then hope to combine them into some ideal phonation. Voice therapy techniques are primarily vehicles of facilitation—that is, we try a particular therapy approach to see if it facilitates the production of a better voice. If it does, then we utilize it as therapy practice material. If it does not, we quickly abandon it. As part of every clinical session, we must probe and search for the patient's best voice. When an acceptable production is produced, we use this "best" voice as the patient's voice target. The easiest achieved and/or best-sounding voice is often used as the patient's target in voice therapy.

Functional voice problems range from producing no voice at all (*aphonia*) to producing a tight, strangled-sounding voice (*spasmodic dysphonia*). In functional aphonia, the vocal folds appear normal on examination. When the patient attempts to produce voice or phonate, the vocal folds separate further. This separation of the vocal folds, which prevents a normal voice from occurring, is not done willfully by the patient; rather, the individual's attempt to produce voice seems to result in a separation (*abduction*) of the folds rather than an approximation or closing (*adduction*). Fortunately, patients with functional aphonia generally have an excellent therapy prognosis, and they usually completely recover their voice after symptomatic voice therapy.

An opposite problem, characterized by the vocal folds adducting too tightly, is observed in spasmodic dysphonia. When the patient is asked to phonate, the entire larynx seems to close down, and structures above the vocal folds close in a sphincteral movement so that the true vocal folds are approximated tightly together (see Chapter 2). The patient struggles to push out the expiratory air against the tight larynx, which results in the strangled, tight-sounding voice of spasmodic dysphonia. Although the literature does report successful management and therapy results for spasmodic dysphonia, the problem is among the most difficult of voice disorders to treat by symptomatic voice therapy.

THE SITES OF VOCAL HYPERFUNCTION

Vocal hyperfunction is defined in this text as the involvement of too much muscle force and physical effort in the systems of respiration, phonation, and resonance. Identification and description of the specific anatomical sites and physiology required for each of these vocal parameters can introduce the reader to the problem of vocal hyperfunction.

Respiration

The regulation of breathing for phonation is basically involuntary and highly automatic in everyday speech; however, public speakers or actors or singers learn to take in quick breaths and then extend them over a prolonged period of continuous voicing. Singers, for example, require an additional supply of air in excess of those obtained in normal inhalation and are able to replenish their air supply quickly and efficiently. Singers must be able to sustain prolonged expiration.

Unusual force or muscle tension (hyperfunction) can be observed in various phases of respiration among both normal persons and clinical voice patients. Although normal speakers without vocal pathology can tolerate vocal stresses related to inadequate and inefficient respiration, patients with vocal pathology usually cannot tolerate such respiratory inefficiency. Perhaps the most common problem of respiration observed among voice patients is the attempt to speak on an inadequate expiration. The inspiratory phase may be inadequate for the phonatory task. Untrained singers may elevate their shoulders, using their neck accessory muscles for inhalation.

Some voice patients literally use chest and abdominal muscles in competition with each other. Rather than contracting or expanding the chest (thorax) in direct coordination with contraction or expansion of the abdomen, these two anatomical sites may be "pulling and pushing" against each other. Lecturers or singers, in their need to get in a "big" breath, to take a maximum inhalation, may display obviously distended abdomens, fixed thoraxes, elevated shoulders with the associated neck accessory muscles in a hypertonic state, and possibly heads thrust forward. Although such "deep breathers" may have increased their air volume, they are in no position to parcel out their exhalations for a controlled sustained phonation. More commonly, perhaps, we see patients who suffer not from too little or too much inhalation, but from improper utilization of their expirations. A speaker may let out so much expiration early in a verbal passage that by the end of the sentence, he or she is short of breath.

Normal speakers demonstrate adequate inspiration–expiration for the daily needs of voice, generally speaking. Professional users of voice demonstrate much more vigorous respiration and show much muscular participation in large, quick inspiration followed by steady expiration that can produce vocal beauty and intensities not possible from untrained speakers or singers. Many voice patients have problems with inspiration–expiration movements as well as poor timing and control of sustained expiration—symptoms of voice that are related to lack of respiratory control.

We discuss normal respiration and its role in supplying expiratory air pressures and volumes needed for normal phonation in Chapter 2; there, we also consider some of the respiration problems of patients with voice disorders. In Chapter 5, we demonstrate several therapy approaches that have been found helpful in improving respiratory function and control for voice.

Phonation

Voice, or *phonation*, is produced by vibration of the vocal folds. This phonation is produced by expiratory airflow coming from the lungs, passing between the approximated vocal folds, and setting the vocal folds into vibration. How elastic or tense these folds are, indicated by their elongation and thickness, determines their frequency of vibration; the faster they vibrate (higher frequency), the higher the perceived pitch of the voice. How vigorously the vocal folds vibrate, caused by the air pressure below them and the velocity of air passing between them, determines the intensity of phonation or the perceived loudness of voice. Although respiration problems may obviously contribute to faulty voice, the majority of voice problems seem to result from faulty approximation of the vocal folds.

The space between the vocal folds is known as the *glottis*. Many vocal problems originate at this glottal level, particularly along the inner membranous border of each vocal fold. The vocal folds are brought together muscularly for phonation; likewise, they are separated by active muscle contraction of a pair of muscles (described in Chapter 2) whose primary function is to abduct the vocal folds. The glottal posture of the vocal folds, their thickness, elasticity, and degree of approximation, has much to do with the quality of the sounds of phonation. Many functional voice disorders are the result of faulty physiology of laryngeal muscles, particularly in the faulty approximation or bringing of the two vocal folds together.

Sometimes the vocal folds are approximated too tightly together. The membranes that cover the vocal folds are placed so firmly together that the larynx acts as a valve, preventing the flow of air that normally sets the vocal folds into vibration. The resulting voice is tight and sounds at times almost like the strained voice of the laryngeal "stutter" or spasmodic dysphonia. An opposite problem may be observed when the vocal folds are brought together in such a lax manner that far too much breath escapes between them, which produces a whispered or very breathy voice.

Voice authorities disagree about the influence of inappropriate pitch level or fundamental frequency on the development of various vocal pathologies. For some patients an inappropriately low or high pitch level might appear as a primary etiologic factor in a vocal disorder, but for other patients faulty pitch levels have developed secondarily from the increase of vocal fold mass due to early polypoid or nodule growth. That is, sometimes the inappropriate pitch level produces the dysphonia, and sometimes the prolonged dysphonia produces vocal fold tissue changes and thus alters pitch. It is important for any speaker or singer to use the vocal mechanism optimally with regard to fundamental frequency. Speaking or singing at an inappropriate pitch level requires excessive force and contraction of the intrinsic muscles of the larynx, which leads to vocal fatigue or the hoarseness related to a tired vocal mechanism.

A common pitch deviation may be the inappropriately low pitch of young professional males, such as teachers or clergy members, who speak at the bottom of their pitch ranges in an attempt to convey some extra authority through their voices. Young professional women may also speak at fundamental frequency values well below the normative values of the average adult female. An inappropriate pitch level, whether too low or too high, requires unnecessary muscle energy to maintain the necessary vocal fold adjustments of length and mass to produce the "artificial" voice. Of the many variables we identify as hyperfunctional voice behaviors, inappropriate pitch level is one of the easiest of the disorders to remedy. Sometimes just by raising or lowering the fundamental frequency slightly, patients will experience a lessening of the energy they employ to speak, which will result in a noticeable decrease in their dysphonia.

Initiation of phonation at the beginning of words is known as *glottal attack*. We often hear *easy* or *soft glottal attack* in voicing patterns that are considered typical of a southern accent, or in what may be called a legato in music—the soft, uninterrupted voicing pattern that seems to flow without break. Words begin softly, and a blend of unvoiced air gradually becomes voiced. In southern dialect the words not only begin softly, but most of the vowels in the utterance are prolonged as well. Soft glottal attack as a vocal style appears to be easy on the vocal mechanism; however, a politician or performer with such an easy attack may sound a "bit boring and too passive" in overall presentation.

The opposite type of voicing mode is known as the *hard glottal attack*. Phonation is abruptly initiated, so that often each word sounds like an individual entity with its own initial stress and stresses put on the beginning of words. We often hear hard glottal attack in the voicing patterns of people in such large eastern cities as New York or Philadelphia. Their overall speaking patterns appear much faster, for example, than what we hear in southern speech. Speaking with hard glottal attack is often characterized as vocal hyperfunction. Voice therapy may entail a patient's deliberately attempting an easier vocal attack to take the "work" out of voicing.

Vocal abuse and vocal misuse can contribute to voice problems. By *vocal abuse* we mean that the laryngeal mechanisms are used excessively in various nonverbal abusive ways, such as continuous coughing, throat clearing, laughing, crying, or smoking. Such abusive behaviors can have negative effects on laryngeal function and sometimes on vocal production as well. Vocal misuse may consist of excessive or inappropriate voicing, such as speaking with excessive vocal hard attack, speaking at the wrong voice pitch, speaking too loudly, or speaking too much. The additive nature of the vocal fold edema (swelling) or tissue engorgement that may result from excessive voicing, such as screaming or yelling, enlarges the vocal folds. This vocal fold enlargement changes the sound of the voice. The patient, in turn, reacts to the vocal change and begins to employ other vocal behaviors to compensate for the changed vocal mechanism. These compensatory behaviors further contribute to what is perceived as some kind of voice problem.

Coughing and excessive throat clearing frequently contribute to dysphonia and laryngeal pathology and sometimes add edema and irritation to an already pathological condition. True infection of the larynx is often the primary etiologic factor in dysphonia, and patients experience acute or chronic laryngitis; instead of imposing upon themselves temporary periods of voice rest during the infectious stage of the disease, patients may continue to phonate, which compounds vocal fold irritation. Lecturing or serious singing on top of an existing laryngeal infection can have disastrous aftereffects and perhaps damage the vocal mechanism permanently. External irritants, particularly once laryngeal pathology has been established, may exacerbate certain vocal pathologies; smoking, excessive alcohol consumption, smog, and dust have all been identified as culprits that help maintain various laryngeal disorders. It would appear that once any kind of vocal abuse has been identified, intelligent efforts by the patient to reduce such abusive behavior might noticeably lessen vocal symptoms.

Resonance

Much of the beauty or the quality of the voice is produced by the resonating chambers that begin within the larynx itself, extend into the pharynx, the oral cavity, and the nasal cavity above. Fant (1960) introduced an acoustic theory of voice, often called the *source-filter theory,* which in effect says that the voice we hear emitted from the mouth or nose is composed wholly of the original vocal fold phonation that has been modified by successive supralaryngeal structures. Each vowel produced has its own unique vocal tract configuration, as described by Sever (1982):

> Specifically, for voiced sounds, the glottal signal is the input to the vocal tract. Due to the ability of the vocal tract to assume different three-dimensional shapes for the production of different vowels, the resonance characteristics of the vocal tract will change accordingly. It follows that, as the glottal signal is transmitted through the vocal tract, it will be modified in a manner that will be different for each vowel. (p. 26)

The voice, originating by the airstream vibrating the vocal folds, is amplified in the upper airway cavities of the neck and head. This amplification is called *resonance.* In normal voicing, the vocal fold vibrations produce the source of sound that flows into the resonating tubes of the vocal tract (the hypopharynx, the oral pharynx, and the nasal cavities, all described in Chapter 2). The vocal tract is much like an extended tube starting immediately within the larynx and extending up the throat into the oral cavity, which is, in turn, coupled with the nasal cavity. Certain sounds or voice frequencies are amplified selectively, depending on the surface, shape, and restrictions of the resonating cavities. The resonating cavities have particular compatible natural vibrations that respond optimally to certain frequencies of the sound spectrum, known as *resonance frequencies.* If the sound wave frequencies in the upper airway are compatible with the natural resonances, natural amplification and resonance will occur. Many cavity resonators, however, are altered by changes in surface and shape so that natural resonant frequencies are changed. This may alter natural frequency of vibration and result in a dull voice lacking amplification and resonance. Some speakers alter or diminish their natural resonance potential by using various hyperfunctional behaviors. Where the individual places the voice, low or high in the resonating tract, has much to do with ease of phonation and how the voice sounds to the listener.

The first resonating cavity that has immediate influence on the glottal voice is within the larynx itself. Viewing the larynx from above with various viewing procedures, such as through the nasoendoscope (explained in subsequent chapters), we can observe muscle effects within the supraglottal larynx (false folds and aryepiglottic folds) changing the opening within the superior larynx by their contraction and relaxation. The superior laryngeal opening is continually changing shape. From within the larynx, the glottal tone (at this point, a sound wave) travels into the lower pharynx (hypopharynx). The hypopharynx itself is continually changing shape by muscle contraction and relaxation, which, in turn, change the topographic surface (soft-relaxed versus taut-tense) of the hypopharyngeal cavity (Pershall & Boone, 1986). The hypopharynx and the oropharynx continually change shape, both horizontally and vertically, during speaking and singing (Laver, 1980). The pharynx appears to change its shape continually during speech and singing, and these pharyngeal shapings contribute greatly to the resonance of the voice.

In normal speaking and singing, the oral opening within the mouth is continually changing. In fact, the production of each vowel demands a unique positioning of tongue and lips and opening of the mandible. One form of vocal hyperfunction is seen in the patient who speaks with severe mandibular restriction, or "talking through one's teeth," which forces all vowels to be produced primarily by tongue movement alone. The mandible is locked shut, and the molars are clenched tightly together.

For the various adjustments required in producing vowels, the patient changes the dimensions of the oral cavity by flattening or elevating the tongue, with little or no size change contributed by the movement of the mandible. Many patients with mandibular restriction complain of symptoms of vocal fatigue, pain, or fullness in the hyoid area after prolonged speaking or singing. The entire burden of articulation is on the tongue. Mandibular restriction is a common diagnostic entity in many patients with hyperfunctional voice disorders. Recognizing this, Froeschels (1952) developed the *chewing approach* in voice therapy. Voice clinicians using the chewing approach for selected voice patients generally report that it not only promotes greater mobility of the mandible, but that it also reduces other oral hyperfunctional postures.

The overall positioning of the tongue within the oral cavity influences the resonance of the voice. Laver (1980) describes "neutral lingual settings" where the normal individual carries the overall tongue mass within the oral cavity most of the time. In normal speech, the tongue makes obvious phonetic adjustments, such as moving the tip to touch behind the gum ridge behind the upper, central teeth, but more often the main tongue body remains in a "neutral" position. Occasionally speakers have thin, baby-sounding voices; such individuals generally produce this baby-sounding voice by carrying the overall tongue body in a high, forward position. If such an anterior tongue position is identified (by testing) as a cause of a baby-sounding voice, it can often be changed to a more neutral position by voice therapy. An opposite problem, carrying the tongue excessively posterior, produces back voice resonance (Boone, 1991). Posterior tongue carriage, as a hyperfunctional tongue position, can often be eliminated using some of the voice therapy techniques we discuss in Chapters 5 and 7.

Some patients display problems of nasal resonance that are related to variations in coupling the oral and nasal cavities together. In spoken English, only the nasal consonants (*m, n, ng*) are given nasal resonance by relaxing the velum and allowing the velopharyngeal port to be open. The sound waves then pass into the nasal cavity for further resonance. Although most patients with excessive nasalization have structural problems (cleft palate, short velum, severe head cold), occasional voice patients produce nasal voices for wholly functional reasons.

Most hyperfunctional resonance behaviors alter the size, shape, and surface of the resonating cavities. The best-sounding voice is often one with the best resonance because of compatibility between the frequency of vibration of the vocal folds and the resonant frequencies of the supraglottal resonators. Voice therapy is often effective in identifying unnecessary force and tension at the various sites of the upper airway. Once such hyperfunctional behavior is identified, such as speaking through clenched teeth, the patient should be made aware of the forceful behavior and its negative effect on voice. The clinician asks the patient to produce the hyperfunctional behavior on purpose, and then contrasts it with an easy behavior (such as voicing while the teeth are clenched followed by a wide-open mouth). The patient is then asked to hear the difference in the sound of the voice between the two contrasted behaviors, effort versus ease. When natural resonance is uncovered, often by using a more natural or neutral setting of oral structures, the improvement of the voice is often marked.

SYMPTOMATIC VOICE THERAPY

Patients with vocal complaints often show symptoms related to the improper functioning of respiratory, phonatory, and resonance systems. These symptoms often appear to be related to abuse and/or misuse of the vocal mechanisms, with or without the development of laryngeal pathologies. Some voice problems are created solely by abuse and misuse. Other voice problems may be the result of organic or physical problems. In most cases, however, *how* the patient uses the vocal mechanisms has much to do with how the patient sounds. The focus of *symptomatic voice therapy* is helping the patient optimally use the systems of respiration, phonation, and resonance for the easiest-produced and best-sounding voice possible.

Although the original causes of voice problems may never be identified (identifying laryngeal disease is easier), why vocal problems continue or maintain themselves is often a complex issue. For many voice patients the original cause of the initial dysphonia may be long past—that is, patients may speak the way they do today because this is the way they spoke yesterday. Respiration, phonation, and resonance are the result of highly automatic motor behaviors. It appears, therefore, that improper vocal production quickly becomes automatic and involuntary, often resisting an individual's attempt to overcome it. Direct modification of the symptoms is not always recommended. For example, if it were determined at the time of a voice evaluation that a patient with functional dysphonia spoke with excessively hard glottal attack, direct work on such sudden-onset vocalization might not be the desired target behavior in voice therapy. Rather, reducing loudness and slowing down the speaking rate might soften glottal attack without ever working directly on it.

Sometimes a voice problem serves a patient well, either consciously or subconsciously, and the patient may resist changing the sound of the voice by symptomatic voice therapy. In his classic work *Voice of Neurosis* P.J. Moses (1954) argued that to eradicate the vocal symptom is only to encourage the patient to develop another symptom, perhaps more maladaptive than the voice disorder was. For various problems of maladaptive function and neurosis, however, behavioral therapy has been successful in reducing aversive symptoms without observable symptom migration (Wolpe, 1987). In reviewing voice cases over time, it would appear that more often the emotional or psychological problem that may have precipitated the voice problem has disappeared. Much of the continuing dysphonia thus appears to be related to a habit set of faulty phonation. Often, then, a direct attempt at vocal symptom modification is warranted, sometimes supplemented by some counseling and support provided by the voice clinician. In addition to voice therapy, some voice patients will require professional counseling by a psychologist or psychiatrist who works closely with the voice clinician.

To be effective, symptomatic voice therapy first requires the identification of any kind of vocal abuse or misuse that may contribute to the voice problem. Once such abuse-misuse is identified—for example, continued throat clearing—the clinician must help the patient develop methods for reducing the behavior. Taking the "work" out of phonation is often a primary task in therapy. In symptomatic therapy, the clinician and the patient attempt various voice-producing tasks (see Chapter 5) that seem to produce optimal respiration, phonation, and resonance. Sometimes, reducing vocal effort will initially result in a poorer-sounding voice; for example, a child with vocal nodules who begins to produce voice with minimal unneeded effort may initially sound more dysphonic. In time, the voice may sound much better. Sometimes, too, the easiest-produced voice is often the one that sounds better, such as what we frequently observe in functional dysphonia.

In this text we call the techniques that work in voice therapy *facilitating approaches.* When particular facilitating approaches are identified as helpful in therapy, much of symptomatic voice therapy is devoted to practicing the approach for reestablishing a more optimal method of voice production.

SUMMARY

The thesis of this chapter and the rest of the text is that most voice disorders appear to be related to laryngeal abuse and vocal misuse. Such disorders, whether they are wholly functional or organic in origin, can be successfully treated by symptomatic voice therapy. Thorough evaluation of a voice problem and possible identification of abuse-misuse are important requisites for the successful treatment of people with voice disorders.

Chapter 2

The Normal Voice

Few things are so difficult to define or understand as what is normal and what constitutes normal limits. Voice therapy is often "antagonistic" therapy. We are trying to undo what patients have done to their voice through overworking the mechanism. To be effective in voice evaluation and therapy, clinicians must have a good working knowledge of the structures involved in phonation. Also, they must have a knowledge of the normal function of these structures. This chapter presents the structures and functions necessary for respiration, phonation, and resonance with a current view of the clinical physiology of these events.

Separating the normal speaking voice into three individual parts (respiration, phonation, and resonance) for purposes of study is helpful, but we must remember that the three components of voice are highly interdependent. For example, without the expiratory phase of respiration there would be no voice phonation or resonance. Also, these three processes are constantly changing simultaneously. Let us first consider the structures and function of respiration, particularly as they relate to production of voice.

RESPIRATION

Humans have learned to use respiration for speech by sustaining their exhalations for phonation. Both speaking and singing require an outgoing airstream capable of activating vocal fold vibration. When "training" their voice, speakers or singers frequently focus on developing conscious control of the breathing mechanism. This conscious control, however, must always be consistent with the physiological air requirements of the individual. When a problem occurs with respiration, it is often the conflict between the physiological needs and the speaking/singing demands for air that causes faulty usage of the vocal mechanism. Our dependence on the constant renewal of the oxygen supply imposes certain limitations on how many words we can say, how many phrases we can sing, or how much emphasis we can use on one expiration.

Respiration Structures

Inspired air enters through the nostrils and passes into the nasal cavities into the nasopharynx through the open velopharyngeal port into the oropharynx. For mouth breathers, the air would enter through the open mouth and pass through the oral cavity over the surface of the tongue and into the oropharynx. The air would then flow through the hypopharynx. From the hypopharynx the inspiration would flow into the larynx (Figure 2–1), pass between the ventricular or false vocal folds, and pass between the true vocal folds down into the trachea or windpipe. At the bottom end of the trachea, the airway divides into the two bronchial tubes shown in the accompanying photograph of the lungs and tracheal bifurcation (Figure 2-2). The bronchial tubes further branch into divisions known as the bronchioles, and they eventually terminate in the lungs in little air sacs known as the alveolar sacs. Some of the bronchioli are visible in the upper picture of Figure 2–2, but most of the bronchioli and all the alveoli are covered by the pleural membrane that covers the lungs.

The ribs connected to the 12 thoracic vertebrae and their connecting muscles play an important role in respiration, as we shall see when we discuss respiratory function. The thorax can move in several ways. For example, the rib cage wall expands for inspiration of air and collapses for

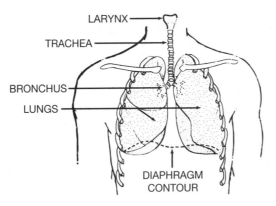

FIGURE 2–1   The Respiratory Tract
Note the resting level of the diaphragm as outlined in the diaphragm contour.

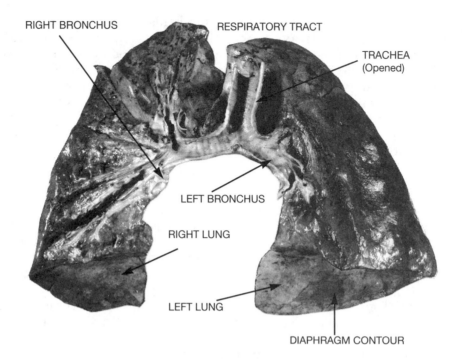

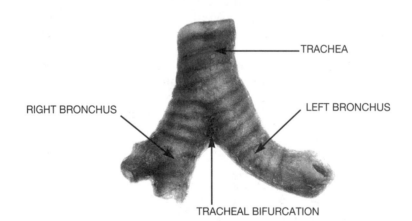

FIGURE 2–2 Lungs and Tracheal Bifurcation

An illustration of the tracheal bifurcation that introduces air into the lungs by way of the left and right bronchi. At the bottom end of the trachea, the airway divides into the two bronchial tubes. The bronchial tubes further branch into divisions known as the bronchioles, and they eventually terminate in the lungs in little air sacs known as the alveolar sacs. Some of the bronchioli are visible in the upper picture, but most of the bronchioli and all the alveoli are covered by the pleural membrane that covers the lungs.

expiration. Sometimes the accessory muscles in the neck assist in deep inspiration when they contract because they elevate the shoulders and increase the vertical dimension of the thorax. At the base of the thorax is the important diaphragm, a composite of muscle, tendon, and membrane that separates the thoracic cavity from the abdominal cavity. As the diaphragm contracts, it descends and increases the vertical dimension of the thorax; as the diaphragm relaxes, it ascends back to its higher position. The diaphragm has direct contact with the lungs, and only the pleural space comes between the lungs and the diaphragm; the shape of the diaphragm, its superior contour, can be seen on the lower surface of the cadaver lung in Figure 2–2. The relaxed diaphragm is high in the chest within the rib cage, and the stomach and liver lie directly below it. As the diaphragm contracts and descends, it pushes from above on the contents of the abdomen below, often displacing the abdominal wall by pushing it outward on inspiration. The abdominal wall is composed primarily of the abdominal muscles that sometimes play an active role in expiration. This is especially true in singing, in loud speech, when laughing (thus the term *belly laugh*), or when producing a very long phrase. We identify those muscles of the thorax and the abdomen that relate to respiration as we discuss respiration.

Respiration Function

The respiratory tract functions much like a bellows. When we move the handles on the bellows apart, the bellows become larger; the air within it becomes less dense than the air outside it. The outside air rushes in due to the lower pressure of the less dense air in the bellows and the greater pressure of the more dense outside air. The inspiration of air into the bellows is achieved by active enlargement of the bellows' body. Similarly, in human respiration the inspiration of air is achieved by active movement of muscles that enlarge the thoracic cavity. When the thorax enlarges, the lungs within the thorax enlarge. The air within the lungs becomes less dense than atmospheric air, and inspiration of air begins. The air is expired from the bellows by bringing the handles together, decreasing the size of the bellows' cavity, thus compressing the air and forcing it to rush out. In human respiration, however, much of expiration is achieved by passive collapse of thoracic size and not by active muscle contraction. This is an extremely important fact and can be valuable information for voice clinicians. Much of expiration is passive. Hixon, Mead, and Goldman (1976) have described human respiration as having two types of forces that are always present: passive forces (such as the elastic lungs) and active, volitional force (such as contraction of muscles of inspiration). The pleural membrane that covers the lungs clings almost adhesively to the inner wall of the thorax. As the thorax expands by muscular contraction, the lungs within it expand. The inherent elastic force of the lungs is always there. Their elastic recoil will be as fast as thoracic collapse allows. In fact, in at-rest expiration (e.g., the expiration during the quiet breathing of sleep), the expiratory phase of respiration is wholly accomplished by the elasticity of the inherent or passive forces.

Passive Components

Much of the air pressure or "power" required for normal speech can be supplied by the passive factors of respiration (passive exhalation). This is desirable because no muscle action is required to supply this breath power, and thus there is no tendency to "overdo" (hyperactivity) the effort. When a long phrase or other speaking task (such as increased loudness or singing) requires more effort or "breath power," we make up the difference between the power provided by passive factors and the needed amount of breath power by using the abdominal musculature.

Active Components

A key problem for many voice-disordered patients is the tendency to "squeeze" the glottis closed in order to produce the needed power, rather than to increase air pressure by contracting the abdominal muscles. We can better understand this "mistake" by a simple analogy. If we are watering flowers in a garden and we want to reach the far row of plants, we can either place a thumb over the end of the hose and squirt the water further (increase the power), or we can increase the water power by turning the faucet on further. When we squeeze the glottis closed, we are "putting a thumb over the end of the hose." When we contract the abdominal muscles, we are "turning the faucet on further" and increasing the airflow. Even though squeezing the glottis tends to increase the vocal power, vocal quality is diminished because the voice sounds strained. If this method is habitual, the excessive effort becomes the basis of a hyperfunctional voice disorder. Such effort may lead to vocal nodules, contact ulcers, vocal polyps, recurring laryngitis, or loss of voice. We often see this type of voice production in politicians who are campaigning and frequently speak loudly to make a point. If they use too much effort in overadducting the larynx to achieve the loudness, vocal strain and laryngeal swelling edema will likely result. This occurred during President Clinton's campaign speaking. He frequently resorted to voice rest between speeches to allow his swelling in the larynx to reduce and the resultant laryngitis to subside. When we need increased power to speak louder, to stress words, or to extend a phrase when singing or speaking, we should use the larger muscles of the abdomen and "turn on the faucet" controlling the source of air. Thus, the pressure at the valve (the larynx) is not excessive, and vocal quality is improved with delicate laryngeal tissue not subjected to stress and strain, which produces laryngeal edema and laryngitis. Vocal quality is not diminished, and adverse tissue change is avoided. Voice clinicians may use this water analogy to teach patients how to monitor breath control by properly using expiratory reserve volume (see definition of terms below) via the abdominal muscles, rather than using excessive glottal valving in the larynx.

Relaxation Pressure

The best (most efficient and most pleasing vocal quality) voice is produced at mid air-pressure levels and mid lung-volume levels of air, as shown in the relaxation pressure curve in Figure 2–3. To demonstrate this, simply take about a half-breath and produce an /i/ vowel for 5 seconds at a medium loudness level. Then listen to the vocal quality. Now take a very deep breath and produce the same /i/ vowel for 5 seconds at medium loudness. The vocal quality will generally be poorer with the effort required to control the greater air volume and higher air pressure, thus contributing to the perception of poorer voice quality. Finally, produce the same /i/ vowel for 5 seconds at medium loudness immediately after releasing three-fourths of your air supply. Again, the vocal quality will suffer as you try to compensate for the low air pressure and low lung volume. The excessive muscular contraction required to phonate at this low lung volume will also be seen in the "overvalving" in the larynx giving rise to the rougher voice quality.

This exercise demonstrates how vocal quality is affected by extremely high or low air pressure at high or low lung volume. It translates into an excellent clinical-stimulation technique. We can often change the vocal quality of our dysphonic patients by instructing them to use the midrange of air pressure and lung volume. Teaching a shortened phrasing pattern may be important to teaching breath-stream management. Except in singers or actors this generally is all the "respiration training" that needs to be given by the speech-language pathologist. All of the emphasis placed on breathing exercises and respiration training, in the past, seems unproductive and unnecessary for nearly all of our patients with dysphonias.

We frequently use glottal fry to improve vocal quality in hoarse patients. We instruct patients to (a) let out half the air, and (b) produce an "ah" and let it die away in a popping sound. The glottal fry requires a very low amount of airflow and can be sustained with little air pressure. Thus, we can operate in the most efficient range of the relaxation pressure curve with modest lung volume and modest air pressure. The voice, thus produced, with little muscular effort (mainly passive respiratory forces) is the exact opposite of the typical hyperfunctional voice of the dysphonic patient. After producing a glottal fry of about 60 to 75 Hz for 10 seconds, repeated five or six times, the patient is told to

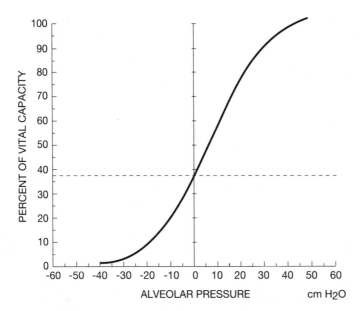

FIGURE 2-3   The Relaxation Pressure Curve
The passive forces of exhalation tend to generate force during
inhalation that works to restore the lung and rib cage system to the
normal resting state or equilibrium. After active inhalation, these
passive forces of exhalation rebound to provide some of the expiratory
force needed for speech. There is a nearly linear relationship between
relaxation pressure and lung volume in the range between 20 % and
70 % of the vital capacity. This curve represents the pressure
generated by the passive factors of the respiratory system.

repeat the phrase "Easy does it." The quality of the voice is almost
always better than the typical voice produced by a patient with nodules,
a polyp, or cord thickening. During this procedure, we are ready to
record the voice. We immediately ask the patient's name (which the
patient nearly always makes with a habitual or typical dysphonic voice),
and we also record the response. Thus, we have a comparison on tape of
the voice with vocal improvement ("Easy does it") and the typical
dysphonic voice (the name). When we ask patients to listen to both tape-
recorded samples and tell us which sounds better, they invariably answer
the "Easy does it." This procedure is an important step in clinic because it
demonstrates (a) the ability to improve the voice and (b) a self-
monitoring skill for initiating better breath-stream management while
reducing laryngeal effort. We now need to consider the muscles of
respiration that contribute active, volitional force in inspiration, as shown
in Figure 2–4. The primary muscle of inspiration is the diaphragm, as
already noted. Perhaps the external intercostals play the next most
important role in inspiration; because of their oblique angulation, when

they contract, they lift the rib below, enlarging the rib cage on a somewhat horizontal plane. Slight elevation of the upper thorax is achieved with contraction of the pectoralis major and minor, the costal elevators, the serratus posterior, and the neck accessory muscles (primarily the sternocleidomastoid). The primary inherent elasticity and recoil of thoracic structures come into play when the active muscles of inspiration cease contracting and relax, but some muscles of expiration can assist in expiration. These muscles of expiration may contract in some conditions of talking, singing, and forced expiration such as we use in playing wind instruments. The primary muscles of expiration are the four abdominal muscles, the internal oblique abdominal, external oblique abdominal, transverse abdominal, and the rectus abdominal. Some thoracic decrease can also be achieved by active contraction of the internal intercostals (they slant upward in the opposite direction of the external intercostals) and the posterior inferior serratus.

In passive respiration, the kind of breathing we do when sleeping, the active contraction of inspiratory muscles produces the inspiration, and the expiration phase of the respiratory cycle is wholly related to the passive (nonmuscular) collapse properties of the thorax. These passive factors may include lung elasticity, rib untorquing, visceral recoil, and gravity's pulling the ribs down to a resting position. When we add the function of expiratory muscles to the passive expiration, we alter the duration and force of the expiration. For example, while speaking long passages, we may well begin with passive expirations; active contraction of expiratory muscles comes after passive expiration has begun. Any time we prolong the expiration beyond a simple tidal volume (see definitions below), we have added some active muscle contraction of the expiratory muscles. When patients tell us that they "have to work hard to talk" or that "it is such an effort to speak," we should be alerted to hyperfunction in the respiratory and phonatory (laryngeal level) processes.

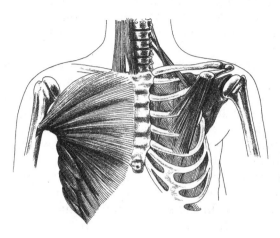

FIGURE 2–4 The Thoracic Surface Muscles of Respiration
Muscles shown include the pectoralis major, the external and internal intercostals, the scalene, pectoralis minor, and the sternocleidomastoid muscles. Bones readily identified include the clavical, sternum, scapula, and ribs 1 to 8. *(J. M. Palmer,* Anatomy for Speech and Hearing. *[New York: Harper & Row, 1972], p. 149. Used with permission.)*

Figure 2–5, the simple tracings of a pneumotachometer, shows the relative time for inspiration-expiration for a passive, tidal breath, for saying the numbers "one, two, three, four, five" and for singing the musical passage "I don't want to walk without you, baby." Note that the inspiratory time during normal tidal breathing is much longer than the quick inspiration for speech and singing. This is noted by the rapid rise of the tracing from a resting base line in an almost vertical move. In the tidal breath the rise from the base line is gradual and sloped rather than vertical. In subsequent discussions we use the following terms to describe aspects of respiration. Methods for evaluating respiratory volumes and capacities will be discussed in Chapter 4.

Lung Volumes and Capacities

Tidal volume (TV) is the amount of air inspired and expired during a typical respiratory cycle; it is determined by the oxygen needs (not the speaking or singing needs) of the individual.

Inspiratory reserve volume (IRV), known also as complemental air (Comroe, 1956), is the maximum volume of air that can be inspired beyond the end of a tidal inspiration.

Expiratory reserve volume (ERV), known also as supplemental air, is the maximum volume of air that can be expired beyond the end of a tidal expiration.

Residual volume (RV) is the volume of air that remains in the lungs after a maximum expiration. No matter how forceful the expiration, the residual volume cannot be forced from the lungs.

Vital capacity (VC) is the total amount of air that can be expired from the lungs and air passages from a maximum inspiration; it represents the total volumes previously listed, with the exception of residual volume (which cannot be expired).

Total lung capacity (TLC) represents the total volume of air that can be held in the lungs and airways after a maximum inspiration. It can be measured only by special volume displacement tests (not by measuring the total expiratory volume).

In the normal inspiratory–expiratory cycle of tidal volume, the relative timing of inspiration–expiration, as shown in Figure 2–5, is only slightly longer for expiration. Human beings appear to have a slight bias toward longer expirations, which is apparently quite compatible with the need to extend expiration for purposes of communication. The respiratory system supplies the power for phonation, as described in the myoelastic theory of phonation later in this chapter.

Influencing types of respiration are the interactions and pragmatics between the speaker and the listener, the type of utterance being produced, the background noise in the setting, the relative arousal level of the autonomic nervous system, the comfort of the speaker, and so

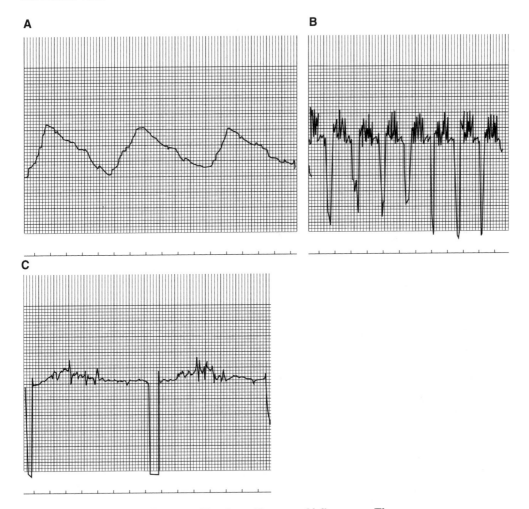

Figure 2-5 Pneumotachometer Tracings Measure Airflow over Time
Note the relative time for inspiration as opposed to expiration for three conditions: tracing A (three tidal breaths) produces an inspiration-expiration time ratio of about 1:2; tracing B (counting from one to five on eight trials) produces a ratio of about 1:3; tracing C (singing twice, "I don't want to walk without you, baby") yielded an inspiration–expiration ratio of approximately 1:10.

forth. Therefore, some of the ensuing descriptions of the physiology of respiration, when lifted out of speaking or singing context, often appear to be deceptively simple. For example, when an individual begins to speak or sing, the inspiration time unit is often shortened (by employing more vigor to the muscles of inspiration) and the expiration time is obviously extended. Hixon et al. (1976) have studied the dynamics and function of the thorax, rib cage, diaphragm, and abdomen during speech and have concluded that there are marked differences in respiratory function according to body position and type of speech task. For example, utterances that required near-total use of a patient's vital capacity activated different activity zones, depending on whether the patient was in an upright or supine body position; the inspiratory activity "was governed predominantly by the rib cage and the abdomen in the upright body position and the diaphragm in the supine position" (Hixon et al., 1976, p. 297). It appears that during the inspiratory phase preceding speech, we shorten our inspiration and then use the chest wall and the abdomen in different ways for the expiratory phase (when we are actually speaking). We renew inspiration and catch up on inspiration during conversational passages, tucking in the abdomen with a slight elevation of the rib cage. Hixon and Abbs (1980) have written that the "importance of this shape is that it forces the diaphragm—our major inspiratory muscle—into a highly domed position where its action results in the development of great amounts of inspiratory force very rapidly" (p. 63).

Bless and Miller (1972) and Otis and Clark (1968) have written that normal speakers adjust inspiration–expiration to match the linguistic utterances they wish to make. Inspiration during conversation, public speaking, and even singing happens quickly, and it is usually masked from the view of all but the searching eye. After a quick inspiration, normal speakers then begin the passive expiration, quickly using the tidal volume and adding the sustained expiration of the expiratory reserve. Fluctuations of expiratory air flow, to meet a speaker's demand for stress and changes in vocal intensity, are apparently made by slight chest wall adjustments. Increases in airflow and subglottal pressure are made quickly and with little visible effort to match the linguistic or artistic needs of speakers or singers. Gifted talkers or singers also learn to take little, quick catch-up inhalations sandwiched within what appears to listeners to be a continuous expiratory flow. When breath support or perhaps breath control is a problem in a voice-disordered patient, it is often related to failure to take these catch-up breaths at appropriate places. At other times, the tendency to push too hard in extending the expiratory reserve volume produces the strained vocal quality discussed earlier.

PHONATION

The airway requires various protective structures to prevent the infiltration of liquids, the aspiration of food particles and fluids during deglutition (swallowing), and the inhalation of foreign bodies during respiration. In most higher mammals, particularly humans, the larynx serves as the basic valvelike entryway to the respiratory tract. All incoming and outgoing pulmonary (lung) air must pass through the valving glottal opening of the larynx. Negus (1957) wrote that the primary biological roles of the larynx are, first, to prevent foreign bodies from moving into the airway and, second, to fixate the thorax by stopping the airflow at the glottal level, which permits the arms to perform heavy lifting and extensive weight-supporting feats. This primitive, valvelike action appears to be the primary function of the human larynx. Using the laryngeal valving mechanism for phonation has required the development of intricate neural controls that permit humans to use the approximating valvelike vocal folds for the precise phonations required in speaking and singing. The valving action of the larynx functions first because we have a fixed framework (the laryngeal cartilages); second, we are able to open (abduct) and close (adduct) the valve, primarily by using the intrinsic muscles of the larynx; and third, the valving mechanism receives external support from the extrinsic muscles of the larynx.

Laryngeal Structures

Prominent above the trachea (wind pipe) is the larynx, with its large, protective thyroid cartilage housing the individual cartilages, muscles, and ligaments that compose the total laryngeal structure. In some people, particularly in adult males, the thyroid cartilage (called the Adam's apple) is so prominent that it can easily be seen rising high in the neck during swallowing, dropping low during conversational speech, and rising slightly on high notes during singing.

Photographs of the five primary laryngeal cartilages (cricoid, thyroid, paired arytenoids, and epiglottis) are shown in Figures 2–6 through 2–10. Two other small paired cartilages, the corniculates (small cone-shaped bodies that sit on the apex of the arytenoids extending into the aryepiglottic folds) and the cuneiforms (tiny cone or rod-shaped cartilage pieces under the mucous membrane covering the aryepiglottic folds), apparently play only a minimal role in the phonatory functions of the larynx. Read the legends under each of the cartilage photographs thoroughly, observing some of the other structures that are also identified.

The three major cartilages seem to play separate roles, and each one is dependent on the others, primarily by muscle action and ligament attachment. The cricoid appears almost as an enlarged and complete tracheal ring, forming the solid base of the larynx (other tracheal rings are incomplete or three-quarter rings). It is circular in shape, and the two pyramid-shaped arytenoids sit on top of its high posterior (signet-shaped) wall. We shall see later, that the arytenoids rock, slide, and rotate on their articular facets on the cricoid by action of the intrinsic laryngeal muscles. Partially surrounding the cricoid and arytenoids, on three sides, is the U-shaped thyroid cartilage, which has two points of articulation with the cricoid cartilage below. All the laryngeal cartilages (similar to cartilage throughout the skeletal system are coated with a tough, leathery covering (the perichondrium), which gives the lateral view of the larynx in Figure 2–6 such a waxy look. This perichondrium covering has been removed in the subsequent photographs of the separate cartilages.

There are two main groups of muscles of the larynx: the extrinsic and the intrinsic. The extrinsic muscles have one attachment to the larynx and another attachment to some structure external to the larynx. The extrinsic muscles give the larynx fixed support and elevate or lower its position in the neck. Functionally, the extrinsic muscles (all but the cricopharyngeus) may be divided into two groups, elevators and depressors.

Elevators	Depressors
digastrics	omohyoids
geniohyoids	sternohyoids
mylohyoids	sternothyroids
stylohyoids	thyrohyoids

The extrinsic elevators lift the larynx high during swallowing and

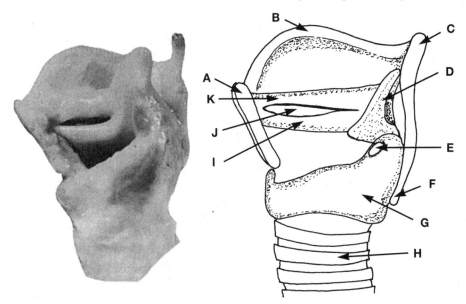

FIGURE 2–6   A Lateral Left View of the Larynx, with the Left Half of the Thyroid Cartilage Removed

The unretouched photograph shows a remarkable view of the ventricle opening between the true folds and the false folds. (A) Cut edge at lamina of thyroid cartilage; (B) arch of the thyroid cartilage; (C) superior horn of the thyroid cartilage; (D) arytenoid cartilage, right; (E) articular facet of the cricoid and arytenoid cartilage; (F) inferior horn of the thyroid cartilage; (G) cricoid cartilage; (H) tracheal ring; (I) vocal fold, right; (J) ventricle; (K) ventricular fold or false fold.

slightly during production of high singing notes. The depressors lower the larynx after deglutition and after high-note singing; they also lower the larynx a bit for production of low singing notes. Actually, normal

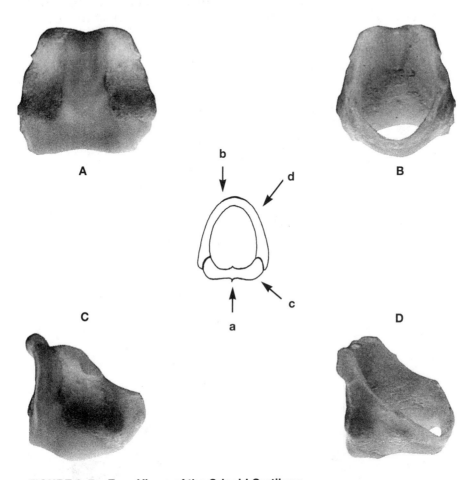

FIGURE 2–7 Four Views of the Cricoid Cartilage
In all photographs, ligament and muscle attachments and the membranous covering have been removed, showing the bare cartilage. The line drawing shows the overall superior contour of the cricoid, and the anatomical site of the four cricoid photographs indicates that photograph A was taken from that view. (A) Posterior surface of the cricoid; the difference in texture (smooth and rough) is related to ossification; the smooth portions represent the ossification; (B) anterior view; (C) right lateral view of the cricoid ring with the cartilage tipped upward, exposing the superior rim of the signet portion of the cartilage; upon this clearly defined rim rotate the two arytenoid cartilages; (D) right lateral view of the cricoid; note the contrast in thickness between the thin anterior portion of the ring and the high signet posterior portion. This difference in size is also shown in (B).

speakers should experience only minimal vertical excursion of the larynx. Trained singers keep the height of the larynx nearly constant while singing a range of high and low notes (Sataloff, 1981).

The other extrinsic laryngeal muscle (other than the elevators and depressors) is the cricopharyngeus, which is a part of the lower portion

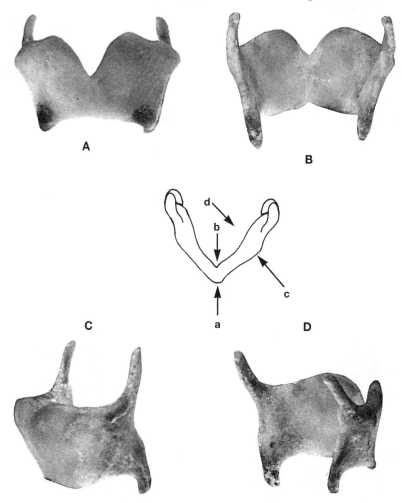

FIGURE 2–8   Four Views of the Laryngeal Thyroid Cartilage
The letters in the line drawing of the superior view of the thyroid cartilage indicate the side of the cartilage photographed. (A) Direct frontal view of the thyroid; (B) posterior view of the cartilage (note the clear extension of the inferior and superior horns on each side); (C) primarily the thyroid cartilage wall; (D) the thyroid posteriorly from a three-fourths view. The size and shape of the thyroid cartilage can be extremely variable in normal individuals (Dickson & Maue-Dickson, 1982). Asymmetry is often seen in normal individuals (Kahane, 1983).

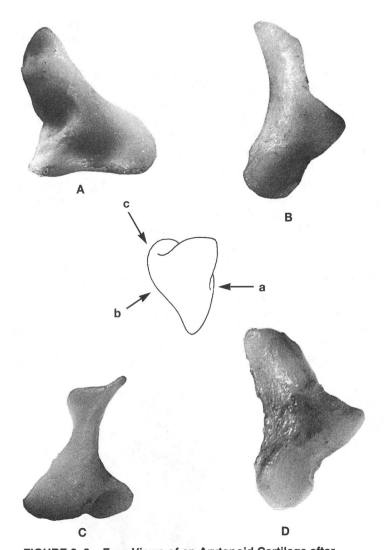

FIGURE 2–9   Four Views of an Arytenoid Cartilage after Removal of Ligament, Muscle, and Membrane Attachments
(A) Lateral view of the indentation (fovea) toward the base, which receives the attachment of the thyroarytenoid muscles (vocal fold); the higher indentation on the left margin receives the ventricular fold; the muscular process to which the posterior and lateral cricoarytenoids are attached is visible at the right base; (B) medial view of an arytenoid that has been tilted up slightly to the left; the right angular corner is the vocal process; (C) posterior-lateral view of the muscular process at the base; note toward the right base the cricoarytenoid articular facet (point of joint articulation); (D) camera lens picks up the base of the cartilage as well as its medial wall; the curving base of the arytenoid allows it to rotate, slide, and rock upon the cricoid rim below during adduction and abduction and tensing of the vocal folds.

of the inferior pharyngeal constrictor. This cricopharyngeus muscle serves as the new source (neoglottis) of vibration in esophageal speech production. The sphincterlike fibers of the cricopharyngeus, originating from the posterior wall of the cricoid cartilage, help to anchor the larynx in the fixed position in which it usually lies. In *The Voice and Its Disorders*, Greene (1980) writes that "the steadying influence of the cricopharyngeus on the larynx during phonation is of importance" and that the cricopharyngeus "is in fact an antagonist to the cricothyroid muscle" (pp. 36, 38). The distance between the larynx and the hyoid bone, as determined by the function of the extrinsic muscles, is often the focus of instruction by singing teachers in the production of a good singing voice. However, it does not appear that the good speaking voice requires much active muscle movement from either elevators or depressors. The sphincteral action of the larynx and its phonatory capabilities appear to be the function of the intrinsic muscles of the larynx, which we consider in more detail than we did the laryngeal extrinsic muscles. The larynx has six pairs of intrinsic muscles. Four of them are clearly identifiable in the photographs and drawings in Figure 2–11. One pair of muscles, the posterior cricoarytenoids, is known as the lone vocal fold abductor (these muscles open the glottis by separating the folds at the posterior larynx). The other five intrinsic muscles can be classified as adductors (they close the glottis by bringing the posterior portion of the vocal folds together),

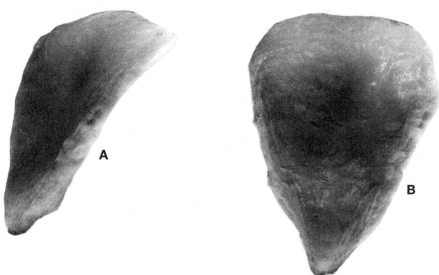

FIGURE 2–10   Two Views of the Epiglottis
The epiglottis has been removed from its attachment on the lower, internal surface of the anterior portion of the thyroid cartilage. For purposes of photography, the cartilage has been denuded, excising away its ligament and muscle attachments and its membranous covering. (A) Epiglottis from a frontal-lateral view; the rotation of the cartilage permits us to see the concave epiglottal contour; (B) epiglottis in its whole anterior dimension, which represents the lingual surface.

although they have other functions. The following brief descriptions identify each muscle in Figures 2–11 and 2–12.

Posterior Cricoarytenoids   This lone abductor muscle (E in Figure 2–11) is the largest laryngeal intrinsic muscle. The fibers originate from a middle depression on the posterior surface of the cricoid and angle up, inserting in the muscular process of the arytenoid on that side (right-sided fibers go to the right muscular process, and so on). This paired muscle is innervated by the recurrent laryngeal nerve. Its primary function is to abduct the folds by rotating laterally the vocal process of the arytenoids.

Lateral Cricoarytenoids   This paired muscle (F in Figure 2–ll) functions as a direct antagonist to the posterior cricoarytenoid as it plays its adductor role. The lateral cricoarytenoid originates from the upper border of the arch of the cricoid cartilage and inserts into the muscular process of the arytenoid on the same side. Innervation is also the recurrent laryngeal nerve. When this muscle contracts, it rotates the muscular process forward and at the same time causes the vocal process of the arytenoid (and the attached posterior part of the vocal fold) to "toe in" at the midline.

Transverse Arytenoids   These muscle fibers (H in Figure 2–11) originate from the lateral margin and posterior surface of one arytenoid and insert on the same sites on the opposite arytenoid. The transverse arytenoids are not paired muscles, per se. They transverse the distance between the two arytenoids. Innervated bilaterally by the recurrent laryngeal nerves, when these muscles contract, they approximate the bodies of the arytenoid cartilages together, functioning as adductor intrinsics as well as vocal fold compressors.

Oblique Arytenoids   This muscle (G in Figure 2–11) originates from the muscular process of one arytenoid and courses obliquely upward and across to the apex of the opposite cartilage. The fibers actually continue obliquely to the lateral border of the epiglottis and are known as the aryepiglottic muscles after they leave the arytenoid apex. The aryepiglottics become part of the aryepiglottic folds, which also include some cuneiform cartilage and membrane; these folds are active in the swallowing mechanism. The oblique arytenoid muscles are innervated bilaterally by the recurrent nerves and are active in bringing the vocal folds closer together by approximation of the apex of each arytenoid cartilage.

Thyroarytenoids   The paired thyroarytenoids, shown in Figure 2–12, form the bulk of the muscular portion of the vocal folds. The inner section of the thyroarytenoid is known as the vocalis section, and the larger, more lateral fibers are known as the thyromuscularis, or external thyroarytenoids (Zemlin, 1988). As Figure 2–12 shows, the fibers

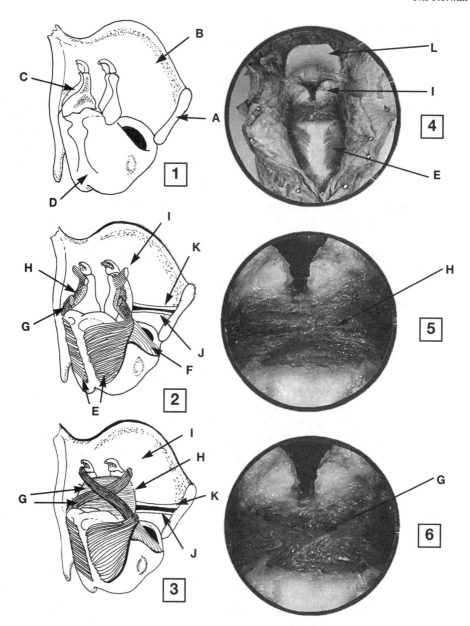

FIGURE 2–11 Intrinsic Structures of the Larynx

Basic laryngeal cartilage structures: (A) cutaway of right thyroid wing; (B) left thyroid cartilage wall; (C) left arytenoid cartilage; (D) posterior of cricoid cartilage. *Intrinsic muscles*: (E) posterior cricoarytenoid; (F) lateral cricoarytenoid; (G) oblique arytenoid; (H) transverse arytenoid; (I) aryepiglottic; (J) thyroarytenoid (vocal fold); (K) ventricular fold. (L) The epiglottis.

originate on the inner surface of the thyroid cartilage and extend posteriorly to where they insert in the vocal process (vocalis fibers) and the lateral surface (external thyroarytenoid) of the arytenoid cartilages. The inner border of the vocal fold contains the vocal ligament that originates at the anterior commissure and extends to the vocal process end of the arytenoids.

In summary, the vocal folds include both sections of the thyroarytenoids, the inner surface of the arytenoid cartilage, and the vocal ligament. The whole apparatus is covered with a tough, white membrane known as the conus elasticus. Figure 2–12 shows the individual components of the vocal folds, and Figure 2–13 shows the white membranous covering of the vocal folds (as they appear to the eye), with the folds in an open abducted position. The muscular aspect of the folds, the thyroarytenoids, are also innervated by the recurrent laryngeal nerve, and they seem to have a dual function. They shorten themselves as required for producing lower phonation frequencies, and, by their own muscular tension and elasticity, they work as glottal adducting structures.

Cricothyroids Figure 2–12 shows the anteriorly placed paired cricothyroid muscles that lie external to the laryngeal cartilages. This muscle pair is made up of two parts or portions: the obliqua and the recta. The fibers originate from the anterior-lateral arch of the cricoid cartilage and end in two distinctly different insertions. The lower fibers (obliqua portion) insert near the lower horn of the thyroid cartilage, and

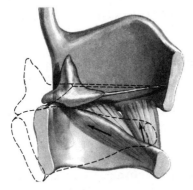
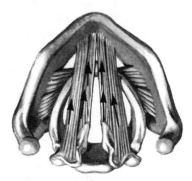

FIGURE 2-12 The Cricothyroid Muscles
The cricothyroid muscles can be seen in the drawing on the left, obliquing from the inner superior surface of the cricoid cartilage up to the thyroid cartilage. The medial fibers of the vocalis section and the lateral section of the thyroarytenoids are seen in the drawing on the right. (Reprinted with permission from *The CIBA Collection of Medical Illustrations*, illustrated by Frank H. Netter, M.D. All rights reserved. Copyright © 1964, CIBA Pharmaceutical Company, Division of CIBA-Geigy Corporation.)

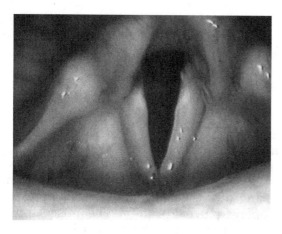

FIGURE 2–13   Normal Vocal Folds in Abducted Expiratory Position

Normal vocal folds in abducted expiratory position, as viewed with oral video endoscopy: The anterior commissure (V) is at the bottom of the picture, the glottis is the dark V portion, and the right vocal fold is on the left side of the picture.

the more superior fibers (recta portion) course to the lower margin of the lateral thyroid cartilage wall. This pair of muscles is innervated by the superior laryngeal nerve. When they contract, they increase the distance between the thyroid and arytenoid cartilages, thus contributing to pitch elevation by stretching the vocal folds; the tensing of the vocal folds (by elongating them) is an adducting action.

Phonation Function

It is difficult to discuss the cartilages and the muscles of the larynx without some description of laryngeal function. Before we describe function and laryngeal physiology, we should review the various laryngeal structures that have been presented.

Hirano (1981) has described the *functional* structure of the vocal folds in such a way as to explain the *mucosal wave* that is responsible for vocal fold vibration. The cover (epithelium and superficial lamina propria, Reinke's space) and the transition (intermediate and deep layers of lamina propria) over the vocal fold body (vocalis muscle) slide and produce a wave that moves or travels across the superior surface of the vocal fold about two-thirds of the way to the lateral edge of the fold. The wave will generally dissipate before reaching the inner surface of the thyroid cartilage. The moving cover over the body produces this mucosal wave. Without a mucosal wave there is no vibration and no phonation. This can be seen in the postsurgical (stripped) vocal folds of patients who present with aphonia following removal of large portions of vocal fold mucosa. While the cords may look white and the medial edge may be straight, they do not vibrate. The mucosa that has recovered the folds after surgery is adherent to the underlying tissue and is also stiff. Without the cover and body relationship described by Hirano (1981), vibration does not occur. When vocal folds that have been overinjected with Teflon as a treatment for unilateral paralysis are viewed stroboscopically they frequently may also fail to vibrate (Watterson, McFarlane and Menicucci 1990). When there is a disruption in the cover of the vocal fold from scarring, a mass such as a nodule from underlying carcinoma or from swelling (edema), there is a visible alteration of the normal mucosal wave. Table 2–1 shows the functional organization of the vocal folds with the tissue density increasing as we move deeper into the vocal fold. The surface is less dense while the body of the vocal fold muscle is most dense.

Table 2–1   Functional Structure of the Vocal Folds

Vocal Fold Physiology

Cover

Epithelium
Superficial lamina propria
(Reinke's Space)

Transition

Intermediate and deep layers of lamina propria
(Vocal ligament)

Body

Vocalis muscle

We subscribe to the myoelastic aerodynamic theory of phonation (Van den Berg, 1968). It begins basically with an expiration (air volume and air-pressure changes), setting the approximated (closed) vocal folds in vibration as the airflow passes between the folds (transglottal pressure drop). In the prephonation period, the vocal folds may be abducted in the expiration position (Figure 2–14A). The folds approximate one another for phonation as phonation begins (Figure 2–14B). The five laryngeal adductor muscles contract to bring the vocal folds together.

Two of the adductors—for example, the lateral cricoarytenoid and the thyroarytenoids—have very rapid contraction times, sometimes as fast as 15 msec, which Martensson (1968) has written is "exceedingly fast and surpassed only by the extrinsic eye muscles" for speed. It would appear that vocal fold adduction is achieved in milliseconds, prior to the onset of voicing. As the folds approximate, they begin to obstruct the airflow passing through the glottal level of the airway. Zemlin (1981) states: "It is extremely important to note that complete obstruction of the air passageway is not necessary to initiate phonation. If the glottal chink

A

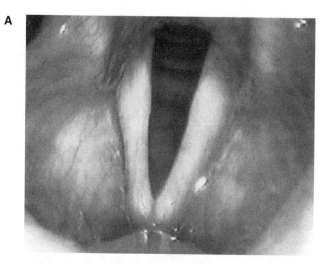

B

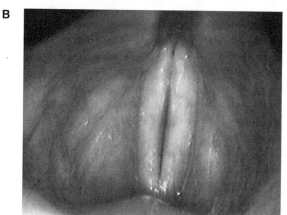

C

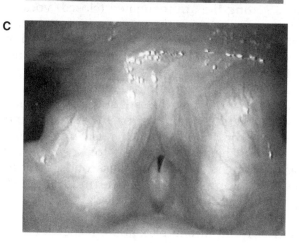

FIGURE 2–14 Three Photographs of the Vocal Folds

In (A) the vocal folds are open (abducted) in the expiratory position. In (B) the folds have approximated (adducted) and are in the phonation position. In (C) the vocal folds are in the typical Y position for whispering, with the muscular portion of the folds approximated laxly and the posterior one-third of the cartilage portion rotated apart. (The vocal folds in photographs A and B appear larger than the vocal folds in C, because the false vocal folds overlap and partially cover the true vocal folds during production of a whisper.

is narrowed to about 3 mm, a minimal amount of airflow will set the folds into vibration" (p. 183).

The subglottal pressure builds up when the folds are approximated. The volume of expired air leaving the lungs is impeded at the level of the glottis, resulting in an increased velocity of airflow through the glottis. Subglottal pressure increases (with respect to the supraglottal air pressure), and the vocal folds are blown apart, equalizing supraglottal and subglottal pressure (the opening phase of one cycle of vibration). Because of the mass of the folds (their muscle and ligament are covered with a membrane) and the Bernoulli effect, they come back together again to their previous approximation line (the closed phase of the phonatory cycle). The Bernoulli effect is the "sucking" attraction of the vocal folds toward each other, caused by the increased velocity of air passing between the approximated folds. This results in a "suction action" (negative pressure under the vocal lips relative to a positive pressure above the vocal lip) that draws the folds together.

The vibratory cycle of the vocal folds can be summarized as follows: The intrinsic adductors approximate the folds as expiration begins. Subglottal pressure increases. The airflow passes through the glottal opening and blows the folds apart. The static mass of the folds and the Bernoulli suction effect bring them back together again. The vibratory cycle then repeats itself. This is repeated approximately 125 times per second in the phonation of an adult male and 215 times per second in an adult female.

During normal phonation, the vocal folds approximate each other along their total anterior–posterior dimension. Some normal females sometimes demonstrate a slight posterior glottal chink or gap during phonation. The photographs in Figure 2–14 show the relative approximation of the vocal folds during normal phonation and also during normal expiration and whispering. The vocal folds appear slightly shorter during phonation and whispering in the photographs; that is, the vocal folds are always longer in the open abducted position than in the closed adducted one. The configuration of the glottis for whispering is characterized by an open, posterior chink, with the arytenoid cartilages and their vocal processes angled in an open Y position. Although the vocal folds are parallel to each other during whispering, they do not firmly approximate. This lack of adduction, particularly in the posterior chink, produces frictional sounds when the outgoing airstream passes through, producing what we perceive as turbulence or whispering.

The vocal folds appear to be maximally long during at-rest breathing and shortened somewhat during phonation. In fact, at the lower end of an individual's pitch range, at the level where conversational phonation is generally found, the vocal folds are considerably shortened as compared to their length during expiration. When we speak about the length and thickness of the folds, we refer to the mechanism that controls fundamental frequency, or the pitch of the voice that we hear. Fundamental frequency is directly related to how many vibratory closings and openings (cycles) the vocal folds make in one second. The rate of vibration is related to their thickness-length-elasticity. A short, thick, somewhat lax fold vibrates at a much slower rate (thus producing a low pitch) than a long, thin, tense fold, which will produce a higher pitch. The length of the vocal folds increases almost in a

Table 2–2   Normal Fundamental Frequency (F_0) and Pitch Range for Four Voices (Bass, Tenor, Alto, and Soprano)

		Typical F_0 and Pitch Range			
Note on Piano	*Physical Hz*	*(Bass)*	*(Tenor)*	*(Alto)*	*(Soprano)*
C_6	1,024				1,040
B	960				
A	853				
G_5	768				
F	682			700	
E	640				
D	576				
C_5	512		550		
B	480				
A	426				
G_4	384				

		Typical F_0 and Pitch Range			
Note on Piano	*Physical Hz*	*(Bass)*	*(Tenor)*	*(Alto)*	*(Soprano)*
F	341	340			
E	320				
D	288				
C_4	256				F_0 256
B	240				
A	213			F_0 200	
G_3	192				
F	170				170
E	160				
D	144		F_0 135	140	
C_3	128				
B	120				
A	106	F_0 100			
G_2	96		95		
F	85	80			

"stair-step" fashion, corresponding to increases in frequency. By using X-ray laminagraphy, which permits cross-sectional, coronal viewing of the vocal folds, Hollien (1962) found that the mean thickness, or mass, of the folds systematically decreased as voice pitch increased. It appears, then, from the multiple studies conducted on vocal fold length and thickness by the Hollien group, that fundamental frequency, or voice pitch level, is directly related to the length and thickness of the individual's vocal folds.

The relative differences between men and women in vocal fold length (approximately 17–20 mm for men and 12–17 mm for women) and vocal fold thickness appear to be the primary determinants of differences in voice pitch; the typical fundamental frequency for men is around 125 Hz; for women, around 215 Hz. Table 2–2 shows examples of normal pitch values, including pitch range and fundamental frequency. When individuals phonate at increasingly higher pitch levels, they must lengthen the vocal folds to decrease their relative mass and increase their tension. Increases of pitch, therefore, appear to be related to lengthening of the vocal folds, with a corresponding decrease of tissue mass and an increase of fold tissue elasticity. Lowering the pitch is directly related to shortening the folds.

It would appear that both the cricothyroids and possibly the cricopharyngeus play active roles in elongating the vocal folds, which in turn increases their elasticity. The vocal folds are stretched by the action of the cricothyroids, which increase the distance between the arytenoids and the thyroid cartilage by drawing the cricoid cartilage up toward the thyroid, which in effect lowers the posterior cricoid rim upon which the arytenoids sit. The cricopharyngeus, when contracted, can pull the cricoid slightly posterior, adding to vocal fold stretching and thus increased elasticity. For a detailed description with accompanying drawings of the elongation functions of the cricothyroid muscles, see the phonation chapter in *Speech and Hearing Science* (Zemlin, 1988). Relaxation of the cricothyroids with the simultaneous contraction of the thyroarytenoids appears to be essential for shortening and thickening the folds, which lowers the pitch of the voice. Greene (1980) has suggested that the cricopharyngeus may play an antagonist (shortening) role to the cricothyroids.

It appears that at the upper end of the natural pitch range increased elasticity of the vocal folds results in increased glottal resistance, requiring increased subglottal air pressure to produce higher-frequency phonations. Increased tension of the vocal folds requires greater air pressure to set the folds into vibration. Van den Berg (1968) has written that the average person must slightly increase subglottal air pressure in order to increase voice pitch; however, because increasing subglottal pressure has an abducting effect on the vocal folds, the folds must continue to increase in tension to maintain their approximated position. Although the primary determinant of pitch appears to be the length, mass, and tension of the vocal folds, increases in pitch level are usually characterized by increasing subglottal pressures, increased medial compression, and increased glottal airflow rates.

The vocal folds can elongate and stretch only so far. If singers want to extend their pitch range beyond what normal vocal fold stretching can do, they are forced to produce a falsetto voice. We might describe the production of the falsetto voice in this manner: The folds approximate with tight, posterior vocal process adduction. The posterior cartilaginous portion is so tightly adducted that little or no posterior vibration occurs while the anterior portion vibrates rapidly. The lateral portions of the thyroarytenoid do not actively vibrate to produce the falsetto voice. The mucosal wave is confined to the medial edge of the vocal folds. The amplitude and height of the mucosal wave are greatly reduced in high pitch and even more reduced in the production of falsetto. The inner vocalis segment of the muscle is extremely contracted (and thus thinned out) along the vocal ligament. As the membrane wraps the ligament, the membrane itself becomes the primary vibrating structure during falsetto. In falsetto the vocal folds may remain somewhat open, although parallel, which gives falsetto its characteristic "breathy" quality. At times there may also be a posterior chink during the production of falsetto, which contributes to the breathy quality of falsetto voice. Judson and Weaver (1965), Rubin and Hirt (1960), and Hollien (1962) have all described the falsetto (called the "loft" register by Hollien) as a production of the vibrating membrane of the anterior two-thirds surface of the glottal margin. This limitation of the mucosal wave to the anterior two-thirds of the vocal folds has the effect of making the cords functionally shorter and thus the higher pitch of falsetto.

The kind of pitch opposite from the falsetto in both quality and airflow rate is the low glottal fry. Greene (1980) described the fry as the pulse register, the "lowest range of notes and synonymous with vocal fry, glottal fry, creak and strohbass" (p. 81). The glottal fry sounds something like the sputter of a low-powered out-board motor or as we tell our patients the sound of a stick being dragged along a picket fence. Zemlin (1988) wrote that fry is produced when the folds are approximated tightly with a flaccid appearance along the glottal margin. Moore and von Leden (1958) found that during fry a double vibration of the folds is followed by a prolonged period of approximation (almost two-thirds the duration of the vibratory cycle). Vocal fry may well be the normal vibratory cycle we use near the bottom of our normal pitch range. It is normally produced near the end of a long phrase when subglottal air pressure and airflow rate are both low and lung volume is less. The normal nontense larynx makes use of this last end of the air supply by relaxing the vocal fold medial margins to phonate on the last available air. Some speakers may add fry to their phonation to give, in their minds, an authoritative quality to what they are saying. Although glottal fry does not appear to be a vocal abnormality, some voice patients successfully work to eliminate it by elevating their pitch levels slightly and increasing subglottal air pressure slightly.

Related to the production of voice pitch and the pitch range of any individual is *voice register*. It appears that a particular register characterizes a certain pattern of vocal fold vibration, and the vocal folds are approximated in a similar way (vibratory mode) throughout a particular pitch range. Once this pitch range reaches its maximum limit, the folds adjust to a new approximation contour (or mode of vibration), which produces an abrupt change in vocal quality. Van den Berg (1968) describes three primary forms of voice register: chest, midvoice, and falsetto. We would add to these three the vocal fry register at the lower end of the normal pitch range.

The frontal, coronal view of the folds sketched in Figure 2–15 shows the thickened folds of the chest or normal register contrasted with the thin folds of the falsetto register. From the perceptual viewpoint, voice register is confined to the similar sound (quality) of an individual's voice at various pitches. Although this similar quality is undoubtedly related to the similarity in vocal fold approximation and vibration characteristics (mode of vibration), voice teachers strive to blend the various registers, so that the difference in quality of voice becomes almost imperceptible as the singer goes from one register to the next. Some singers seem to have only one register; no matter how they change their pitch, their voice

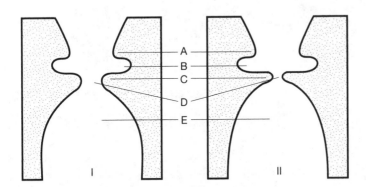

FIGURE 2–15 Line Tracing on a Tomogram

A line tracing on a tomogram that presents an X-ray frontal view of the vocal folds showing vocal fold approximation contours for (I) chest register, and (II) falsetto register: (A) Ventricular fold; (B) open ventricle; (C) vocal fold; (D) glottis, opening between folds; (E) trachea. Note the thicker fold approximation for the chest register, as opposed to the thinner, superior approximation of the two folds during the production of the falsetto register.

always seems to have the same quality, with no discernible break toward the upper part of the pitch range. This is no small accomplishment and requires considerable voice training. It is a highly regarded attribute in the professional singing voice. Such persons' frontal X-rays would probably show a relatively stable contour in the approximations of the vocal folds. An excellent review of the literature and detailed description of voice register may be found in Luchsinger and Arnold (1965). The intensity of the voice, perceived as loudness of the voice, is directly related to changes in subglottal and transglottal air pressures drops. Hixon and Abbs (1980) have written, "Sound pressure level, the primary factor contributing to our perception of the loudness of the voice, is governed mainly by the pressure supplied to the larynx by the respiratory pump" (p. 68). It appears that the trained voices of actors or singers increase in intensity by increasing both subglottal pressure and airflow rate (similar to the water hose analogy mentioned earlier), with only minimal increase of glottal tension (Bouhuys, Proctor, & Mead, 1966). At very loud levels untrained voices often increase in pitch as part of the loudness. It is difficult for untrained voices to produce loud sounds at very low pitch levels. The trained voice of the bass singer has no trouble being very loud indeed.

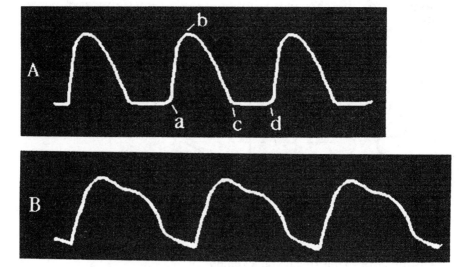

FIGURE 2–16 Laryngograms

The two laryngograms represent (A) a prolonged vowel /i/ at 125 Hz normal intensity and (B) at a louder intensity. The letter a represents the beginning of the closing phase as the cords come together; at b the cords are completely together and beginning to open; at c the cords are open; at d the open phase is completed and another cycle begins. The closed phase (b to c) is much longer in the louder production (B). The open phase (c to d) is shorter in the louder production (B).

As voice intensity increases, the vocal folds tend to remain closed for longer periods of time during each vibratory cycle (see Figure 2–16), and the greater intensity of voice is characterized by greater excursion of the vibrating folds. It would appear that, as intensity increases, increased glottal tension impedes the rate of airflow, increasing subglottal pressure. At lower pitch levels this tension during intense phonations is minimal. It causes singers, for example, to run out of air sooner when producing varying intensities at low pitches than at high ones. Evidently, speakers or singers who continually require a loud voice could use their vocal mechanisms more optimally by developing their expiratory skills and relying more on increased subglottal air pressure and increased airflow rates, and less on increased glottal elasticity, to achieve louder intensities. Besides pitch, loudness, quality, and register as measurable dimensions of voice, Perkins (1983) has added constriction and vertical as well as horizontal focus to the concept of the production of voice. He describes the feeling of constriction on a continuum of open (the yawn) to closed (the swallow). Imagery or feeling is used to determine the vertical focus of the voice, "the perception associated with the placement of the focal point of the tone in the head" (Perkins, 1983, p. 113). At the low end of the vertical focus, speakers or singers feel their voice is being squeezed out of the throat, whereas at the high end the focus seems to be high in the head. The sensation is described as if the tone were "floating in the head." Vocal efficiency seems to occur best at the higher end of the vertical placement. It has been our experience that subjects given these instructions relative to the imagery of constriction and verticality produce voices with greater aperiodicity (hoarseness) at the low end of the vertical scale and greater vocal clarity at the high end. In time the Perkins construct of constriction and horizontal as well as vertical focus may well have greater measurement potential and utilization. Vocal quality may well be related primarily to supraglottal resonance, but important components of the spectrum of the laryngeal tone have their origins at the level of the glottis. How the vocal folds are approximated together, laxly or tightly, in part determines the quality of the voice. Many individuals can produce several different voices, all at the same pitch level, by varying the approximation characteristics of the vocal folds. A breathy voice is often produced by adding phonation to the ongoing expiration, with the folds only laxly approximating one another. Spectrographic analysis of the breathy voice shows us that noise and aperiodicity produced by the turbulent airflow typify the first part of the utterance, and that phonation (greater periodicity) comes in after some delay. The four spectrograms in Figure 2–17 contrast the breathy voice (with much aperiodicity and noise) with the harsh voice (with hard glottal attack) and the normal voice and hoarse voice.

Each of the spectrograms was produced by the same normal speaker

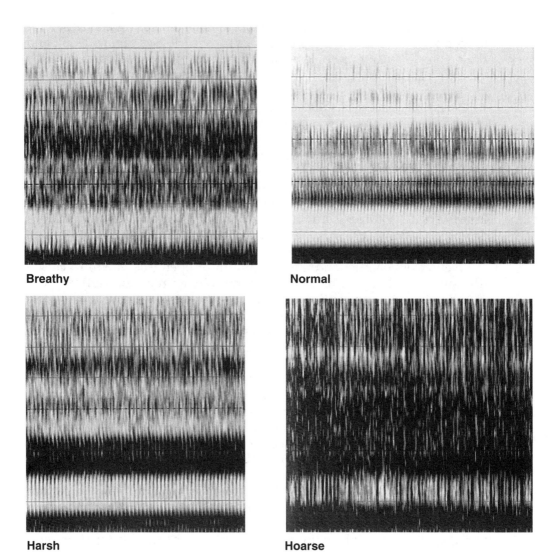

Breathy

Normal

Harsh

Hoarse

FIGURE 2–17   Spectrograms
Four spectrograms of the same speaker producing the /i/ vowel under four conditions: breathy, normal, harsh, and hoarse. The relative spacing of the formants stays the same as the signal source changes.

prolonging an /i/. In hard glottal attack, the opposite kind of vocal onset is observed. Here the first voicing patterns begin abruptly with the onset of expiration. The glottis seems to be held tightly until a sudden release of air sets the folds into vibration. Faulty positioning of the vocal folds is also characteristic of patients with adductor spasmodic dysphonia. (While we use the term *adductor spasmodic dysphonia*, Watterson &

McFarlane, 1992, make a case that the abductor and adductor types are actually different disorders, not two types of the same disorder.) These patients bring the folds so tightly together that they act like a valve, almost totally preventing the flow of air from traveling through the glottis. The patient's voice is strained and has a strangled quality. How the folds are approximated has much to do with how voices sound. Study of the vocal fold "set" aspect of phonation has been limited to such methods as high-speed film, viewing the larynx through indirect laryngoscopy, or employing spectrograms that visually display the voices that we hear. Even though we know something about the extreme of breathiness and hard glottal attack, our knowledge of vocal fold physiology for most of the voices we hear is relatively lacking in regard to vocal fold approximation and its effect on quality. The development of flexible videoendoscopy and glottographic instruments has allowed us to study the production of these aspects further. McFarlane and Lavorato (1984) have discussed the use of videoendoscopy in the study of voice disorders. We discuss this topic in detail in Chapter 4, where we present evaluation procedures. Likewise, Watterson, McFarlane, and Menicucci (1990), McFarlane (1988), McFarlane and Watterson (1991), and Tyler and Watterson (1991) have all addressed aspects of glottal closure and its effect on voice quality.

RESONANCE

The fundamental frequency produced by the vocal folds would be a weak-sounding, "reedy" voice without the additional component of resonance. Years ago one of the authors observed a patient who had been cut from ear to ear with a massive wound that opened immediately superior to his thyroid cartilage. Before the wound was sutured, we heard the patient's feeble attempts at phonation. Much of his airflow and sound waves escaped through the wound opening. The result was a voice that was truly unique. Someone even likened it to the thin bleat of a baby lamb. Apparently, what is perceived as the quality, timbre, richness, and loudness of the voice is largely produced by the supraglottal resonators. Even though the structures of the chest and trachea may play some role in resonance, this role is not as clearly defined as that of the supraglottal resonators of the pharynx, oral cavity, and nasal cavity.

Structures of Resonance

The vocal tract begins, for all practical purposes, at the level of the glottis. The airflow and sound waves probably have some beginning passage in the ventricular space (B in Figure 2–18) between the true folds (A) and the ventricular folds (C). In Figure 2–18 the cavities of the vocal

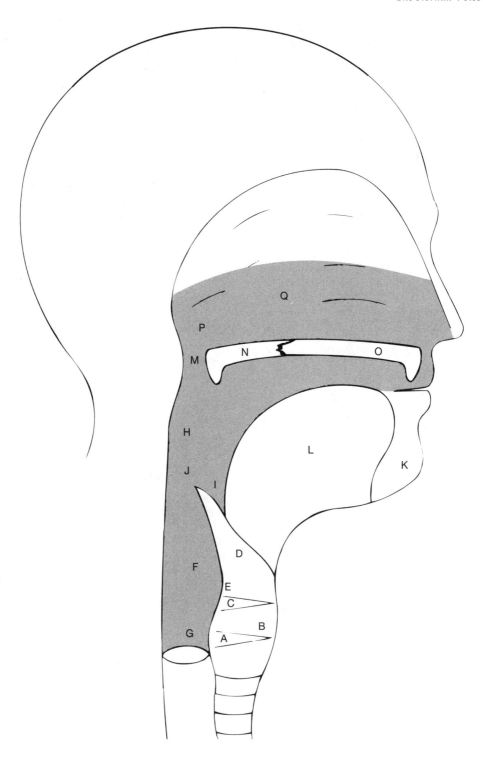

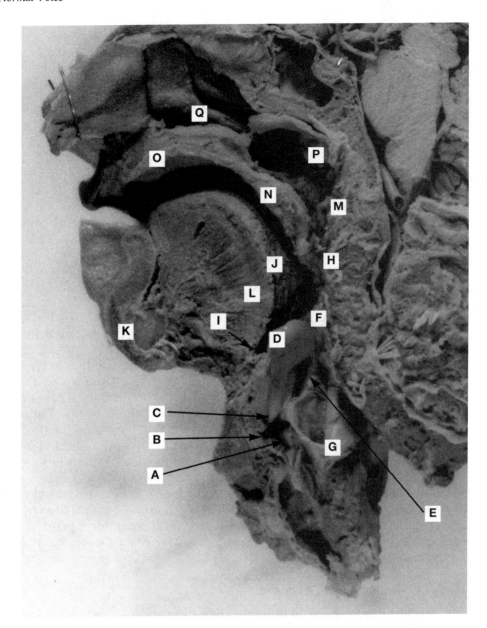

FIGURE 2–18   The F-Shaped Vocal Tract

The F-shaped vocal tract is shown in both the line drawing on the left and the photograph of a cadaver head on the right. Letters A through O identify various structures of the vocal tract: (A) True folds; (B) ventricular space; (C) ventricular folds; (D) epiglottis; (E) aryepiglottic folds; (F) hypopharynx; (G) lower pharyngeal constrictors; (H) middle pharyngeal constrictors; (I) vaculae; (J) oropharynx; (K) mandible; (L) tongue; (M) Passavant's pad; (N) soft palate (velum); (O) hard palate; (P) nasopharynx; (Q) nasal cavity.

tract have been shaded in black. The epiglottis (D), by its concavity, probably serves as a deflector or sounding-board resonator as sound waves travel between the aryepiglottic folds (E) into the hypopharynx (F). The hypopharynx is the cavity directly above the esophagus. Its anterior border comprises the structures and opening of the larynx; its sides and back wall are composed of the lower pharyngeal constrictors (G). The oropharynx (J) is just before the tip of the epiglottis. The small angular spaces between the front of the epiglottis and the back of the tongue (L) are called the vaculae (I). Cutting away the mandible (K) in a lateral view is the great body of the tongue, which occupies most of the oral cavity and forms the constantly changing floor of that cavity. The hard palate is designated (O), with the soft palate, or velum (N), forming the roof of the oral cavity. The lips, teeth, and cheeks play obvious front and lateral roles in shaping the oral cavity. The middle and superior pharyngeal constrictors form the lateral and posterior muscular wall of the oropharynx (J). The site of the velopharyngeal closure, necessary for the separation of the oral and nasal cavities required for oral resonance, is the Passavant's pad (M) area of the superior pharyngeal constrictor; most subjects do not have much Passavant area enlargement. As shown in Figure 2–18, superior to the velopharyngeal contact point, the posterior pharyngeal wall makes a sharp angulation forward, forming the superior wall of the nasopharynx (P) and continuing on as the superior wall of the nasal cavity. We make no further structural breakdown of the nasal cavities (Q) as a prelude to our discussion of resonance. Note that Figure 2–18 also shows the lateral walls, pillars of fauces, muscles of the palate, pharynx, and tongue. If we look again at the overall lateral view of the vocal tract, we see that the total darkened areas look slightly like a large letter F. The vocal tract in the photograph resembles an F because the velopharyngeal port is open, connecting the oral and nasal cavities. If the port were closed at the velopharyngeal contact point, the vocal tract opening available for voice resonance would resemble a printed letter r, formed only by the pharynx and the oral cavity opening above the surface of the tongue.

Mechanism of Resonance

A vibrator, such as the string of a violin or the vocal folds, originates a fundamental vibration (or sound waves), which by itself produces weak barely audible sounds. This vibrating energy is usually amplified by a resonating body of some type. For example, a violin string, when plucked, will set up a fundamental vibration; this vibration becomes resonated by the bridge to which the strings are attached, which then sets into vibration the sounding board below and in turn the main resonating body of the violin (the chest), which provides open-cavity resonance.

When all the violin parts are working together in harmony, the fundamental tone of the involved string becomes louder, richer, and fuller in quality. The same string stripped out of its mount on the violin and then plucked (even with the same amount of tension to the string) will sound less intense and thinner in quality.

The violin provides a ready example of the two main types of resonance, the sounding-board effect and the open-cavity effect. When a particular string of the violin is bowed, the airwaves that develop are low in amplitude and barely audible; however, because the vibrating string is stretched tightly over the bridge of the violin, it sets the bridge itself into vibration. The bridge functions as a sounding board. The sounding board then vibrates, setting into vibration the air over a much larger area, increasing the loudness of the tone. The sounding-board vibration also introduces the sound waves into the violin cavity itself. The main body, or chest, of the violin provides cavity resonance to the source sound of the vibrating string. The string vibrating alone, which is similar to laryngeal vibration without supraglottal resonance, produces a barely audible tone. The cavity resonance provided by the body of the violin increases the volume of the vibrating string. The size and overall shape of the resonating cavity have an obvious relationship to the resonance of a vibration.

Every frequency of vibration has an ideal resonating cavity size and shape. The ideal is represented by the cavity that seems to give the loudest tone and the tone with the fullest amount of amplification to its overtones. This may be thought of as acoustic efficiency. This observation can be easily tested by placing a tuning fork over a large glass and varying the amounts of water in the glass. At a particular level of water, the glass will provide optimum resonance, heard as increased loudness and richness of the sound. The lower the frequency of the vibrating wave, the larger the size of the resonating cavity. The thinner string of the violin requires a much smaller resonating body than the larger string of the bass viola, which requires a resonating body as tall as the person who plays the instrument.

The human vocal tract is continually changing. As Minifie (1973) has written:

> During the production of vowels the vocal tract may be viewed as a tortuously shaped tube open at one end (the opening between the lips) and bounded at the other end by a vibrating valve (the vocal folds) which has the effect of closing off the tube at the larynx. The three-dimensional geometry of this tube may be altered through the contraction of muscles which regulate the movements of the tongue, velum, pharynx, mandible, lips, epiglottis, and larynx. These structures may be moved individually or in various combinations. The combination of structures which move during the production of a particular speech sound will determine the

unique vocal tract configuration, and hence, the unique acoustical filter for that sound. (p. 243)

Some areas of the vocal tract, depending on their configuration, are compatible with the periodic vibration coming from the vocal folds and amplify the fundamental frequency and its harmonics. For example, a fundamental frequency of 125 Hz will resonate harmonic frequencies at 250, 375, 500 (each subsequent harmonic frequency is a whole number multiple of the fundamental), and so on. The continuous vocal tract tube is constantly interrupted at various sites from the intrusion and movement of various structures. Some of the interruptions or constrictions may be severe, such as carrying the tongue high and forward in the oral cavity. Any movement of mandible, tongue, or velum, for example, will greatly alter the opening of the oral cavity. Some of the movements have no effect on the fundamental or sound source; some of them filter or inhibit the fundamental. What finally emits from the mouth or the nasal cavity perceived as voice has become a complex periodic signal with the same fundamental frequency as the vocal fold source, but highly modified in its overall sound characteristics. We can hear several familiar voices all saying the same few words at the same fundamental frequency, and still be able to differentiate each voice and assign it to each familiar person. Perhaps even more importantly, by filtering the glottal tone we can tell if the person has a cold, is upset, angry, tired, frightened, or the meaning could even be changed by the change in quality or emphasis while saying the same words. The vocal characteristics related to the individualization of each person's vocal tract will have given each voice its own unique characteristics (vocal quality) as the result of the amplification and filtering unique to each vocal tract.

The F configuration of the supraglottal vocal tract is constantly changing. What happens in any one portion of the tract influences both the total flow of air and sound wave through the total tract and the sound that eventually emits from the mouth (or nose). By action of the pharyngeal constrictors and other supraglottal muscles, the overall dimensions of the pharynx are always changing. The membranes of the pharynx and the degree of relaxation or tautness of the pharyngeal constrictors have noticeable acoustic filtering effects. Higher-frequency vocalizations seem to receive their best resonating effects under a fairly high degree of pharyngeal wall tension. Lower frequencies appear to be better amplified by a pharynx that is somewhat relaxed. This may be related to the short wave length of high-frequency sounds and the long wave length of the low -frequency components.

The oral cavity, or mouth, is as essential for resonance as the pharynx. Of all our resonators, the mouth is capable of the most variation in size and shape. It is the constant size/shape adjustment of the mouth that permits us to speak or, more accurately, allows us to be understood. Our vowels and diphthongs, for example, are originated by a laryngeal vibration, but shaped and restricted by size/shape adjustment of the oral cavity. The mouth has fixed structures (teeth, alveolar processes, dental arch, and hard palate) and moving structures. We are most concerned with the moving structures, primarily the tongue, velum, and mandible, in our study of voice resonance. It is the mouth and other supraglottal resonators that give us the perception of a regional dialect to help identify the speaker.

The tongue is the most mobile articulator, and it possesses both extrinsic and intrinsic muscles to move it. Each of the extrinsic muscles can, upon contraction, elevate or lower the tongue at its anterior, middle, or posterior points and extend it forward or backward. The intrinsic muscles control the shape of the tongue by narrowing, flattening, lengthening, or shortening the overall tongue body and elevating or lowering the tongue tip. The various combinations of intrinsic and extrinsic muscle contractions can produce an unlimited number of tongue positions with resulting size/shape variations of the oral cavity. In addition to the tongue movements, the lowering and closing of the mandible contributes to the formation of specific vowels. The relationships of these cavities to vowel formants have been well described in several references, such as the Peterson and Barney study (1952), and in chapters by Netsell (1973) and by Daniloff (1973) in *Normal Aspects of Speech, Hearing, and Language.*

The structural adequacy and normal functioning of the velum are also important for the development of normal voice resonance. The elevation and tensing of the velum, as well as some pharyngeal wall movement, are vital for achieving velopharyngeal closure. A lack of adequate palatal movement, despite adequacy of velar length, can cause serious problems of excessive nasality. Although the velum probably serves as a sounding-board structure in resonance, it plays an obviously important role in separating the oral cavity from the nasal cavity. The movement and positioning of the velum change the size and shape of three important resonating cavities: the pharynx, the oral cavity, and the nasal cavity. Therefore, any alteration of the velum (such as a soft-palate cleft or velar weakness) may have a profound influence on resonance. Velar movement is only one component contributing to velopharyngeal closure (Zwitman, Gyepes, & Ward, 1976). Closure patterns that separate the oral and nasal cavities from one another may include velar action coupled by posterior pharyngeal wall movement, or velar action with active lateral and posterior pharyngeal wall movement. Watterson and McFarlane (1990) describe five classes of velopharyngeal closure and their various effects on speech and voice. Regardless of the type of closure pattern (velar-posterior-lateral pharyngeal wall), the site of closure is generally in the Passavant's area (designated as M in Figure 2–18).

The fundamental frequency that comes from the vocal folds is modified throughout the vocal tract. Movements and constrictions within the tract contribute to the overall amplifying or filtering or modification of the voice signal produced by the vibrating vocal folds. Faulty use of the structures of the vocal tract often leads to disorders in quality and resonance.

SUMMARY

In our review of the respiratory aspects of phonation we found that the outgoing airstream is the primary driving force of voice. The efficient user of voice develops good expiratory control. A description of the physiology of phonation reviewed the structures and mechanisms of normal phonation, including frequency and intensity. Supraglottal structures and functions specific to quality and resonance were also reviewed. The entire vocal tract contributes to the amplification and filtering of the fundamental frequency into the final unique voice of any speaker. The understanding of these normal processes provides the underpinning for providing effective voice therapy for patients with a variety of dysphonias.

Chapter 3

Voice Disorders

Voice disorders result from faulty structure or function somewhere in the vocal tract: in respiration, in phonation, or in resonance. A traditional, although artificial, way of looking at voice disorders is to divide them into two etiologic (causative) categories: functional or organic. Functional voice disorders are usually caused by faulty use of vocal mechanisms. Organic voice problems are related to some physical abnormality in structure or function at various sites of the vocal tract. As we consider different functional-organic voice disorders in this chapter, we also look at the various sites of the vocal tract to see how they may be contributing to the voice disorders.

When the voice changes in any negative way the voice is said to be disordered or dysphonic. Such changes have many different common names, *hoarseness, harshness, huskiness, stridency*, to name only a few. Unfortunately, there is little common agreement about what these terms mean among listeners. In this text, we use a more generic term, dysphonia, which means any alteration in normal phonation. This lack of a common vocabulary for the various parameters of voice production and voice pathology is perhaps related to the number of different kinds of specialists who are concerned with voice—the laryngologist, the singing teacher, the speech-voice scientist, the speech-voice pathologist, and the voice-and-diction teacher. The laryngologist is primarily interested in identifying the etiologic and pathological aspects for purposes of treatment; the singing teacher uses imagery in an attempt to get the desired acoustical effect from the voice student; the speech-voice scientist has the laboratory interest of the physiologist or physicist; the speech-voice pathologist often attempts to use the knowledge and vocabulary of all three of these disciplines to bring about treatment; and the voice-and-diction teacher assesses the dynamics of voice production and uses whatever is necessary to "get" the best voice. It is no wonder that interdisciplinary communication among voice specialists breaks down.

The general public tolerance of an indifference to voice problems makes the early identification of voice pathologies difficult. Hoarseness that persists longer than several days is often identified by the laryngologist as a possible symptom of serious laryngeal disease. And it may be. Hoarseness is certainly the acoustic correlate of improper vocal fold functioning, with or without true laryngeal disease. The distinction between organic disease of the larynx and functional misuse has been a prominent dichotomy in the consideration of phonatory disorders. It is important for the laryngologists, in their need to rule out or identify true organic disease, to view the laryngeal mechanism by laryngoscopy in order to make a judgment about organic-structural involvement. In the absence of observable structural deviation, the laryngologist generally describes the voice disorder as functional. It has become important for the speech-voice pathologist to view the larynx as part of the voice evaluation and in designing the voice therapy (McFarlane & Lavorato, 1984; McFarlane, Watterson, & Brophy, 1990; Watterson & McFarlane, 1991).

Functional aphonia, for example, may be a wholly functional voice problem. The patient may exhibit normal breath flow and an adequate open pharynx and oral cavity for normal resonance but totally lack voice. When a functionally aphonic patient attempts to use voice he or she may whisper through very incompletely approximated vocal folds or may make a very weak shrill, high-pitched breathy whistle of a voice. The result is basically a form or variation of a whisper. As a result, some have called functional aphonia *whisper aphonia*. A patient can also functionally misuse the vocal tract (such as by inadequate breath support or excessively hard glottal attack or by closing down the supraglottal mechanisms), which, in time, may lead to organic changes of structure, such as bilateral vocal nodules or contact ulcers. Such nodules might well have been caused by excessive vocal abuse and misuse. Once the nodules develop, however, they contribute to the poor voice that is often characterized by low pitch, excessive breathiness, and severe hoarseness. Many structural organic alterations of the larynx (such as cancer or granuloma or web) can have profound effects on the larynx and the vocal folds in particular, which can result in serious alterations of voice.

A normal voice requires relatively normal usage of respiratory, phonatory, and resonance mechanisms. Conversely, poor use of these mechanisms can produce faulty voice. Some poor voices result from faulty respiratory timing and control; for example, the patient may "run out of air" in the middle of a verbal passage. Instead of renewing the breath with some kind of catch-up inspiration, the patient continues to attempt to vocalize. The resulting insufficient air flow, low lung volume, and inadequate subglottal air pressure can be heard in the dysphonic voice toward the end of the utterance. Changes in the mass-size-tension of the vocal folds result in changes of frequency, also characterized by fluctuations in voice pitch.

As described in Chapter 2, normal phonation requires that, in addition to proper mass-size adjustments, the two vocal folds approximate each other optimally along their entire length (from the anterior commissure up to, and including, the vocal process). The easy imitation of voices by some actors suggests that individuals are able to vary the strength of fold approximation. Consistent with this observation is the further observation that most functionally caused dysphonias are related directly to underadduction or overadduction of the vocal folds and to alterations in airflow. In underadduction, the folds are too laxly approximated, resulting in a breathy type of phonation. Sometimes, after prolonged hyperfunctional use of the voice, the folds will show an open chink posteriorly; actually, this posterior chink is the incomplete adduction of the vocal processes. Overadduction of the folds results in the tight valving of the glottal mechanism, so much so that the individual may be unable to phonate for speech.

Spasmodic dysphonia (adductor type) is a severe overadduction problem. The voice sounds strained, like the kind of phonation we hear from someone attempting to talk while lifting a heavy object; the valving action of the larynx (fixed, tight adduction) overrules the individual's desire to phonate, and phonation becomes nearly impossible. Often, conditions that increase the mass-size of the vocal folds—that is, cord thickening, nodules, or polyps—will, by their size and the irregular shape of the vocal fold edge, make the optimum adduction of the vocal folds impossible. Glottal growths, such as nodules (McFarlane & Watterson, 1990), and polyps, interfere with the approximating edges of the vocal folds, and they often produce open chinks between the approximating folds on each side of the growth. Any structural interference between the approximating edges of the vocal folds usually results in some degree of dysphonia and air wastage. However, some patients may actually attempt to cope with this air wastage by overadducting the folds and thus produce too little airflow. This gives rise to a strained, tight, squeezed-off voice rather than a breathy voice quality. Occasionally, unilateral or bilateral paralysis of intrinsic muscles of the larynx results in paralysis of one or both of the vocal folds, producing obvious voice problems related to faulty approximation and air wastage.

On nasoendoscopy (McFarlane, Watterson, & Brophy, 1990), we often observe resonance being altered by surprisingly large movements of supraglottal structures (false folds, aryepiglottic folds, pharyngeal walls, tongue). For example, the tight voice of spastic dysphonia is not only produced by tight sphincteral closure of the vocal folds, but by pronounced supraglottal shutoff or valving as well. By watching the movements of the oro- and hypopharynx during nasoendoscopy (McFarlane & Lavorato, 1984; Pershall & Boone, 1986), we have come to appreciate the dynamic role that these structures have in both vocal quality and resonance. Supraglottal structures play an important role in the production of both normal and abnormal voice.

Table 3–1 lists 27 voice disorders, some *primarily* the result of misuse of vocal mechanisms, and some the direct result of organic changes of vocal mechanisms. The left column lists 13 voice disorders whose etiology appears to be primarily functional; the names of many of these functional voice disorders describe, in effect, the vocal changes they cause. The right column lists 14 organic conditions of the vocal tract that may contribute to various vocal pathologies. The organic disorders are more often labeled by etiology or the tissue change they may cause than by the acoustic alterations they may produce.

Table 3–1   Twenty-Seven Voice Problems Related to Either Faulty Usage of the Vocal Mechanisms or to Organic Changes of Vocal Mechanism

Functional Disorder	Organic Disorder
Contact ulcers	Cancer
Diplophonia	Dysarthria
Falsetto	Endocrine changes
Functional aphonia	Granuloma
Functional dysphonia	Hemangioma
Phonation breaks (abductor spasms)	Hyperkeratosis
Pitch breaks	Infectious laryngitis
Spasmodic dysphonia*	Laryngectomy
Thickening (vocal fold)	Laryngofissure
Traumatic laryngitis	Leukoplakia
Ventricular dysphonia	Papilloma
Vocal nodules	Pubertal changes
Vocal polyps	Vocal fold paralysis
	Webbing

*The etiology of spasmodic dysphonia is unknown. It may be classified as a functional disorder by some authors (for a discussion of this disorder and its subtypes, see Watterson & McFarlane, 1992; Karnell, 1992).

VOICE DISORDERS RELATED TO FAULTY USAGE

In this section, we consider the voice problems listed in the left-hand column of Table 3–1. These voice disorders result from using the vocal mechanisms in a faulty manner. For reader convenience, we consider separately each of these functional voice disorders, including their possible etiology and management, in alphabetical order, as they appear in Table 3–1.

Contact Ulcers

As we mentioned in Chapter 2, the total length of the glottis can be divided into thirds: the anterior two-thirds is muscular (vocalis portion of the thyroarytenoids) and covered by a membrane; the posterior third is cartilaginous (arytenoids) and covered by a membrane. Contact ulcers, which generally form along the posterior third of the glottal margin, seem to result from one of three causes. The first is excessive slamming together of the arytenoid cartilages during production of low-pitched phonation coupled with excessively hard glottal attack and perhaps increased loudness and frequent throat clearing and coughing. The speaker is usually a hard-driving person who speaks in a loud, controlling low pitch, often with words punctuated with sudden onset. However, Watterson, Hansen-Magorian, and McFarlane (1990) found that hard glottal attack was reported only 26% of the time by diagnosing clinicians, while pain was reported in 56% of the total of 57 cases studied. The second etiology for contact ulcer is gastric reflux, where stomach acid may be forced up the esophagus and irritate the area between the arytenoids or the vocal fold covering (Koufman, 1991). Koufman feels that this gastroesophageal reflux disease (GERD) may account not only for many contact ulcers but also for many cases of so-called functional dysphonia, and thus he advocates ambulatory 24-hour pH monitoring for patients suspected of having this disorder. Third, intubation for surgery is a cause of contact ulcer, especially where bilateral rather large granulomas are the presenting picture following any type of surgery.

The typical symptoms of contact ulcers are deterioration of voice after prolonged vocalization (vocal fatigue), accompanied by pain in the laryngeal area or sometimes pain that lateralizes out to one ear. Watterson, Hansen-Magorian, and McFarlane (1990) also found hoarseness/roughness reported 75% of the time and throat clearing in 65% of the 57 cases of contact ulcer they studied. Laryngoscopy usually reveals bilateral ulcerations with heavy buildup of granulation tissue along the approximating margins of the posterior glottis. Greene (1980) labeled the toughened membranous tissue changes on the posterior glottis as *pachydermia*, citing the work of Kleinsasser (1979); Greene (1980) wrote that "contact ulcers are not actually ulcers or granulomas but consist of 'craters' with highly thickened squamous epithelium over connective tissue with some inflammation (edema)" (p. 147).

The diffuse irritation of the posterior glottis often associated with contact ulcers may be the result of esophageal reflux, sometimes associated with diaphragmatic or hiatal hernia and disease of the lower esophageal sphincter (LES). The patient experiences esophageal reflux while sleeping, which results in the pooling of acid secretions in the vocal process (posterior) end of the glottis (Cherry & Margulies, 1968). In studying the sensitivity of the posterior larynx to gastric juices, Delahunty and Cherry (1968) were able to produce, experimentally, contact ulcers and granulation tissue in dogs by swabbing gastric juices on their vocal folds. It now appears that patients with contact ulcers who also demonstrate marked irritation of laryngeal/pharyngeal tissue are candidates for a thorough examination of the gastrointestinal tract (Koufman, 1991). If a hiatal hernia, for example, is found with contact ulcers, the patient may best be treated with antacids, acid-inhibiting agents, diet management, and voice therapy. Other behavioral changes such as elevating the head of the bed and reducing the size of meals and eating several hours before going to bed are helpful in reflux management. The focus of voice therapy for patients with contact ulcers is to take the effort out of phonation. The patients must learn to use a voice pitch level that can be produced with relatively little strain (which usually means pitch needs to be elevated), to speak with greater mouth and jaw relaxation, to speak at lower levels of volume, and to eliminate all traces of excessively hard glottal attack. Contact ulcers are rare today. According to Watterson, Hansen-Magorian, and McFarlane (1990) these cases comprise about 1% of total voice cases. Those patients who do have contact ulcers, however, seem to respond fairly well to voice therapy that is systematically employed. Surgery is usually not helpful, since the ulcers generally return postoperatively.

Diplophonia

The term *diplophonia* means "double voice." A diplophonic voice is produced with two distinct voice sources, each voicing simultaneously with the other. Occasionally, someone may produce a double voice with one vocal fold in a different mass-size-tension mode than the other fold— that is, one fold vibrates at a different vibratory speed than the other one. For example, a woman with a large unilateral vocal polyp was observed who spoke with a diplophonic voice. Her normal vocal fold vibrated at its normal frequency, while the involved fold (much enlarged with a broad-based polyp) vibrated more slowly and produced the diplophonic voice. Other possible causes of diplophonia that have been reported are laryngeal web, vocal-cord paralysis, ventricular fold vibration simultaneous with true fold vibration, and aryepiglottic vibration added to normal fold vibration and also strictly functional maladjustments of the folds. Theoretically, any bodies (folds or structures) that can approximate in the vocal tract, through which outgoing airflow can pass, have the potential for producing a sound (or voice) when set into vibration.

The treatment of diplophonia is aimed at eliminating the source of the second voice. Sometimes, surgical removal of a unilateral mass or elimination of a laryngeal web will result in a single voice. More often, diplophonia is corrected by voice therapy (which we discuss in Chapters 5 and 6). This is accomplished by reducing the hyperfunction or laryngeal tension that is producing the second sound source.

Falsetto

Other names for falsetto are *puberphonia* , *mutational falsetto*, and *incomplete mutation* of voice (discussed later in this chapter). The sound of falsetto is both high pitched and breathy in quality. There are frequent downward pitch breaks by the person using falsetto voice. The high pitch is produced as discussed in Chapter 2 with the anterior portions of the vocal folds only vibrating and the posterior part of the folds open or gapped. The folds approximate with thin vocal lips and do not completely touch in the midline. The result vocally is a voice that is too high for the speaker and that draws attention to itself. The perception is of a small, young, immature speaker. Males with falsetto voice are often mistaken for females on the telephone or in situations where the listener is unable to see the speaker. Falsetto is the upper end of the normal range and represents the highest register of voice. It is a voice disorder when used as the major mode of vibration or voice by either male or female adults. Use of this voice projects a female quality for male speakers and a juvenile or immature impression when used by female speakers. However, the social penalty for this type of voice is greater for the male speaker. Falsetto is nearly always due to functional causes and is generally very responsive to treatment by voice therapy. An ENT (ear-nose-throat) examination is always in order to rule out the unlikely possibility of an endocrine or structural etiology. We have very rarely felt the need to refer these patients for counseling or psychotherapy. McFarlane (1988) reports an exception of a patient who was undergoing psychotherapy simultaneously with voice therapy and whose response to voice therapy was less successful. We have never had a patient relapse into a falsetto voice after completion of voice therapy.

Therapy for falsetto voice takes the general approach of lowering the pitch and improving the vocal quality. This is accomplished by digital pressure to produce a lower pitch, using "glottal fry to a tone," extending the cough or throat clearing, which are almost always at a dramatically lower, more appropriate pitch level. Other techniques that are helpful are inhalation phonation and half-swallow boom. Aronson (1990) advocates massage of the larynx and manual lowering of the high tense laryngeal position during falsetto production.

Functional Aphonia

Patients with *functional aphonia* speak with a whisper. In order to rule out some form of organic laryngeal involvement, such as vocal fold paralysis, these patients must be examined by either indirect laryngoscopy or videoendoscopy of the larynx (McFarlane, 1990). When functional aphonic patients are requested to say "ah," their vocal folds simply are not set adequately in vibration.

Functional aphonia has no organic cause. In fact, it is frequently described as a *hysterical* or *conversion* symptom, according to Aronson, Peterson, and Litin (1966), who found these two terms used by various laryngologists for 20 functional dysphonic and aphonic patients they had observed. Although functional aphonia may well be a form of conversion hysteria, Brodnitz (1971) recommends that we avoid using the term in the "presence of the patient because of the social stigma attached to it" (p. 65). Usually patients have had several temporary losses of voice before the disorder becomes permanent. In our experience, they may also have had a recent bout of the flu or an upper respiratory infection (URI) prior to onset of functional aphonia. Aphonic patients may derive some temporary reinforcing gains from their loss of voice, such as not having to give speeches or not being able to preside over meetings. Aphonia may even become permanent after moments of acute stress by maintaining itself for various reasons. Aronson, Peterson, and Litin (1966) report that in 10 out of 27 patients they studied the onset of functional dysphonia or aphonia was associated with an event of acute stress; in 13 of the 27 patients, it was associated with stress over a longer period of time. The onset of functional aphonia is sometimes related to the patient's having experienced some laryngeal pathology or other disease. For example, Boone (1966b) described the physical origin of functional aphonia in two patients, one who became aphonic after a meningitis attack, and the other after a laryngeal operation, when she could not end the voice rest imposed upon her by the laryngologist. Both of these aphonic patients were highly responsive to voice therapy. We once successfully treated a patient who developed functional aphonia suddenly during his testimony as a witness in a courtroom trial.

Patients with functional aphonia communicate well by gesture and whisper or by a high-pitched shrill-sounding weak voice. Typical aphonic patients whisper with clarity and sharpness. Aphonic patients rarely avoid communication situations; conversely, they communicate effectively by using facial expressions, hands, and highly intelligible whispered speech. What they lack in communication is voice.

Embarrassed and frustrated by lack of voice, aphonic patients generally self-refer to a physician or speech-language pathologist. Despite Greene's (1980) warning that many patients with functional aphonia may require psychological counseling, most aphonic patients, in our experience, completely recover their normal voice with voice therapy (usually in the first session of therapy). Aphonic patients as a group, in fact, have an excellent prognosis. It is almost as if for whatever reason the patient has lost the "set" for phonation. The voice clinician's task is to help the patient "find" his or her voice primarily by helping the patient use vegetative phonations, such as coughing or inhalation phonation or sometimes using masking noise (Chapter 5). The patient then extends the vegetative phonation into the production of a vowel, into nonsense syllables, then into single words, then phrases, and so on. Aronson (1990) suggests digital manipulation of the larynx of these patients.

By using behavioral modification approaches, such as those suggested by Eysenck (1961), Sloane and MacAulay (1968), and Wolpe (1987), we have had excellent success in directly working on voice. Typical aphonic patients experience restoration of normal voice in the first, or at least, in very few voice therapy sessions (McFarlane, 1988; McFarlane & Lavorato, 1984; Lavorato & McFarlane, 1988). Wilson (1987) described the "sudden and complete recovery" of several teenage girls who responded well to symptomatic voice therapy. Suggested methods of symptomatic voice therapy for functional aphonia will be presented in Chapter 6.

Functional Dysphonia

Some of the most disturbed voices we hear may have no organic or physical cause. Patients may approximate the vocal folds in a lax manner, producing breathiness, or in a tight manner, producing symptoms of harshness or tightness. In addition, patients may close off their voice by bringing the ventricular folds together or by pursing off the larynx by firm, sphincteral-like closure of the aryepiglottic folds. Voice problems that do not result from an organic pathology may be called *functional dysphonia*, a term that conveys very little to the voice clinician other than the important implication that there is no structural pathology present. In fact, the common usage of the term *functional dysphonia* is confined to those dysphonias where the problem persists independent of any kind of pathology observed on laryngoscopy. After a history of continuing dysphonia, the typical patient is finally examined by laryngoscopy and found not to have any neurological or additive lesion, such as nodules or papilloma or granuloma (or whatever). In many cases of functional dysphonia, we can hardly visualize the vocal folds by nasoendoscopy because they are often covered by an almost complete supraglottal shut-off (ventricular and aryepiglottic fold adduction). Functional dysphonia appears to be the product of both laryngeal and supralaryngeal shutdown. In addition, patients complain of many vague disorders—throat "fullness," pain in the laryngeal area or chest, dryness of mouth while talking, neck tightness, and so on—that are usually related to vocal fatigue. The voice frequently just gives out.

A functionally caused dysphonia does not necessarily sound different from one that is organically caused. Some of the hoarsest voices are produced by people whose larynges demonstrate no pathology whatsoever; on the other hand, serious organic problems, such as beginning cancer, may produce no alteration of the voice. Anyone with persistent dysphonia (longer than 10 days) ought to undergo a laryngeal examination to determine the possible cause of the problem and to rule out serious laryngeal disease. While developing critical listening skills is important for the voice clinician, since the same voice sound can be produced by several different laryngeal adjustments or conditions, it is essential that the larynx be visually inspected. We suggest that the speech-voice pathologist also visualize the larynx as part of the voice evaluation (ASHA, 1992b; McFarlane, 1990; Watterson, 1991).

Aronson (1990) objects to the term *functional* dysphonia because he thinks that such problems are generally psychogenic in nature:

> A psychogenic voice disorder is broadly synonymous with a functional one but has the advantage of stating positively, based on an exploration of its causes, that the voice disorder is a manifestation of one or more types of psychologic disequilibrium —such as anxiety, depression, conversion reaction, or personality disorder—which interferes with normal volitional control over phonation. (p. 131)

As discussed in Chapter 1, we believe that most functional voice problems may be successfully treated symptomatically, by working on dimensions of voice directly to improve the sounds of the voice. In most cases, however, clinicians should offer patients much psychological support, in an attempt to minimize their anxieties and concern, and should search with the patients for the best voices they can produce.

The first dimension of voice to be evaluated and worked on if necessary is fundamental frequency. If a patient has no organic problem contributing to dysphonia but has a faulty pitch, the clinician should use various facilitating approaches (see Chapter 5) to develop an appropriate pitch. The vocal intensity of the voice is also measured; if the patient has a loudness problem, direct attempts to change the volume can be initiated. For the occasional patient whose voice loudness is directly related to shyness and insecurity, working on respiratory support and loudness per se may be combined with attempting to improve self-concept and interpersonal relationships as well. The majority of voice patients with vocal intensity problems, however, are quite responsive to symptomatic therapy designed to increase their voice loudness. Clinicians help these patients change their pitch and loudness and evaluate how the patients view the changes. The clinicians should observe how the patients respond to direct modification of pitch and loudness. For patients who resist such direct approaches, counseling or concurrent psychotherapy might be appropriate. We have rarely found that professional psychological counseling with the psychologist or psychiatrist is necessary, since the vast majority of these patients' voice disorders yield to a symptomatic voice therapy approach.

Quality of voice is often the primary problem in functional dysphonia. The vocal folds may approximate one another in a faulty manner and produce alterations in quality; words such as *hoarse, harsh, strident,* and *breathy* are applied to these voice-quality dimensions of functional dysphonia. Harshness is often the product of overapproximation (excessive medial compression) of the folds when they come sharply together, producing what is also perceived as hard glottal attack. Sometimes harshness is accompanied by inappropriately high levels of loudness, too high pitch, possible tongue retraction, and contraction of the pharyngeal constrictors. Harshness often indicates a voice that requires a lot of effort and force to produce. The opposite problem may be breathiness, produced by folds that may approximate too loosely. Laxity of approximation generally produces an excessive escape of air, perceived as breathiness. Sometimes, as Brodnitz (1971) suggests, the breathy, tired voice appears only after prolonged hyperfunctional voice use. It may emerge late in the day, after a patient has done a lot of phonating, particularly if such phonation has required a good deal of effort and force and the environment is stressful or presents a high level of background noise.

Functional dysphonia often becomes "the" voice of the person—the way that person talks. For such persons, voice therapy should not be initiated until they are made aware of their ability to change and elect to change their voice. For patients who are motivated to change the quality of their voice, and who are accurately diagnosed as having functional dysphonia, voice therapy is remarkably successful.

Phonation Breaks (Abductor Spasms)

A *phonation break* is a temporary loss of voice that may occur for only part of a word, a whole word, a phrase, or a sentence. The individual is phonating with no apparent difficulty when suddenly a complete cessation of voice occurs. Such a fleeting voice loss is usually situational and it usually happens after prolonged hyperfunction. Typical patients with this problem work too hard to talk, often speaking with great effort, and suddenly experience a complete voice break. Such patients usually struggle to "find" their voice by coughing, clearing their throat, or taking a drink of water. In most cases, phonation is restored and remains adequate until the next phonation break, which may occur in only a few moments or not for days. Other than continued vocal hyperfunction, no physical condition seems to cause these phonatory interruptions. They may result from a variety of physiological sources, ranging from reduced subglottal air pressure near the end of a phrase to the "loading" of the true vocal fold by the ventricular fold or mucus on the true fold. Many times these breaks result from excessive laryngeal muscle tension and inappropriate adjustments of the otherwise normal mechanism.

Voice patients who experience phonation breaks or abductor spasms rarely show them during voice evaluation sessions. In their histories, however, such patients report the occurrence of phonation breaks, often with much embarrassment when they occur. Occasionally patients have been told by their employers that they must learn to use their voices correctly (without voice breaks) or they would lose their jobs. Fortunately, the treatment of phonation breaks is relatively simple: taking the "work" out of phonation and elimination of inappropriate vocal behaviors such as excessive coughing and violent throat clearing. Some of the voice therapy techniques described in Chapter 5, designed to reduce vocal hyperfunction, (tongue protrusion /i/, chant talk, nasal glide stimulation, warble) are most effective in eliminating the phonation break problem. Specific therapy procedures for phonation breaks or more severe abductor spasms are discussed in Chapter 6.

Pitch Breaks

There are two kinds of *pitch breaks*. One is a developmental phenomenon seen primarily in boys experiencing marked pubertal growth of the larynx, and the other is caused by prolonged vocal hyperfunction, particularly while speaking at an inappropriate pitch level.

The rapid changes in the size of the vocal folds and other laryngeal structures produce varying vocal effects during the pubertal years. Boys experience a lowering of their fundamental frequency of about one octave; girls, a lowering of only about two or three notes. This change does not happen in a day or two. For several years, as this laryngeal growth is taking place, boys will experience temporary hoarseness and occasional pitch breaks. Wise parents or voice clinicians witness these vocal changes with little comment or concern. These mass-size increases of puberty tend to thwart any serious attempts at singing or other vocal arts. Luchsinger and Arnold (1965) point out that much of the European literature on singing makes a valid plea that the formal study of singing be deferred until well after puberty. Until a male child experiences some stability of laryngeal growth, the demands of singing might be inappropriate for his rapidly changing mechanism. Laryngeal strain is a real concern when serious singing is attempted during this period. One of the authors was told by Beverly Sills, the most famous of recent sopranos, that she stopped singing altogether for 3 years during puberty. Interestingly, Beverly Sills, unlike any other opera singer we know, had only a single voice teacher for her entire child and adult career.

The age and rate of pubertal development vary markedly. From the pediatric literature we find that the main thrust of puberty for any one child seems to take place in a total time period of about 4 years, 6 months; the most rapid and dramatic changes occur toward the last 6 months of puberty (this is when pitch breaks if they occur, may be observed in some boys). Most pubertal changes begin at age 12 in boys (and a little earlier in girls) and are completed by age 16.

Younger children and adults might experience a different kind of pitch break, related to the voice breaking an octave (sometimes two octaves) up or an octave down when speaking at an inappropriate pitch level. When individuals speak at an inappropriately low frequency, their voice tends to break one octave higher; if they speak too high in the frequency range their voice may break one octave down.

The tracings in Figure 3–1, recorded on a Visi-Pitch, show the inappropriately low fundamental frequency tracings of a 39-year-old minister, suddenly breaking into abrupt upward shifts. His lower F_0 value was 100 cycles and his higher (the pitch break F_0) was 300 cycles. We discuss pitch breaks further in the next chapter when we discuss finding a pitch level appropriate for the mass-size of the individual's vocal folds, which can help to avoid or eliminate sudden, unwanted shifts in vocal frequency. (The Visi-Pitch and other feedback devices and their manufacturers are listed in the references at the end of the book.)

Pitch breaks can also result from overall vocal fatigue. Heavy users of voice, such as actors after prolonged rehearsals or during long running performances, may begin to experience pitch breaks after hours of

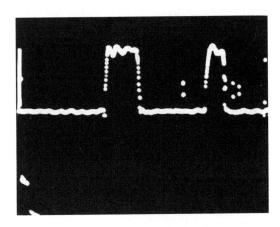

FIGURE 3–1   A Visi-Pitch Tracing of the Voicing Pitch Breaks of a 39-Year-Old Minister
The lower tracing is a prolonged /a/ at about 100 Hz, breaking abruptly to the high tracing at 300 Hz. The pitch breaks occur when he sustains phonation at the lowest voice he can produce.

prolonged voicing. Such continued vocal hyperfunction, speaking with too much effort, will sometimes result in either pitch or phonation breaks. Such pitch breaks are usually warnings that the vocal mechanisms are being overworked and being held at an inappropriate pitch level for a prolonged period of time. We refer to such pitch or phonation breaks as *vocal limping,* just as one limps when walking with an injured foot. With a little temporary voice rest (two or three days) and initiation of techniques of easy phonation (glottal fry, yawn-sigh, etc.), fatigue-induced pitch and phonation breaks usually disappear.

Spasmodic Dysphonia

Probably the most extreme form of a hyperfunctional voice disorder is *spasmodic dysphonia* (SD). Patients' voices sound strained, choked off with the attempts to voice, as if they are trying to push the outgoing airstream through a tightly adducted laryngeal opening. Endoscopic examination (Davis, Boone, Carroll, Darveniza, & Harrison, 1987) shows that the tight voice is indeed produced by hyperadduction (severe approximation) of the true folds, often accompanied by tight closure of the false vocal folds (ventricular folds) with supraglottal constriction of the aryepiglottic folds and contraction of the lower pharyngeal constrictors. The total laryngeal and lower pharyngeal airway appears to close down (McFarlane & Lavorato, 1984; McFarlane, 1988). No wonder we hear a strained, "strangled" voice in such patients.

In addition to the problem of voicing, patients with spasmodic dysphonia complain about the difficulties they experience trying to force expiratory air out whenever they desire to phonate. Aronson (1990) comments that the tight voice during adductor spasmodic dysphonia "occurs only during voluntary phonation for communication purposes and not during singing, vowel prolongation, laughing, or crying" (p. 161). However, in patients who have carried the diagnosis of spasmodic dysphonia for some period of time and who are more severe, we see symptoms of this disorder in prolonged vowels as well. The patients soon learn to expect phonation difficulties whenever they attempt to speak. In this sense, spasmodic dysphonia resembles stuttering. In European writings, in fact, the condition is sometimes called the "laryngeal stutter." McFarlane and Shipley (1979) make a case for spasmodic dysphonia *not* being considered as laryngeal stuttering based on there being a greater number of important dissimilarities than important similarities between the two disorders. Most patients with spasmodic dysphonia experience some normal voice in certain situations. Case histories of these patients reveal that such situations as "talking to my cat" or "speaking to others in a pool while I tread water" are times when patients have experienced normal voice.

The most common type of spasmodic dysphonia appears to be related to tight laryngeal adduction (known as adductor spasmodic dysphonia). Aronson (1990), however, also describes a second form of the disorder, known as abductor spastic dysphonia. Patients with this disorder exhibit normal or dysphonic voices that are suddenly interrupted by temporary abduction of the vocal folds, resulting in fleeting aphonia. After such momentary aphonia, the patients' voice patterns are restored again (until the next aphonic break). Endoscopy shows that the vocal folds of such patients abduct suddenly, "exposing an extremely wide glottic chink" (Aronson, 1990, p. 185). More often than not, the abductor spasms appear to be triggered by unvoiced consonant sounds. The abductor-type disorder is a much rarer form of spasmodic dysphonia. For example, Davis et al. (1987) reported that of 25 successive cases of spasmodic dysphonia observed in a Sydney, Australia, hospital, 24 were adductor type and one was an abductor type. The abductor spasm can often be treated successfully as a phonation break. Watterson and McFarlane (1992) make a strong case for considering the abductor type as a different disorder altogether and not a subtype of spasmodic dysphonia. Colton and Casper (1990) also seem to indicate that the two are different in pathophysiology and require different treatments.

The cause of the disorder is still unknown. In fact, the generic name spasmodic dysphonia includes disorders with several different causes or etiologies. In two studies (Aminoff, Dedo, & Izdebski, 1978; Davis et al., 1987) spasmodic dysphonic patients have been examined by voice scientists, speech-language pathologists, neurologists, otolaryngologists, and psychiatrists. Both studies found some patients with no sign of neurological disease and others with some symptoms of neurological disease (with or without essential tremor). Both studies found no evidence of laryngeal pathology or psychiatric involvement in any of the patients studied that could justify the severity of the voice problems. In the Australian study (Davis et al., 1987), spasmodic dysphonic patients exhibited significantly decreased airflow rates when speaking, as compared to a normal control group. The decreased airflow would seem to be directly related to laryngeal-pharyngeal constriction (which was also observed on endoscopy). What is the cause of such airway constriction? Although the cause of spastic dysphonia is still unknown, more patients than not do seem to exhibit neurologically based problems. Case (1991) agrees with this view. He writes: "Few professionals today consider the majority of adductor [spasmodic] dysphonia patients as having psychogenic voice disorders. Rather, they are classified more often as having a neurogenic etiology with possible psychogenic sequelae" (p. 174). Aronson (1990) states that adductor spasmodic dysphonia "may be of psychogenic, neurogenic or of unknown etiology" (p. 162). He contends that there are several disorders lumped under one perceptual term of spasmodic dysphonia.

Despite the possible neurogenic cause of the disorder, drug therapy has not been an effective method of treatment. Speech-language pathologists tend to treat the disorder behaviorally and also psychologically. In general, however, voice therapy has not been reported in the literature as a particularly successful treatment for spasmodic dysphonia. Voice therapy attempts for spasmodic dysphonia are described further in Chapters 5 and 6 in this text. A surgical approach (described in Chapter 6), cutting the recurrent laryngeal nerve on one side, creating a unilateral vocal fold paralysis, has been reported as helpful (Dedo & Izdebski, 1983). These authors report beneficial long-term results for 306 patients, as determined by voice analysis and patient self-reports. In patients who have undergone recurrent laryngeal nerve sectioning, positive results have been reported but the original voice symptoms have recurred in some of these patients.

The most recent advances in the treatment of spasmodic dysphonia are with the use of Botulinum toxin (Botox) injections directly into one or both vocal folds (thyroarytenoid muscles). This produces a partial weakness of the injected muscles, which decreases the hyperactivity of the vocal folds and eliminates the excessive laryngeal valving. Thus, the vocal qualities associated with spasmodic dysphonia are reduced (Blitzer, Brin, Fahn, & Lovelace, 1988). Injection with botulinum toxin (Botox) has the advantage of not producing a unilateral paralysis as the nerve-sectioning technique does (Dedo & Izdebski, 1983). Ludlow, Naunton, Fujita, and Sedory (1990) have demonstrated that Botox injection is successful in reducing or eliminating the voice symptoms of spasmodic dysphonia patients who have previously undergone recurrent nerve sectioning and suffered a subsequent return of symptoms while the one cord remained paralyzed.

Thickening (Vocal Fold)

Various inflammatory conditions of the larynx, such as infectious and traumatic laryngitis, may produce irritation and swelling (edema) of the vocal folds. Another form of enlargement along the glottal margin of the vocal folds is known as *vocal fold thickening*. Whereas vocal nodules and polyps are more focal lesions (occupying less space) on the vocal folds, thickening is a broader-based lesion that often covers the anterior two-thirds of the glottal margin or the membrane covering the muscular portion of the vocal fold. There are basically two types of thickening. One represents early tissue reaction (swelling) to vocal fold trauma, often a precursor to vocal nodules or polyps; the second is the result of prolonged (chronic) irritation that often results in extensive polypoid degeneration and more advanced changes of the vocal fold tissue. Let us consider each of these thickening changes separately.

In most cases, vocal fold thickening results from continuous vocal abuse. Continuous use of loud voice, screaming and yelling, in time may result in some tissue changes along the glottal margin. We have only to observe vocal fold vibration on videoendoscopy and stroboscopy to appreciate the vigorous adduction of the folds and participation of supraglottal structures (ventricular and aryepiglottic folds) that accompany coughing, yelling, or screaming at higher pitches. As a volunteer subject with videoendoscopy, one of the authors witnessed bilateral tissue changes on the glottal margin (beginning of redness) of his own folds after only five minutes of continuous staccato yelling of the word *peach*. Such yelling is a benign vocal experience compared to the continuous screaming of some young children at play or the performance of some rock singers. The cause of early vocal fold thickening thus seems to be the same as the cause of vocal nodules, primarily vocal abuse and misuse. However, other reported causes of thickening and vocal nodules have been summarized by Andrews (1986, p. 107):

1. Constitutional tendency
2. Chronic upper respiratory problems
3. Psychological living environment—for example, size of family
4. Physical living environment—for example, air pollution
5. Personality and adjustment
6. Endocrine imbalance, especially thyroid
7. Vocal abuse, sudden straining of the voice; continuous abusive practices
8. Vocal misuse: incorrect pitch and loudness

To this list we add another:

9. Post surgical thickening of the vocal folds

Certain children and adults are very sensitive to vocally irritating events. For example, some people can use vocal folds excessively and never develop any tissue changes that result in vocal symptoms. Others, with the slightest allergy, cold, or vocal abuse-misuse, develop aversive glottal margin problems. The emotional and physical environment undoubtedly negatively affects many people. In the case of children or adults with vocal fold thickening, such environmental influences cannot be allowed to continue without some attempt at modification. This makes it absolutely essential to take a careful case history, which will be developed further in Chapter 4. The overwhelming cause of vocal fold thickening, however, is vocal abuse and misuse. Until such vocal excesses are identified and reduced in frequency (they can rarely be totally eliminated), vocal thickening, nodules, and polyps cannot be successfully treated.

Vocal fold thickening can usually be reduced by a voice therapy program that promotes easy and proper use of the vocal mechanisms (vocal reeducation), with heavy emphasis on curbing vocal abuse-misuse. This example of a 6-year-old with vocal fold thickening is, unfortunately, typical:

> Edith was referred for a voice evaluation because of chronic hoarseness. Indirect laryngoscopy found that she had bilateral cord thickening with no demonstrable history of allergy or infection. Her parents were counseled to do what they could to help Edith eliminate unnecessary crying and yelling, and Edith was sent home. On a subsequent visit to the laryngologist, no change in cords was observed by laryngoscopy. It was thus decided to "strip" the thickenings surgically. (We must note here that we never suggest vocal fold stripping except for treatment of malignant tissue that must be removed, and we never suggest this procedure for children.) This was done with excellent results. Three weeks after surgery the child demonstrated clear cords bilaterally, free of thickening. After a postoperative period of approximately three months, the family returned to the laryngologist, complaining of the child's recurring hoarseness. Laryngoscopy found that Edith once again had bilateral cord thickening, with the early formation of a vocal nodule on one fold. It was then decided to begin voice therapy. Special efforts were made to identify particular vocal abuses by the child, and a school playground situation was isolated as the cause of continuous vocal strain. Eliminating this and other adverse vocal behavior gradually eliminated the vocal nodule and nearly eliminated the bilateral thickening, as well.

The preceding case illustrates that surgical treatment of cord thickening or nodules, without removing the abusive cause of the problem, will not usually be a permanent solution to the vocal problem. Reducing the source of the irritation (such as eliminating an allergy, reducing smoking, or curbing vocal abuse) is probably the best management of the problem. Our strong preference is to have a serious course of voice therapy first. This will generally obviate the need for surgery for this problem and for nodules. Voice therapy likely would have made the surgery in this case unnecessary.

A second form of vocal fold thickening is often more diffuse because it frequently indicates a more advanced tissue reaction to prolonged laryngeal abuse and misuse. The vocal fold swelling is broader than the anterior-middle third site that is the typical location of nodules or polyps. Rather, the swelling may extend along the glottis from the anterior commissure to the beginning of the vocal process of the arytenoid cartilages. Much swelling, known as *polypoid degeneration*, is characteristic. If, in addition to vocal abuse-misuse, the patient is a heavy smoker or alcohol consumer, the increased mass of the folds can seriously compromise all attempts at vocalization. The primary treatment of extensive polypoid degeneration may be medical-surgical, supplemented by voice therapy. However, trial voice therapy at first is warranted. The primary thrust of voice therapy is to identify possible laryngeal abuses (such as throat clearing) and voice abuses (such as speaking with excessive glottal attack), and to eliminate abuse such as smoking, then to provide the patient with methods for reducing these aversive behaviors. Many of the voice therapy facilitating approaches presented in Chapter 5 have been effective in reducing overall vocal fold thickening.

Traumatic Laryngitis

In *functional laryngitis* or *traumatic laryngitis*, patients experience swelling of the vocal folds as a result of excessive and strained vocalization. The voice sounds hoarse, lacking in volume. Typical functional laryngitis may be heard in the voices of excited spectators after a football or basketball game. In the excitement of the game, with their own voices masked by the noise of the crowd, the fans scream at pitch levels and intensities they normally do not use. The inner glottal edges of the membrane become swollen (edematous) and thickened, an expected consequence of excessive approximation. The increased edema of the folds is accompanied by irritation and increased blood accumulation. The acute stage of functional laryngitis is at its peak during the actual yelling or traumatic vocal behavior, with the vocal folds much increased in size and mass. Brodnitz (1971) wrote that functionally irritated vocal folds appear on laryngoscopic examination to be much like the thickened, reddened folds of acute infectious laryngitis.

There is an important difference in treatment, however. For functional or acute, nonspecific laryngitis—which is usually the result of continued irritation by such causes as allergy, excessive smoking and alcohol drinking, and vocal abuse—the obvious treatment is to eliminate the vocal irritant whenever possible. In the case of functional laryngitis secondary to yelling or a similar form of vocal abuse, eliminating the abuse usually permits the vocal mechanism to return to its natural state. The temporary laryngitis experienced toward the end of a basketball game is usually relieved by a return to normal vocal activity and most of the edema and irritation vanish after a good night's sleep. Chronic laryngitis may typically produce more serious vocal problems if the speaker attempts to "speak above" the laryngitis. The temporary edema of the vocal folds alters the quality and loudness of the phonation; the speaker increases vocal efforts; this increase in effort only increases the irritation of the folds, thereby compounding the problem; and finally, if such hyperfunctional behavior continues over time, what was once a temporary edema may become a more permanent polypoid thickening, which sometimes develops into vocal polyps (more localized) or nodules. For this reason, functional laryngitis should be promptly treated by eliminating the causative abuse and, if possible, by enforcing a short period (2–3 days) of complete voice rest.

Voice rest in itself is not a "cure" for most voice disorders. This is not true, however, for traumatic laryngitis. Complete or absolute voice rest, which means no phonation or whispering for several days, is usually enough for irritated vocal fold margins to lose their swelling and return to their normal shape. It is important that voice rest designed to promote healing of irritated vocal fold surfaces *not* include whispering; whispering (as most people do it) still causes too much vocal fold movement, and irritation from the rubbing together of the approximating surfaces of each fold is still possible. Studies have shown that during whisper the ventricular folds (see Figure 2–14) often may be brought into function (Pearl & McCall, 1986). The events that cause traumatic laryngitis must be identified and curbed. If such hyperfunctional vocal behavior continues over time, such changes as polypoid thickening, vocal nodules, or vocal polyps may occur.

Ventricular Dysphonia

Ventricular dysphonia, sometimes known as *dysphonia plicae ventricularis* or *false fold phonation*, occurs more often than previously indicated (Boone, 1983). Ventricular dysphonia is produced by the vibration of the approximating ventricular folds. Sometimes the ventricular voice becomes the substitute voice of patients who have severe disease of the true folds (such as severe papilloma or large polyps). The ventricular voice is usually low pitched because of the large mass of vibrating tissue of the ventricular bands (as compared to the smaller mass of vibrating tissue of the true folds). In addition, the voice has little pitch variability and is therefore monotonous. Finally, because the ventricular folds have difficulty in making a good, firm approximation for their entire length, the voice is usually quite hoarse. This combination of low pitch, monotony, and hoarseness makes most ventricular voices sound very unpleasant. If no persistent true cord pathology continues to force patients to use their ventricular voices, this disorder usually responds well to voice therapy. Sometimes, however, *hypertrophy* (enlargement) of the ventricular folds is present; this makes their normal full retraction somewhat difficult. Ventricular phonation is impossible to diagnose by the sound of the voice alone. Laryngoscopic examination during phonation shows the ventricular folds coming together, covering (partially or completely) from view the true folds that lie below. Some ventricular dysphonias display a special form of diplophonia (double voice), whereby the true folds vibrate and also drive the ventricular folds to vibrate, since the false folds are sitting on the true folds (loading the true cords with ventricular folds). In our experience, more often than not, the ventricular folds do not vibrate but the loaded true vocal folds are dampened by the false folds. Identification and confirmation of what vibrating structures the patient is using for phonation can best be made by frontal tomographic X-ray (coronal) of the sites of vibration. Ventricular phonation can also be diagnosed by nasoendoscopy and endoscopic stroboscopy (McFarlane & Lavorato, 1984; McFarlane, 1988; McFarlane et al., 1990). In ventricular phonation, the true vocal folds will be slightly abducted, with the ventricular bands above in relative approximation and very possibly resting on the true vocal folds. In normal phonation, the opposite relationship between the true folds and the ventricular bands occurs— that is, the true folds are adducted and the ventricular bands are positioned laterally from the midline position. Once ventricular phonation is confirmed by laryngoscopy or X-ray, any physical problem of the true cords that might make normal phonation impossible should be eliminated. We consider both the elimination of ventricular phonation and its occasional need to be taught when we present voice therapy for special problems in Chapter 6.

Vocal Nodules

Vocal nodules are the most common benign lesions of the vocal folds in both children and adults. They are caused by continuous abuse of the larynx and misuse of the voice. These causative abuses are well described by Case (1991), who places "yelling and screaming, making a hard glottal attack, singing in an abusive manner, speaking in a noisy environment, coughing and excessive throat clearing" at the top of the list of 24 vocal abuses-misuses (pp. 98–99). Nodules, as shown in Figure 3–2, are generally bilateral, whitish protuberances on the glottal margin of each vocal fold, located at the anterior-middle third junction. However, McFarlane and Watterson (1990) demonstrate in their study of 44 cases of vocal nodules that their can be considerable variation in the size, number, and location of vocal nodules in singers and nonsingers. They also demonstrate variation in the nodules of children. Of the variations that can be observed and documented in vocal nodules perhaps the most striking is that nodules can range from singular to two, three, and even four (quad nodules) in number. While these variations are very interesting, two important facts remain: (a) Nodules are very responsive to voice therapy, and (b) the classic description of number and location (juncture of anterior and middle third) is generally accurate. This nodule site is the midpoint of the muscular vocal fold, involving the membrane that covers the vocal ligament and vocalis muscle inner border of the

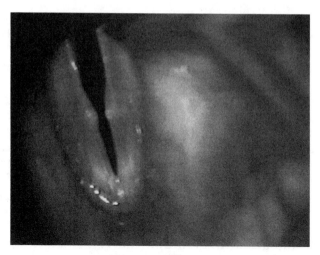

FIGURE 3–2   Bilateral Nodules on the Vocal Folds
Bilateral nodules on the vocal folds are very responsive to voice
therapy.

vocal fold. In the early stages of nodule development, the nodular mass
is soft and pliable. With continuous abuse-misuse the lesion becomes
more fibrotic and may be slightly larger or may become more focused,
smaller and harder.

As the bilateral nodules approximate one another on phonation,
there is usually an open glottal chink on each side of the nodule. This
open glottal chink (produced by the nodules coming together in exact
opposition of one another) results in a lack of complete vocal fold
adduction. This faulty approximation leads to breathiness in the voice
and air wastage. Also the increased mass of the nodules added to the
vocal folds contributes to a lower voice pitch and increased aperiodicity
(usually judged as hoarseness). This leads to a breathy, flat kind of voice
that often seems to lack appropriate resonance. Patients complain that
they need to clear their throat continually and often that they have
excessive mucus or "something" on the vocal folds. Excessive throat
clearing often becomes an identified vocal abuse, which may lead to
further enlargement or further organization and consolidation of the
nodules. Typical patients with vocal nodules complain that their voices
seem to deteriorate with continuous voicing; they may start the day with
fairly good voices that become increasingly dysphonic with continuous
vocal usage. With prolonged speaking and singing, perhaps coupled with
vocal abuse and misuse, phonation rapidly deteriorates. Small nodules

and recently acquired ones can be very successfully treated with voice therapy. Yamaguchi et al. (1986), reporting on voice therapy success with 20 adult females with vocal nodules, found that vocal nodules "either disappeared or were reduced in size" after 3 to 4 months of voice therapy in 65% of the cases. McFarlane and Watterson (1990) reported success in 44 cases presenting both large and small nodules in children and adults, and in both singers and nonsingers. They also document with pictures the before and after therapy conditions of the larynx of a child and an adult singer. The nodules were completely resolved via voice therapy. Boone (1982) developed a four-point program for adults with vocal nodules that focuses on identifying abuse-misuse; reducing the occurrence of such abuse-misuse; searching with the patient for various voice therapy facilitating approaches that seem to produce an easy, optimal vocal production; and using the facilitating approach that works best as a practice method. Although we strongly recommend voice therapy as the primary treatment for nodules, we also acknowledge that larger nodules and long-established ones may be treated by surgery, followed by a brief period of complete voice rest and then voice therapy. However, a trial period of voice therapy is an appropriate conservative course of treatment prior to surgery for nodules in nearly all cases. Since voice therapy must follow if surgery is the treatment, then why not begin with a period of voice therapy? It is not unusual clinically for new nodules to appear several weeks after surgical removal of nodules in both children and adults. Unless the underlying hyperfunctional vocal behaviors are identified and reduced, vocal nodules have a stubborn way of reappearing. Vocal nodules in children before puberty are more common in boys, who are generally aggressive and noisy, busy controlling people with their voices. As boys get older, there is less evidence of nodules, and adolescent females show a higher prevalence of additive lesions related to vocal abuse (Toohill, 1975). The prevalence is also higher in those adult females who, according to Aronson (1990), are "talkative, socially aggressive, and tense, and have acute or chronic interpersonal problems that generate tension, anxiety, anger, or depression" (p. 125). Nodules result from vocal hyperfunction and are therefore often observed in people who in general exhibit "hyperfunctional" personalities. Green (1989) found that children with vocal nodules exhibit more aggressive behaviors than control children as measured with a 50-item problem behavior checklist. Children with nodules demonstrated more aggressive behaviors, acting out and disturbed peer relationships (Green, 1989). Although symptomatic voice therapy has been effective in reducing or eliminating vocal nodules, patients with vocal nodules often require strong psychological support by the voice clinician, and sometimes, in a very few patients, psychological counseling and therapy as well.

Vocal Polyps

Vocal polyps, more often unilateral than bilateral, usually occur at the same anterior-middle third site on the vocal fold(s) as nodules (see Figure 3–3). Polyps and nodules are both related to vocal hyperfunction, and both have some physical similarities. Stone (1982) labels a polyp as a "morbid excrescence, or protruding growth, from mucous membrane" (p. 94). The lesion is usually soft, often fluid filled, and occurs in the inner margin of one vocal fold; because of its softness, it does not irritate the membranous tissue on the opposite fold (as opposed to the bilateral pathology usually observed in vocal nodules). Unlike vocal nodules, which result from continuous or chronic vocal fold irritation, polyps are often precipitated by a single vocal event. For example, a patient may have indulged in excessive vocalization, such as screaming for much of an evening, which produced some hemorrhaging on the membrane at the point of maximum glottal contact. A polyp forms out of such hemorrhagic irritation by eventually adding mass that becomes fluid filled. Once a small polyp begins, any continued vocal abuse or misuse will irritate the area, contributing to its continued growth. A typical polyp lies on the glottal margin, interfering with the approximation of the normal fold.

Polyps, which may be either broad based (sessile-type) or narrow necked on a stem (*pedunculated*), usually occur in the larynx on the inner margin of the affected fold. An excellent description of polyps, their formation, and their treatment was developed by Kleinsasser (1979), who

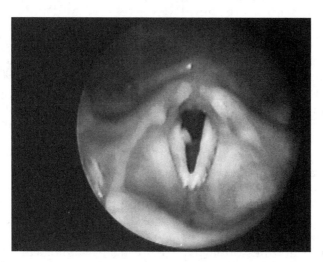

FIGURE 3–3   A Soft, Unilateral Polyp on the Right Vocal Fold

described the lesions as "gelatinous" and responsive to surgery. The goal of modern vocal fold surgery is to preserve as much mucosa as possible and to disrupt the glottal margin as little as possible. Thus, microflap surgery designed to raise a flap of mucosa, remove a cyst or gelatinous material via suction, and then lay the flap back down on the vocal fold is now common and preferred to older stripping techniques. Laser surgery had been thought to be the surgical treatment of choice for vocal fold polyps (Yates & Dedo, 1984). However, it appears that use of the laser for such broad-based tissue lesions does too much damage to the mucosal covering on the vocal fold vibrating edge (Bouchayer & Cornut, 1988). Further, Bouchayer and Cornut (1988) state, "We believe that our insistence on voice therapy for all patients with polyps explains why we have yet to see a single recurrence" (p. 462).

Unless the causative behaviors are identified and prevented from further occurrence, polyps often recur after surgery. With voice therapy and attempts to use the laryngeal mechanisms more optimally, polyps can be permanently eliminated. We have seen even professional singers return to a singing career with an improved vocal hygiene, improved singing technique after surgery, and voice therapy (Lavorato & McFarlane, 1983). We prefer voice therapy as the first approach to treatment of a sessile polyp and surgery followed by voice therapy when initial voice therapy fails to get the desired response. In Figure 3–4 a left vocal fold polyp of the sessile type is shown.

The voices of patients with unilateral polyps are characterized by severe dysphonia. The normal vocal fold vibrates at one frequency while

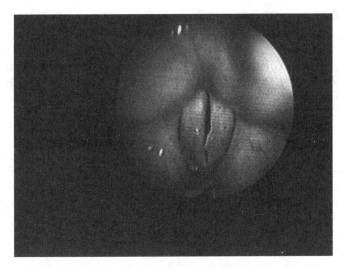

FIGURE 3–4   A Left Vocal Fold Polyp of the Sessile Type

the additive lesion seriously dampens the vibration of the involved fold, resulting in what is perceived as hoarseness and breathiness, often requiring (or so the patient mistakenly thinks) continuous throat clearing. Voice therapy requires identifying and reducing vocal abuse-misuse and searching with the patient for the best voice that can be produced using various voice-facilitating approaches (see Chapter 5). Voice therapy was successful in eliminating a unilateral polyp from this woman:

> Jane was a 29-year-old teacher who was active in competitive sports. She admitted to doing a lot of yelling during her softball season, when she ended up with a hoarse voice that would not go away. Her teaching schedule required her to give 6 hours of lectures each day, supervise a study hall, and assist in girls' field hockey events. Finally, by noon each day she had no voice. Subsequent laryngoscopy found her to have a broad-based polyp (about 5 mm in width) on one fold. Voice therapy was initiated that focused on reducing loudness, developing a soft glottal attack, and opening her mouth more as she spoke. An immediate consequence of the therapy was that when she spoke easily, without effort, her voice at first sounded "more hoarse." She kidded her students and colleagues that she would sound worse in the beginning as she learned to use her voice with less effort. In about 12 weeks, the unilateral polyp completely disappeared, and Jane's voice became normal. She then made continuing efforts to avoid any kind of vocal abuse and misuse and has maintained a trouble-free larynx and normal voice.

VOICE DISORDERS RELATED TO ORGANIC CHANGES OF VOCAL MECHANISMS

In Table 3–1, 14 organic disorders of vocal mechanisms that might cause voice problems were listed. In these disorders, the faulty voice is usually related more to a physical condition than to a vocal abuse-misuse, per se. We now present each disorder in alphabetical order, first considering the etiology of the disorder, and then following with a brief discussion of its overall management.

Cancer

Cancer or *carcinoma* in the vocal tract is a life-threatening disease that requires serious medical-surgical management. Lip and intraoral cancers rarely contribute to changes in voice, but they may have obvious negative effects on articulation and can also be life threatening. Extensive oral lesions involving the tongue, perhaps even requiring partial or total surgical removal of the tongue (*glossectomy*), or palatal and velar cancer can seriously affect articulation and vocal resonance.

The American Cancer Society (1980) reported that in the United States about 15,000 new patients annually develop some form of oral cancer. Some of the identified causes of oral cancer include smoking (particularly pipe smoking), use of smokeless tobacco, chronic infections, herpes, repeated trauma to the irritated site, and *leukoplakia* (whitish plaque). Often patients first experience chronic lesions in the mouth or on the tongue that don't seem to heal. Usually continuous pain near the lesion site brings the patient to the physician. The majority of these oral lesions are treated successfully with microsurgery (removal of small lesions) and radiation therapy. The primary goal of surgery-radiation therapy is to eradicate the primary lesion so that it doesn't spread (metastasize) to another adjacent or remote body site. Sometimes carcinoma is detected in the nasal sinuses and at sites within the pharynx, although such lesions are relatively rare. The most serious vocal tract malignancies, however, are those that involve the larynx, which, by their position in the airway, present a potential threat to airway adequacy. According to Case (1991), "laryngeal cancer comprises 2 to 5 percent of all malignancies diagnosed annually in the United States" (p. 229).

In general, there are three classifications of laryngeal cancers, depending on the site of the lesion: *supraglottal*, involving such structures as the ventricular and aryepiglottic folds, the epiglottis, the arytenoid cartilages, and the walls of the hypopharynx; *glottal*, from the anterior commissure to the vocal process ends of the arytenoids; and *subglottal*, involving the cricoid cartilage and trachea. The treatment combines radiation therapy and surgery for small to moderate lesions; extensive cancer requires perhaps a hemilaryngectomy, a supraglottal laryngectomy, or total laryngectomy. We discuss both of these later in this chapter, and we consider laryngeal cancer, rehabilitation after laryngectomy, and the role of the speech-language pathologist in some detail in Chapter 6.

Dysarthria

Many voice disorders are symptoms of some kind of neurological disease or dysfunction. *Dysarthria* is a motor speech problem that is the result of damage somewhere to the central or peripheral nervous systems. "Dysarthria is the generic name for different motor speech problems that may be caused by a number of nervous-system diseases" (Boone & Plante, 1993, p. 232). Lesions to the recurrent or superior laryngeal nerves involve the peripheral nervous system (they usually cut or traumatize the innervating nerve to the larynx), and they may result in unilateral or bilateral vocal fold paralysis. (We discuss vocal fold paralysis separately later in this chapter.) The vocal problems that are symptoms of a dysarthria are usually related to lesions of the central nervous system, which might be related to such disorders as cerebral palsy, Parkinson's disease, amyotrophic lateral sclerosis (ALS), multiple sclerosis (MS), or multiple strokes. Previous research (Darley, Aronson, &

Brown, 1969) has identified dysarthric symptoms and their associated dysphonias that are related to specific diseases and damage to particular sites of the nervous system. In general, severity of dysarthria is related to the site of the lesion. The lower the lesion in the brain, the greater the severity of the dysarthria; also, bilateral lesions within the hemispheres are more likely to produce dysarthric symptoms than are unilateral lesions. Vocal problems may include inability to control respiration, which causes severe problems in vocal prosody and voice loudness. Changes in vocal fold characteristics may lead to changes in pitch, lack of pitch control, and faulty voice quality related to lack of normal vocal fold approximation and supraglottal interference and *globus* (sensation of lump in the throat). Resonance defects, such as hypernasality, are often part of the voice symptoms of dysarthria and are frequently related to faulty velarpharyngeal closure.

Today dysarthria is treated primarily by various medications (such as L-dopa for the patient with Parkinson's disease) and sometimes by surgery (such as relief of spasticity by cutting appropriate muscles in a spastic extremity). In Chapters 6 and 7 we discuss management by the speech-language pathologist of dysarthria as it affects phonation and resonance .

Endocrine Changes

Occasionally patients are seen whose voice problems are related to some kind of endocrine dysfunction. Endocrine disorders often have a major impact on developing larynges and cause excesses in fundamental frequency, so that an individual's voice is either too low or too high in pitch. For example, in hypofunction of the pituitary gland, laryngeal growth is retarded. A pubescent child with such a problem will experience a continued high voice pitch. Such a pituitary problem can prevent normal development of progesterone by the ovaries (in girls) and testosterone by the testes (in adolescent males). The resulting lack of secondary sexual characteristics (including a change in voice) is treated by endocrine therapy designed to stimulate normal pituitary function. The opposite problem, caused by some tumors of the pituitary gland, results in a "precocious puberty as well as acromegaly" (Strome, 1982, p. 18). Hypofunctioning of the adrenal glands (Addison's disease) can also contribute to lack of secondary sex characteristics, including a prepubescent voice in males. Sometimes tumors in the adrenal system cause adrenal hormone excesses, causing virilization and a deepening of the voice. McFarlane and Brophy (1992) discuss the affect of various medications on voice. Some birth control medications, for example, can cause virilization of the female voice and vocal huskiness as well.

Hypothyroidism, insufficient secretion of thyroxin by the thyroid gland, can produce many physical changes over time, including increased mass of the vocal folds, which, in turn, lowers pitch. Aronson (1990) describes the dysphonia of hypothyroidism as "characteristically *hoarse*, sometimes described as *coarse* or *gravelly*, and of *excessively low pitch*" (p. 60). Such symptoms can usually be well controlled by thyroid hormone therapy. In hyperthyroidism (excessive thyroid function), vocal symptoms are less severe, and the patients experience jumpiness and irritability, which result in a breathy voice that may lack sufficient loudness.

Greene (1980) describes the influence of menstruation on the female voice, particularly at premenstruation, when estrogen and progesterone levels are at their lowest, resulting in a slight thickening of the vocal folds, which can cause a lowering of pitch and some hoarseness (Frable, 1972). Some female opera singers avoid heavy singing obligations several days before and after menstruation. The climacteric (menopause) is another time when some women may experience vocal changes, particularly a lowering of fundamental frequency. Because of the secretion of excessive androgenic hormones after the menopause, the glottal margin becomes thicker, increasing the size-mass of the folds, and producing a lowering of voice pitch (Gould, 1975) and sometimes vocal roughness. It would appear that in any case in which the larynx is under- or overdeveloped for the age and sex of the patient, some endocrine imbalance might be suspected. If some kind of hormonal imbalance is discovered, the primary treatment, if possible, would be hormonal therapy. Voice therapy can be of help to the patient in developing the best vocal performance possible with the changing (because of hormone therapy) mechanism. Most of the techniques presented in Chapter 5 are appropriate when applied to these patients for direct alteration of voice parameters such as pitch, loudness and quality.

Granuloma

There are three kinds of *granulomas*, one resulting from intubation during surgery, another resulting from glottal trauma from abuse-misuse, and a third resulting from gastric reflux. Each of these etiologies suggests a different treatment. These were discussed earlier in this chapter under the heading of Contact Ulcers.

Any patient who is intubated during surgery or for airway preservation risks having a traumatized laryngeal membrane with the subsequent development of granuloma. The risk is particularly greater in children and women, who have smaller airways and are thus more often traumatized by large tubes (Whited, 1979). The physician places a tube down the pharynx into the airway, between the open (it is hoped) vocal folds, and on into the trachea. If the tube is larger than the glottal opening, the patient runs the risk of trauma. Ellis and Bennett (1977) have recommended that in order to prevent intubation granuloma or hemangioma, patients should be intubated with tubes one size smaller than what would be needed "for a snug fit." Some patients, for example, demonstrate sudden changes in voice after general surgery. If the patient who was intubated shows a persistent hoarseness after surgery, indirect laryngoscopy or endoscopy should be performed to confirm or deny the presence of an intubation granuloma. If present, such a granuloma may need to be removed surgically and/or be treated with voice therapy. Another form of granuloma may result from vocal fold trauma related to continuous irritation (such as acid reflux) or sudden accident (such as an external injury to the larynx.) Other than intubation granuloma, the most common form is associated with contact ulcers. The literature suggests, in fact, that contact ulcer and related vocal fold granuloma are probably the same disorder, related to continuous vocal trauma.

Patients with granuloma may experience severe dysphonia, characterized by hoarseness, breathiness, and the felt need to clear the throat frequently. Voice therapy may play a primary role (Perkins, 1977; McFarlane, 1988) in eradication of some granulomas. After surgical removal of the offending lesion, voice therapy is usually needed to help the patient regain a normal voice.

Hemangioma

Hemangiomas are very similar to granulomas, differing only in type of lesion. Whereas a granuloma is usually a firm granulated sac, a hemangioma is a soft, pliable, blood-filled sac. Like granulomas, hemangiomas often occur on the posterior glottis, frequently associated with vocal hyperfunction, hyperacidity, or intubation. This blood-filled lesion, when identified, should be removed surgically (with cold steel or laser). As soon as glottal healing permits, a vocal hygiene program and some voice therapy should be initiated.

Hyperkeratosis

Patients often come to their dentist or otolaryngologist because they are concerned about some oral or pharyngeal lesions they have observed. Once professionally identified, these lesions are often biopsied and found to be either malignant (cancerous) or nonmalignant (benign). Laryngeal examination may also locate and subsequently identify, by biopsy, additive lesions in the pharynx or larynx. *Hyperkeratosis*, a pinkish, rough lesion, is often the identified lesion, a nonmalignant growth that may be the precursor of malignant tissue change. Hyperkeratotic growths are reactive lesions to continued tissue irritation. Therefore, hyperkeratotic lesions must be watched closely over time for any change in appearance. Favorite sites of hyperkeratosis include under the tongue, on the vocal

Laryngeal Lesions

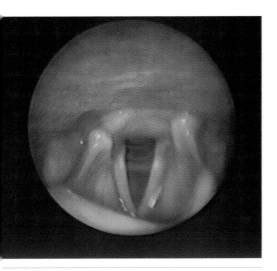

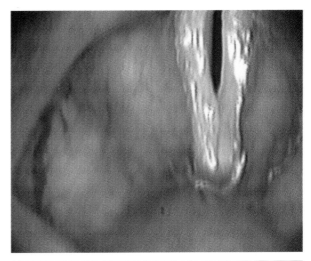

Acute Laryngitis
Note the red swollen vocal cords.

Ventricular Phonation
As is common in many cases of "ventricular phonation" the vibration of the true folds is dampened by the false folds riding on the true folds.

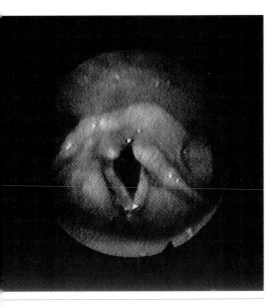

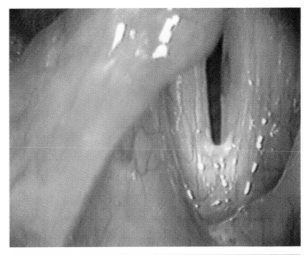

Paralysis and Granuloma/Ulcer
Left vocal cord paralysis and right contact granuloma in 47-year-old male.

Left Vocal Cord Hemorrhage
This 21-year-old singer developed a hemorrhage while singing. The lesion was resolved with rest, and the voice returned to normal.

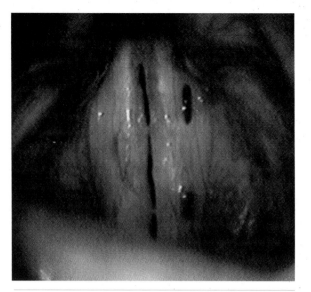

Multiple Left Fold Hemorrhage
This 53-year-old male construction worker and foreman is a heavy smoker and speaks too loudly on the job site.

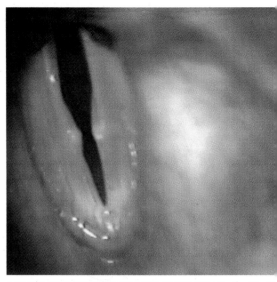

Vocal Nodules
Typical bilateral vocal nodules, which respond very well to voice therapy and abuse reduction.

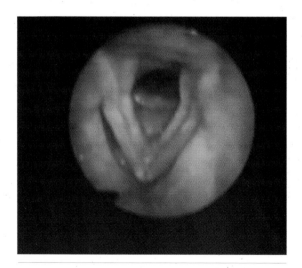

Sulcus Vocalis
This 68-year-old male represents a complete bilateral sulcus vocalis, appearing as a reduplication of the vocal folds, giving him two sets of vocal cords and two ventricles. The arytenoid cartilages appear to be split as well.

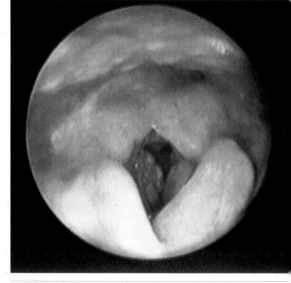

Cancer
Cancer of the larynx in an adult male.

folds at the anterior commissure, and posteriorly on the arytenoid prominences. Their effect on voice may be negligible or severe, depending on the site and the extent of the lesion. We once had an 8-year-old girl voice patient with hyperkeratosis of the vocal folds who had experienced the secondhand smoke of both parents for those 8 years.

It is generally believed that chronic irritation of oral and laryngeal membranes over time—for example, as the result of excessive and continued smoking—is the primary etiology of hyperkeratosis. Consequently, the most effective treatment of the problem is eliminating the source of tissue irritation, possible surgical removal, and voice therapy to improve the voice quality.

Infectious Laryngitis

Some of the same people who experience traumatic laryngitis after only minor abuse-misuse of the voice also experience *infectious laryngitis* when they have a cold. The case histories of such people often contain multiple entries of "loss of voice," or laryngitis. In other individuals, infectious laryngitis is a very rare event that occurs as one of the symptoms of a severe head and chest cold. Infectious laryngitis often develops in a patient who has had a fever, headache, running nose, sore throat, and coughing. Although most problems of infectious laryngitis are viral in origin, the more severe problems (often accompanied by high fever and a very sore throat) may be bacterial infections. Bacterial-caused laryngitis can often be dramatically treated, with relatively quick resolution, through antibiotic therapy. Unfortunately, most laryngitis experienced during a cold (viral in origin) does not respond to antibiotics. The standard treatment is "voice rest, humidification, increased fluid intake (*hydration*), reduced physical activity, and analgesics" (Strome, 1982, p. 12).

From a voice conservation point of view, absolute voice rest—no attempts at spoken communication, including voice or whisper—should be initiated by the patient with such a laryngeal infection. Whispering should be discouraged, because most people produce a glottal whisper by placing the vocal folds in close approximation to one another, which, in effect, produces a light voice. The irritated, swollen tissues continue to touch and to vibrate. What infectious laryngitis patients need is total voice rest for a period of 2 or 3 days, with the vocal folds in the open, inverted-V position and increased fluids (hydration).

Laryngectomy

One of the primary functions of the human larynx is to prevent aspiration into the airway. The larynx contains three valve sites the true folds, the ventricular folds (false folds), and the aryepiglottic folds, each of whose valving action allows them to shut off the airway to prevent the inhalation of liquids, foods, saliva, mucus, and any other stray foreign bodies that may be headed through the larynx into the airway. When the larynx is so compromised by disease (such as advanced cancer) or trauma that it cannot safely perform its valving role, the patient becomes a candidate for a *laryngectomy*, the total removal of the larynx. Without the larynx to protect the airway, an opening is created in the trachea (*tracheostomy*) through which the patient breathes all pulmonary (lung) air in and out. The patient must develop a substitute voicing source, such as an artificial larynx or esophageal speech. Recent modifications of the laryngectomy procedure (Singer & Blom, 1980) permit pulmonary air to flow from the trachea through a prosthetic shunt into the esophagus, facilitating the production of esophageal "voice" without extensive special training. We describe the use of and training for other artificial voicing sources in Chapter 6.

The most common reason to perform a laryngectomy is laryngeal cancer. Small, early detected cancers of the larynx, known as stage I and II cancers, may be treated successfully by radiation therapy and/or minor surgery (Batsakis, 1979). Larger stage III cancers of the larynx can also be successfully treated by radiation therapy and surgery, and require only the removal of involved structures. In more advanced cancers of the larynx (stages IV and V), the most common treatment is total laryngectomy, preceded and followed by radiation therapy. When detected and treated, early laryngeal cancer is 95% successfully treated, making it one of the most curable of all cancers.

Except in cases of traumatic injury to the larynx requiring an emergency laryngectomy, most laryngectomy operations are scheduled only after some counseling has been completed by the surgeon, the speech-language pathologist, and sometimes a laryngectomee (a patient who has had the operation). We describe pre- and postoperative counseling, evaluation, and training of the patient with a total laryngectomy in some detail in Chapter 6.

Laryngofissure

With the development of many innovative laryngeal surgeries for type I, II, and III cancerous lesions, the laryngofissure surgical approach has become more common. The *laryngofissure* is used primarily in exploratory procedures in which the surgeon is investigating the extent of malignancy that may be present. An incision of the thyroid cartilage is made vertically, down from the thyroid notch. The split thyroid cartilage is then extended back on each side, permitting good visibility (particularly of subglottal structures) and easy surgical access. Various surgical procedures are then possible through this large anterior opening of the thyroid cartilage (Tucker, Wood, Levine, & Katz, 1979). If extensive carcinoma is found unilaterally (with normal tissue available to still permit laryngeal valving functions), the patient may then receive a *hemilaryngectomy* (removal of one-half of the larynx). The involved side of the larynx is removed laterally from the midsite where the initial laryngofissure was performed. Structural recovery from a laryngofissure procedure takes about 6 to 8 weeks (Coulthard, 1987).

Patients who receive various surgically reconstructed larynges generally profit from a voice therapy approach that searches with the patient for the best voice possible with those residual structures that are still functional.

Leukoplakia

Leukoplakia are whitish patches that are additive lesions to the surface membrane of mucosal tissue and that often extend beneath the surface into subepithelial space. Although the lesions are classified as benign tumors, similar to hyperkeratosis, they are considered to be precancerous lesions and must be watched closely. Within the vocal tract, common sites for leukoplakia are under the tongue and on the vocal folds. The primary etiology of these white patches is continuous irritation of membranes. The most common cause is heavy smoking; a heroic effort must be initiated to prevent continued irritation, such as absolute insistence that the patient quit smoking and emotional support for the patient. Continued irritation and subsequent growth of leukoplakia often lead to squamous cell carcinoma.

Although leukoplakia on or under the tongue have only minimal effects on voice, leukoplakia on the vocal folds may dramatically alter voice. The added lesion mass to the vocal folds lowers voice pitch and frequently causes hoarseness and sometimes weak loudness. Because leukoplakia are also random in size and location, they often cause the vocal folds to be asymmetrical, which may result in diplophonia as each fold vibrates at a different rate because of its different size or mass. Leukoplakia that occupy space on the glottal margin may prevent optimal approximation of the folds, contributing to a breathiness, reduced loudness and overall dysphonia. The treatment of leukoplakia is medical-surgical, and voice therapy only contributes to developing the best voice possible. In spite of lesion effects, a functional aspect of the dysphonia can often be lessened with therapy. These functional aspects may be the only vocal symptoms, and thus voice therapy is important to restore normal voice.

Papilloma

Papillomas are wartlike growths, viral in origin, that occur in the dark, moist caverns of the airway, frequently in the larynges of young children. They can represent a serious threat to the airway, limiting the needed flow of air through the glottal opening. The majority of papillomas occur in children under the age of 6; for this reason, hoarseness or shortness of breath in preschool children should be evaluated promptly. Although the majority of papilloma stop recurring about the time of puberty, Kleinsasser (1979) wrote that 20% persist beyond puberty. Papilloma of the airway in adolescents and young adults must be considered a serious laryngeal disease, primarily because of its recurrence and persistent threat to the small airway. We have seen adults who developed papillomas in adulthood without ever having them in childhood. When papilloma occur in the larynx, their additive mass often contributes to dysphonia. For this reason, the voice clinician should be particularly alert to any child who demonstrates dysphonia. Any child with continued hoarseness for more than 10 days, independent of a cold or allergy, should have the benefit of a laryngeal examination to identify the cause of the hoarseness. If papillomas are identified, the treatment is medical-surgical; treatment includes laser-beam surgery, conventional excision surgery, radiation therapy, and interferon therapy (Lundquist, Haglund, Carlson, Strander, & Lundgren, 1984). The papilloma should be removed only when they impinge on the airway, since repeated surgery can result in postsurgical webbing of the vocal folds. Eventually, when the individual has developed the immunological state needed to resist the viral-inspired papilloma, the papilloma will no longer recur, according to Kleinsasser (1979).

The surgical and radiation therapy approach to papilloma is required whenever the papilloma growths begin to interfere with the airway. If the lesion mass does not interfere with respiration or voicing, it is usually tolerated. According to Wetmore, Key, and Suen (1985), there may be complications from continued surgical procedures for papillomas. These authors followed 40 patients (26 children; 14 adults) who collectively had received a total of 122 laser surgeries for papillomas over 6 1/2 years. Eleven of twelve patients who had undergone more than six operations over this time period experienced anterior glottal webs with persistent vocal fold edema as complications, and their vocalization was seriously affected. Dedo and Jackler (1982) report that laser surgery was clearly the superior procedure for removal of recurring papilloma in 109 patients; with the laser approach, they report that almost half of their patients eventually reached remission and had no recurrence of the lesions. Despite the possible complications from continuous surgery from recurring papillomas, the lesions must be removed when they begin to impinge on the airway. Lundquist et al. (1984) report a medical approach to the treatment of the viral-caused papillomas: injecting the patients intramuscularly with interferon. In following 17 juvenile patients receiving interferon therapy over a several-year period, Lundquist et al. found that "nine were totally cured, four had no more tumor growth but were still being treated, three experienced diminished tumor growth, and one refused further treatment" (p. 386).

Most recently, interferon drug treatment has been used as a medical treatment for papilloma of the larynx. While this drug has some serious side effects (serious flulike symptoms, etc.) these treatments have produced some good voice results and reduced or eliminated the papilloma. We have seen some patients treated with interferon and have noted significant reduction in the papilloma, and we were able to provide effective voice therapy following drug therapy.

The speech-language pathologist is sometimes asked to see a toddler or young child with an obstructive papilloma who has had to have an open tracheostomy to permit adequate respiration. Developing functional communication with such a child and fostering normal language growth are the primary concerns of the clinician. Teaching the child to occlude the open stoma with a finger or fitting the child with a one-way valve that covers the stoma (to permit vocalization without finger occlusion) usually permits some voicing. In older children or adults who are being treated surgically for a recurring papilloma, helping them to develop the best voice possible with the compromised laryngeal mechanisms is a realistic goal in voice therapy. Some work on respiration control (such as voicing with larger lung volumes of air) or working on loudness and pitch may improve vocal function.

Pubertal Changes

At about age 9, before the onset of puberty, the larynges of boys and girls are anatomically about the same size, and they produce about the same voice pitch (265 Hz). Pubertal growth changes in girls begin around age 9, with the onset of puberty, and gradual pubescent changes occur over a 4- to 5-year period. In boys, puberty begins around ages 11 to 12, and dramatic growth changes occur over the 4- to 5-year pubertal period. However, noticeable laryngeal growth and the dramatic change in vocal fundamental frequency occur in the last year of puberty; the "average time from onset to completion of adolescent voice change is three to six months, one year at most" (Aronson 1990, p. 45). By age 17, adolescents of both sexes have usually reached their full child-to-adult development (Offer, 1980). As we discuss elsewhere (see Chapters 2 and 4), the voice pitch levels of males and females drop dramatically after puberty (the male voice drops at least a full octave; the female voice drops almost half an octave). Laryngeal and airway growth does not happen overnight. Although the changes are gradual, over a 4-year period, marked laryngeal growth (particularly in boys) occurs in the last 6 months of change. During this time of rapid laryngeal growth boys may experience temporary dysphonia and occasional pitch breaks that are not cause for parental or clinical concern. Because these mass changes in puberty tend to thwart any serious attempts at singing or other vocal arts, junior high school is often a poor environment for choral music. A boy who is a soprano in September may well be the choir baritone by June. After reviewing the European literature on vocal pedagogy, Luchsinger and Arnold (1965) make a valid plea that the formal study of singing be deferred until well past puberty. Until children experience some stability in laryngeal and airway growth, the demands of singing might well be inappropriate for their rapidly changing mechanisms. Because of such rapid changes, attempting to develop optimum pitch or modal pitch levels in adolescents should be avoided.

Vocal Fold Paralysis

As presented in Chapter 2, two branches of the vagus (X cranial) nerve, the superior and recurrent laryngeal nerves, have primary motor-sensory functions in the larynx. Laryngeal muscle paralysis can result when either of these two nerves is damaged or severed. The motor component of the superior laryngeal nerve controls the cricothyroid muscles, whose primary role is to change the pitch of the voice by regulating the tension of the vocal folds. The recurrent laryngeal nerve innervates all the other intrinsic muscles of the larynx. Its primary function is the abduction (separation) and adduction (closing) of the vocal folds. If these peripheral nerves (or their central nuclei in the brain stem) are damaged or severed, motor function will be compromised, and the affected muscles will be paralyzed. Figure 3–5 shows a female with unilateral recurrent nerve paralysis.

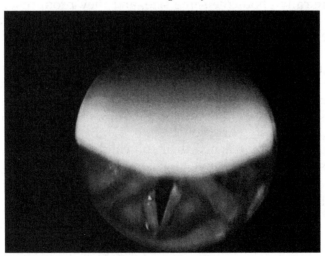

FIGURE 3–5   Unilateral Recurrent Nerve Paralysis
The right cord is fixed in the paramedian position while the left cord moves normally.

Although damage to the superior laryngeal nerve is relatively rare, when it is damaged it produces a paralysis (unilateral or bilateral) of the cricothyroid muscles, so that the patient is unable to make elevations or changes in voice pitch. In the case of unilateral damage, one vocal fold would be normal (able to adjust its length and tension), while the fold on the side of the paralyzed cricothyroid could not change its length or tension. This unilateral kind of involvement that causes canting (tilting) of the larynx often results in a diplophonic voice because one fold vibrates at a different frequency from the other.

Bilateral paralysis of the cricothyroid muscles results in a startling lack of pitch change, and the voice sounds much like a monotone. The result is physiologically and acoustically much the same as cricothyroid joint fixation with its lack of pitch-changing ability. The most frequently observed laryngeal paralysis is a unilateral paralysis with the involved fold paralyzed in the paramedian position. The patient is unable to move the paralyzed fold into the midline for normal vocal fold approximation or away from the midline, which can result in stridor on exercise. This type of paralysis is traditionally called *unilateral adductor paralysis*; the patient is unable to adduct the fold to midline. (The name of the paralysis describes what the involved fold is unable to do.) The cause of unilateral adductor paralysis is usually trauma to the recurrent laryngeal nerve from such causes as neck (particularly thyroid) surgery and accidents. Much rarer is *bilateral adductor paralysis*, whereby both folds are paralyzed in the outer, paramedian position; occasionally, the bilateral positioning is as wide as the glottis can open. Bilateral paralysis is usually caused by a central lesion in the brain stem and is, therefore, a form of dysarthria. The typical voice symptoms of adductor paralysis, particularly the bilateral form, is no voice at all, or *paralytic aphonia*. Unilateral fold paralysis is often temporary because the traumatized nerve can often regenerate. Regeneration is frequently observed within the first 9 months after trauma. Surgical correction of vocal fold paralysis is usually deferred until at least 9 months after onset, and is accompanied by hope for some nerve regeneration with a subsequent return of vocal function. McFarlane, Holt-Romeo, Lavorato, and Warner (1991) found that voice therapy produced superior voice quality in patients with unilateral paralysis when compared to patients treated with Teflon injection. McFarlane et al. (1991) found that voice therapy and muscle nerve reinervation surgery treatment were not significantly different in voice result. Thus, in the interim period, voice therapy can be effective, helping the patient develop some functional or even near-normal voice. Respiration training, the pushing approach, ear training, and promoting hard glottal attack have all been used in helping the patient with unilateral adductor paralysis to develop some voice. We have abandoned the pushing and pulling approach in favor of head turning, half-swallow-boom, and the lateral digital pressure approach discussed in Chapter 5.

Pushing and pulling and the hard glottal attack approach often produce louder voices, but the voice they produce is almost always too vocally rough to be acceptable.

About 50% of patients with peripheral injuries to the recurrent laryngeal nerve experience a return of normal function (Casper, Colton, & Brewer, 1986). If, after 9 months, the involved nerve(s) have not regenerated, or voice therapy has not improved the voice, various medical-surgical approaches are available to develop better laryngeal function, including a useable, functional voice. The most common surgical approach for unilateral adductor paralysis (with the paralyzed fold in the open, paramedian position) is Teflon injection (Weber, Neumayer, Alford, & Weber, 1984). Of 111 patients with unilateral paralysis followed by Weber and his group, 85% had marked improvement in voice function after injection; 2 patients developed airway obstruction secondary to edema requiring temporary tracheostomy. Another surgical approach, implanting Silastic in the anterior commissure end of the paralyzed fold, "fattened" the paralyzed fold sufficiently to bring it into approximation with the normal fold and produced satisfactory voice (Koufman, 1986). Isshiki (1989) reported a type 1 thyroplasty, which repositions the paralyzed vocal fold nearer the midline using an implant set in the side of the thyroid cartilage. This has become an important and popular approach that produces very good voice results. Another procedure for unilateral paralysis, reported by Crumley and Izdebski (1986), involves reinnervating the paralyzed muscles by nerve grafts from the phrenic nerve, or by grafting a section of the superior laryngeal nerve with a portion of the hypoglossus nerve into the vocal fold adductor muscles. Laser surgery has been successful in decreasing open glottal space (Prasad, 1985) for bilateral adductor fold paralysis, and laser arytenoidectomy for bilateral abductor paralysis has successfully opened the glottis (Lim, 1985). Most surgical attempts at reducing the symptoms of unilateral or bilateral vocal fold paralysis need to be supplemented by voice therapy designed to produce optimum phonation with whatever glottal configuration is found after surgery.

Webbing

A laryngeal web growing across the glottis between the two vocal folds inhibits normal fold vibration, which often produces a high-pitched rough sound as it vibrates, and seriously compromises the airway and the open glottis. Webs may be congenital (see Figure 3–6) or acquired (see Figure 3–7). A congenital web, which is detected at the time of birth, is the result of the glottal membrane failing to separate in embryonic development. Depending on the size of the web, the baby will produce stridor (inhalation noises), shortness of breath, and often a different high-pitched (squeal) cry. Approximately three-fourths of all laryngeal webs

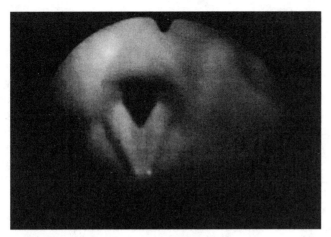

FIGURE 3–6   A Congenital Web
This web produced some shortness of breath on exertion and a
hoarse voice. Voice therapy restored the voice.

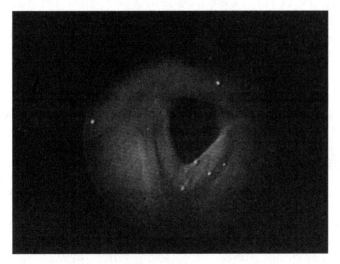

FIGURE 3–7   An Acquired Web
This is a postsurgical web, which produces a hoarse voice. In this
case the voice was responsive to voice therapy.

cross the glottis (Strome, 1982). The presence of a congenital web requires
immediate surgery, often followed by a temporary tracheostomy because
an infant larynx will recover over a period of 4 to 6 weeks.

Acquired webs result from some kind of bilateral trauma of the
inner edges of the vocal folds. Anything that might serve as an irritant to

the mucosal surface of the folds may be the initial cause of the webbing. Because the two vocal folds are so close together at the anterior commissure, any surface irritation due to prolonged infection or trauma may cause the inner margins of the two fold surfaces to grow together. To explain further, one principle of plastic surgery is that, when approximated together, offended tissue surfaces will tend to grow and fuse together. This same principle explains why webbing occurs. The offended surface of the two approximated folds tends to grow together, in this case forming a thin membrane across the glottis. Webbing grows across the glottis in an anterior to posterior fashion, usually ceasing about one-third of the distance from the anterior commissure, where the distance between the two folds becomes too great. Severe laryngeal infections sometimes cause enough glottal irritation to precipitate web formation. Bilateral surgery of the folds, perhaps for papilloma or nodules, can also be followed by a web (Wetmore et al., 1985). External trauma to the folds, such as a direct hit on the thyroid cartilage that causes it to fracture, may damage the folds behind it, thus creating enough glottal irritation for a web to develop. Laryngeal surgery is the most frequent event that produces the postsurgical acquired web. Figure 3–7 is a postsurgical web. Whatever causes the original bilateral irritation, as a part of healing, both folds grow together anteriorly, forming a glottal web sometimes called a *synechia*.

Laryngeal web may cause severe dysphonia as well as shortness of breath, depending on how extensively the webbing crosses the glottis. The treatment for the formation of a web is surgery. The webbing is cut, freeing the two folds. To prevent the surgically removed web from growing again, a vertical keel is placed between the two folds and kept there until complete healing has been achieved. The laryngologist fixates the keel, which is shaped very much like a boat rudder and is about the size of a fingernail, between the folds, preventing them from approximating together. The patient is then on voice rest as long as the keel is in place because its presence inhibits normal fold vibration. When the keel is removed, often in 6 to 8 weeks, the patient generally requires some voice therapy to restore normal phonation. If there was extensive damage to the larynx from the trauma, it may well be impossible after healing and voice therapy to ever develop the same kind of normal voice the patient had before the accident. The prognosis for voice recovery after webbing and its surgical treatment is highly individualized, depending on the extent of the trauma and the size of the resulting web. We have had patients who were able to speak and sing with a normal voice following surgical reduction of the web and a course of voice therapy.

SUMMARY

The majority of voice disorders are related to vocal hyperfunction. Vocal excesses, such as voicing too long and excessive throat clearing, contribute to symptoms of dysphonia or aphonia. Sometimes continued vocal hyperfunction leads to tissue changes of the vocal folds so that such disorders as vocal fold thickening, nodules, polyps, or contact ulcers develop. Organic changes of the vocal folds that may not be directly related to vocal hyperfunction may result from cancer, papilloma, granuloma, and webbing. Various neural problems (such as the cutting of the recurrent laryngeal nerve with a resulting vocal fold paralysis) or neurological diseases produce vocal and resonance changes as part of a dysarthria. In subsequent chapters we examine diagnostic and therapy approaches for these various functional and organic voice disorders.

Chapter 4

The Voice Evaluation

Voice evaluation is the first step in the treatment of a voice disorder. Although identification of a deviant voice may come from several sources (parents, teachers, school nurse, employer, or co-worker), the voice evaluation must be a carefully and scientifically conducted procedure performed by a competent speech-language pathologist. Voice evaluation may either precede or follow a complete examination of the patient by the laryngologist. However, the laryngological results must be considered with the findings of the voice evaluation in order for the voice clinician to make a tentative voice diagnosis and a treatment plan. It is the province of the voice clinician to make the voice diagnosis (analysis of the acoustic and perceptual factors) and to plan voice treatment, just as it is the province of the laryngologist to diagnose laryngeal pathology. These two diagnoses are combined to guide in the best management of the patient's voice disorder.

Successful voice therapy is highly dependent on how well the voice clinician can identify what the patient is doing vocally. The typical voice evaluation is completed after someone else, such as the laryngologist, has already diagnosed the presence or absence of laryngeal pathology that may be contributing to a voice disorder. The speech-language pathologist must make a detailed analysis of what the patient is doing relative to respiration, phonation, and resonance (Blakeley, 1991; Lavorato, 1991). To do this, he or she makes good use of whatever medical descriptions of the problem may be available, takes a detailed case history, observes the patient closely, uses the testing tools and instrumentation (including visualization of the larynx via videoendoscopy and stroboscopy by the speech-voice pathologist) necessary to make an accurate assessment, and introduces to the patient various therapeutic probes (clinical stimulation) to obtain clues about what direction the voice therapy should take.

Although we present the voice evaluation here in a separate chapter, it is important for the reader to appreciate that voice evaluation and voice therapy cannot be separated. Effective voice therapy requires continuous, ongoing assessment. Evaluation and therapy overlap. What is found at the evaluation and given back to the patient as a form of feedback may also have great therapeutic value. Using various therapy approaches as diagnostic probes in an attempt to identify a patient's best possible voice can be an important part of every therapy session. Many of the evaluation procedures and tools described in this evaluation chapter are also used by clinicians in voice therapy. Finally, while we believe in the value of using appropriate instrumentation to evaluate and diagnose voice disorders, the best instrument remains the scientific and clinically trained mind, followed closely by the trained ear.

VOICE SCREENING

Speech-language pathologists in the public schools (see Chapter 8) are in an excellent position to develop voice screening procedures for the early identification of children with voice problems. Most school programs have speech screening programs for new children and for all children in certain grades at specified times of the year. For example, in the fall clinicians may screen all children in kindergarten and third grade. By using some kind of voice screening form, clinicians are able to make better judgments about the parameters of voice. With very little additional testing time per child (perhaps 60–90 seconds), a voice screening program can be added to existing speech and language screening measures.

Different clinicians in various settings have developed various screening forms. The items on the form usually represent the aspects of voice that the clinician considers important for identifying children who may be having voice problems. The screening form helps clinicians focus and organize their listening observations. Wilson (1987) recommends that clinicians use the following tasks in voice screening: counting from 1 to 10; giving a connected speech sample (1 minute); reading a sample (1 minute); and prolonging for 5 seconds each of five selected vowels (high to low). Previous screening forms published by Boone (1973, 1977) have included observations specific to rating the parameters of pitch, loudness, quality, and resonance. These forms have generally been modified as they are field-tested and utilized in various settings. We have found, over time, for example, that the rating task must be as focal as possible to be useful. The more parameters to be rated and the more gradations of the rating, the poorer the reliability in using the form. Nonetheless, McFarlane, Holt, and Lavorato (1985) and McFarlane et al. (1991) have reported that even lay listeners can be nearly as accurate as speech pathologists or ENT physicians in rating voice disorders if the vocal parameters are well defined and limited in number. These authors used a 10-point scale for each of six vocal parameters (pitch, loudness, hoarseness, breathiness, roughness, and overall vocal quality).

The form in Figure 4–1 offers clinicians the information they need for a screening test (Boone, 1986). The single criterion for each of the scale judgments (pitch, loudness, quality, nasal resonance, oral resonance) is whether or not the child's voice on that particular parameter sounds like the voices of peers of the same age and sex. If a child's voice appears lower in pitch than that of peers, the − is circled on the form; if pitch appears normal, the N is circled; if the pitch level is higher than the child's peers, the + is circled. This simple three-point scale is especially useful for rating the parameter of pitch because, as McFarlane et al. (1985) point out, all of their listeners had the most difficulty making consistent and accurate judgments of the pitch parameter.

Inadequate loudness is specified as −; normal loudness as N; and excessive loudness as +. Any deviation of quality is represented by − or +; a breathy, hoarse voice is marked as −, and a tight, harsh voice as +. If denasality (insufficient nasal resonance) is noted, the form is checked −; normal nasal resonance is marked N; and hypernasality is characterized by +. Oral resonance deviations do not occur as often as other problems; however, excessive posterior tongue carriage that produces inadequate oral resonance is marked as −; no problem in oral resonance is (N); and excessive front-of-the-mouth resonance characterized by a baby voice (thin vocal quality) is marked as +. If the child receives either − or + on any of the five clinical parameters, he or she should be rechecked. If problem areas are again identified, a complete voice evaluation (McFarlane,1990; Watterson, 1991) would be recommended (Boone, 1980a). The s/z ratio is included as a screening measure (Eckel & Boone, 1981; Tait, Michel, & Carpenter, 1980). The s/z ratio is a measure of how well a child can sustain a prolonged /s/ phoneme as compared with the /z/ phoneme. The /s/ is a measure of expiratory control, and the /z/ sound adds the laryngeal component to the task. Normal speakers yield about the same maximum duration values of both /s/ and /z/; however, there is a slight skewing of longer duration for the /z/ rather than for the /s/. Apparently, when the laryngeal valving contributes to the task, as in voicing, the glottal structure inhibits the air flow, contributing to a longer duration. Individuals with larynges with glottal lesions (such as nodules or polyps) exhibit significantly shorter /z/ durations than normal subjects, although their maximum /s/ durations appear of normal length

VOICE SCREENING FORM
The Boone Voice Program for Children

Name_____   Sex M F   Grade_____

School_____   Teacher_____

Examiner_____   Date_____

VOICE RATING SCALE

Circle the appropriate symbol(s)

Pitch   — N +   Describe:

Loudness   — N +   Describe:

Quality   — N +   Describe:

Nasal Resonance — N +   Describe:

Oral Resonance   — N +   Describe:

S/Z RATIO

Record 2 trials of [s] and 2 trials of [z] expirations

s = _____seconds

s = _____seconds
                                  Longest s ÷ by Longest z = S/Z Ratio:_____
z = _____seconds

z = _____seconds

DISPOSITION:

☐ Complete voice evaluation required
  (one or more ratings of + or – or an
  S/Z ratio of greater than 1.2)

☐ No further evaluation required

☐ Second screening required_____
                       (Date)
  Comments:

Additional copies of this form (#2350) may be purchased from PRO-ED,
8700 Shoal Creek Blvd., Austin, Texas 78758 512/892-3142

FIGURE 4–1   A Voice Screening Form
(*The Boone Voice Program for Children*, Austin, Texas. Copyright © 1986 by PRO-ED, Inc.)

(Eckel & Boone, 1981). The s/z ratio is computed by dividing the maximum /z/ time into the maximum /s/ time. Eckel and Boone found that more than 95% of their patients with laryngeal pathologies demonstrated s/z ratios in excess of 1.4. The s/z ratio thus seems to provide a quick measure that might identify those people with dysphonia who have possible laryngeal lesions. Most screening forms allow a brief space for comments examiners may want to add to the screening data. For example, the notation "she had a bad cold" would be helpful information for a follow-up visit with someone previously noted as exhibiting "denasality." At the second visit, screening data are compared with present observations. Arrangements should be made for full voice evaluations for those individuals who on follow-up continue to show some departures in voice from their age-sex peers.

THE VOICE EVALUATION AND MEDICAL INFORMATION

Voice patients evaluated by speech-language pathologists have either been "discovered" in voice screening programs, or referred by teachers and other professionals in the schools, referred by physicians (usually laryngologists), or self-referred. Regardless of the referral source, in early contacts with the patient the speech-language pathologist will arrange for a full voice evaluation. For those patients not referred by laryngologists, part of the evaluation process may include a medical evaluation. Occasional voice patients, such as those who do not talk loudly enough or those who use aberrant pitch levels for what appear to be functional reasons, may not require medical evaluation. Patients with voice quality and resonance problems generally require some medical evaluation of the ears, nose, and throat as part of the total voice evaluation.

The most effective voice rehabilitation programs seem to have close team cooperation between the speech-language pathologist and the laryngologist (McFarlane, 1990; Watterson, 1991). Unfortunately, some rural areas of the country have no laryngologists, and it is not uncommon for speech-language pathologists in these areas to report that there are no medical doctors available who can perform *indirect laryngoscopy* (mirror view of the vocal folds). The speech pathologist in such a situation should confer with the patient's local physician, saying, for example, "Tom seems to be hoarse every day. Could you please see that his vocal folds are examined?" Rarely will a physician not appreciate such a request. Physicians who feel that they do not possess the skills required for indirect laryngoscopy will refer the patient to a laryngologist. It is not unusual for patients living in remote areas of the United States to travel several hundred miles for an examination by a laryngologist.

A laryngeal examination must be completed before a patient can begin voice therapy for problems related to quality or resonance. As part of the diagnostic process the speech-language pathologist may wish to use therapy approaches as diagnostic probes; for example, asking a patient to turn the head, or receive digital manipulation may provide important diagnostic information about how tighter vocal fold approximation affects voice quality (see Chapter 5). Voice therapy efforts should be deferred until the medical examination (which would include laryngoscopy) is concluded, because there are occasional laryngeal pathologies, such as papilloma or carcinoma, for which voice therapy would be strongly contraindicated. In such cases, the delay of accurate diagnosis of these pathologies could be life-threatening.

The laryngologist's examination includes an assessment of the larynx and related structures. The vocal folds are assessed by indirect mirror, or, more commonly now, by endoscopic laryngoscopy, and their color, configuration, movement, and position are noted. During the patient's quiet respiration, the laryngologist looks for the normal inverted-V position of the cords. For phonation, the patient is often asked to phonate a relatively high pitch, perhaps by extending an e-e-e (/i/) for several seconds. The higher the pitch, the further the epiglottis and root of the tongue are extended upward, permitting a relatively unobstructed view of the vocal folds. A judgment is made on the adequacy of fold approximation during phonation. Other structures that may be examined include the ventricular folds, laryngeal ventricle, pharynx, tonsils-adenoids, nasal cavities, velopharyngeal mechanism, glands and muscles of the neck. The laryngologist's examination is directed at finding the cause of the patient's presenting voice problem and evaluating the overall status of the larynx and related mechanisms. If the laryngologist wants additional information about how the patient uses his or her voice, or if the laryngologist feels voice therapy may be needed, the patient will be referred directly to the speech-language pathologist. Such referral usually requires a written statement by the laryngologist describing the patient's problem. In actual practice, the written referral may be supplemented by a conversation further describing the problem. The laryngologist's referral usually includes an abbreviated statement of the patient's history, a descriptive statement of the presenting problem, what was told to the patient, and a statement describing the results of evaluation and treatment direction and probable prognosis. It should also request an evaluation and voice diagnosis by the speech-voice pathologist and his or her suggested course of treatment.

The following letter of referral from a local laryngologist who placed strong and continued emphasis on voice therapy for most of his patients with hyperfunctional voice problems was taken from a clinic file:

I have asked Pearl to see you for your voice evaluation at the earliest opportunity. This 44-year-old woman works as a secretary to an insurance executive, a position that requires much talking on the telephone. In the past 6 months she reports continued hoarseness, usually worse at the end of the day, and she complains of occasional pain in the general hyoid region after prolonged speaking. She is married, the mother of three young adult sons. Until 6 months ago, there was no history of vocal distress.

On mirror laryngoscopy, I found the patient to have small bilateral nodes at the anterior one-third junction. Areas immediately adjacent to the nodes were characterized by increased vascularization, suggesting much irritation at this site. On cord adduction, there is noticeable open chinking on each side of the approximated nodes. Her voice, as you might suspect, is quite breathy with an audible escape of air, probably escaping through the open chinking. Inadequate voice loudness, also, appears to be a problem for her.

I am referring her to you for your ideas on what she may be doing wrong with her voice. If you feel she would benefit from voice therapy, please schedule her. I told her that if you felt voice therapy were indicated, we would begin there. If not, we might attempt surgical removal of the nodules and then instruct her on proper voice usage to prevent their recurrence. She appears strongly motivated to improve her voice and will, I'm sure, gladly accept whatever you recommend.

Physicians develop different methods of describing their findings for the speech-language pathologists. Their descriptions may range from a brief "normal vocal folds" to a multipage written evaluation. Typically, the speech-language pathologist may receive statements from the laryngologist similar to these:

Large tonsils and adenoids; no need to remove at this time. Larynx normal. Bilateral thickening runs from the total AP [anterior-posterior] distance on both folds. Could well be related to voice abuse. Could you take her on for voice therapy? No physical basis for the tight voice. Cords show good mobility and normal function. No cord lesions. Do you think she'd be a good candidate for nerve resection? A short, relatively immobile velum. Good symmetry. VP [velopharyngeal] distance looks too excessive for normal closure. Recommend a pharyngeal flap. Could you do pressure-flow study and endoscopic photography? We'll staff her next month.

The laryngologist and the speech-language pathologist work together in planning both the evaluative procedures and remediation steps to be followed. Other professionals sometimes included in the evaluation, which we outline in Chapter 7 when we discuss problems of nasal resonance, may include a pediatrician, plastic surgeon, a neurologist, an orthodontist, a prosthodontist, and a psychologist. Specialization today requires a team of professionals for the effective management of some patients with voice disorders.

We firmly believe in the advantages of a team approach; for example, we very rarely recommend removal of nodules even in adults because voice therapy is generally effective for complete reduction of the nodules (McFarlane & Watterson, 1990). Even in cases of long-standing vocal nodules, we have been able to eliminate the nodules or, in some cases, normalize the voice with some residual (nonsymptomatic) nodules left. Note that it is possible to have normal vocal quality with some small remaining nodule tissue. In such cases, however, the ENT physician, should be advised not to remove the remaining nodule tissue when the voice is normal in quality. Surgical removal of this small remnant is unnecessary and may actually jeopardize the newly established vocal quality, due to scarring. Such treatment philosophies and observations are best shared when there is a good team relationship between the laryngologist and the voice clinician. McFarlane, Fujiki, and Brinton (1984) have discussed this team relationship from the view of the speech-language pathologist:

> The most desired goal is to be regarded by these professional practitioners as peer professionals. This means that we must be able to talk intelligently about their field (be "bilingual," using our jargon and theirs) and their clients, provide a valuable and effective treatment service to their patients, and possess a knowledge and skill base somewhat unique from these other specialties. (pp. 133–134)

Some laryngologists prefer an evaluation form containing a glottal figure. This allows them to make their statements quickly and to accompany them with a line sketch of the pathology (if present) specific to its site and size. Figure 4–2 shows part of such a form (Boone, 1985) that would be completed by the examining physician and returned to the speech-language pathologist.

Community health centers and university clinics routinely obtain medical information and some case history data from patients when the initial appointment is made and, if a voice problem is indicated, schedule the patient first for a medical diagnostic evaluation. Sometimes, however, a voice patient will make the initial appointment without identifying the problem as one of voice. If, for whatever reason, a patient arrives to be treated for some form of dysphonia but has not had a previous medical examination, the speech-language pathologist will want to defer final disposition of the patient until the medical information is obtained. The voice evaluation by the speech clinician may begin, however, even in the absence of the medical information. The case history can be taken, and respiration-phonatory-resonance observations and test data can be obtained; only the decision about whether to begin voice therapy need be deferred until the data base is complete with the ENT exam results.

The ethics and efficacy of speech-language pathologists themselves doing indirect laryngoscopy are worth discussing at this point (ASHA,

VOICE REFERRAL TO PHYSICIAN
The Boone Voice Program for Children

To the physician: This child was recently seen for a voice evaluation. Voice therapy has been deferred until a medical diagnosis has been made. Please complete Section 2 of this form and return it with your recommendations.

Name_____Sex M F Birth Date_____Age_____

School_____ Referring Clinician_____ Telephone_____

SECTION 1
Voice Evaluation Summary
(to be completed by Speech-Language Pathologist)

SECTION 2
Summary of Medical Findings
(to be completed by examining Physician)

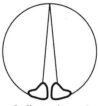

Indicate site and
extent of lesion

Recommendations:
_____ Voice therapy recommended

_____ Voice therapy not recommended

Comments:

Return this form to:

_____

_____   _____

_____   Physician's Signature

_____

_____   _____

                                       Date

Additional copies of this form (#2353) may be purchased from PRO-ED, 8700 Shoal Creek Blvd., Auslin, Texas 78758, 512/451-3246.

FIGURE 4–2   A Voice Referral to Physician Form
(*The Boone Voice Program for Children*, Austin, Texas. Copyright © 1985 by PRO-ED, Inc.)

1992b; Watterson & McFarlane, 1991; Watterson, McFarlane & Brophy, 1990). Some speech-language pathologists are trained to perform endoscopy or mirror laryngoscopy, procedures that are not difficult to master; these persons use indirect laryngoscopy primarily to teach students laryngeal function and to observe the folds directly to determine any changes during therapy. As speech-voice pathologists we use videolaryngoscopy and stroboscopy for research, for teaching purposes, for voice evaluation and voice diagnosis, to provide patients with feedback, and to develop new and more effective voice therapy treatment techniques. Appropriately trained speech-voice pathologists may employ laryngeal visualization techniques in accordance with ASHA (1992b) Guidelines for Vocal Tract Visualization and Imaging. Primary identification of laryngeal pathology is the clear responsibility of the laryngologist, who is also equipped with the medical techniques required to treat the pathology, once it is identified. For the ethical and legal protection of the speech-language pathologist, the voice patient who comes in for evaluation without prior medical examination should be given an ENT laryngeal examination before beginning treatment by the speech-language pathologist. A diagnostic examination of the vocal cords must be done by the laryngologist. The speech-language pathologist trained in videolaryngoscopy may also use mirror laryngoscopy or endoscopy to view the folds for voice diagnosis; this will facilitate the voice therapy treatment of the patient by allowing the clinician to make judgments about vocal fold response to voice therapy techniques. Since the ENT physician is looking for laryngeal disease and the speech-voice pathologist is looking for function related to clinical stimulation this is not a duplicate procedure and is wholly justified and necessary. While on the surface these examinations may seem redundant, they are proper since both specialties have different concerns and goals. Both the ENT physician and the speech-voice pathologist, for example, have the patient phonate but with different goals in mind and with different procedures or vocal maneuvers for the patient to perform. Further, detailed discussion of the ethics of the speech-language pathologist performing videolaryngealendoscopy is presented by Watterson, McFarlane, and Brophy (1990) and in ASHA Guidelines (1992b).

THE VOICE EVALUATION AND THE CASE HISTORY

To understand patients with voice disorders and to understand their problems, it is necessary for clinicians to assemble a case history. Most texts and manuals dealing with diagnosis and appraisal of communicative disorders present general strategies for history taking (Darley, 1965; Dickson & Jann, 1974; Nation & Aram, 1977; Perkins, 1977). Recent texts on management of voice disorders that offer suggestions for history taking include Aronson (1990), Boone (1980), Case (1991), Greene

(1980), and Wilson (1987). Many individualized voice evaluation forms are available for clinicians. Most history forms include major headings that include a description of the problem, the cause of the problem, consistency or variability of the problem, and voice usage. The form shown in Figure 4–3 is typical.

Description of the Problem and Cause

It is valuable for understanding patients to ask directly what they feel are the problems and what might have caused them. It is often effective to ask the same questions of family members or teachers. The different views about what the problem may be and the various guesses about probable causation may offer tips for management. Patients' descriptions often reveal much about their own conceptualization of the problem. What a patient feels the problem is may not be consistent with the opinions of the referring physician or the speech-language pathologist—a discrepancy that may be due to what we call the patient's reality distance. This distance may be the result of the patient's lay background and inability to understand adequately what had been explained. Often we hear highly discrepant reports of "what the doctor said" as a patient recounts the diagnoses of previous clinicians. More often this distance is primarily the result of the inability to accept and cope with the real problem. An individual's defenses may force him or her to describe the problem in a way that is not consistent with the perceptions of others. What a patient says about a problem may, however, provide the clinician with insights that no amount of observation or testing can match. This sort of reality distance is well illustrated by the following excerpts from the clinic records of a 28-year-old computer programmer:

> *Physician's Examination Statement:* George was an extremely hard man to examine with indirect laryngoscopy. He was very fearful during our exam and gagged with the slightest touch to the posterior tongue. His vocal folds show broad-based bilateral polyps, about 4 mm wide along the anterior-middle third junction. Trial voice therapy is indicated.

> *Speech-Language Pathologist's Statement:* Patient voices with much audible strain, characterized by diplophonia, hoarseness, and severe glottal attack. Patient participated in all phases of our evaluation with a fixed smile on his face, contrasted with tight, clenched fists. We may well need here a combined voice therapy–counseling approach.

> *Patient's Statement of the Problem:* Now that I have recently found the Lord, I want to serve Him. Whenever I go to teach at the church, I seem to lose my voice. My computer work presents no problem, because I don't need the voice much there. It's a problem of going hoarse and even losing the voice when I work with the groups at the church.

VOICE EVALUATION FORM
The Boone Voice Program for Children   by Daniel R. Boone, Ph.D.

Name_____   Sex M   F   Date of Birth_____ Age_____

School_____   Teacher_____ Grade_____

Referral Source: Screening_____ Teacher_____ Physician_____ Self_____ Other_____

Examiner_____ Date of Evaluation_____

SECTION 1 ■
History of the Voice Problem

	Child's Report	*Parent's Report* (Informant_____)	*Teacher's Report*
Description of Problem			
Cause of Problem			
Onset of Problem			
Prior Voice Therapy			
Variability through Day			
Voice Usage			

*Abuses:*_____

Misuses:_____

Comments:_____
_____
_____

Additional copies of this form (#2342) may be purchased from PRO-ED, 8700 Shoal Creek Blvd., Austin, Texas 78758, 512/451-3246

FIGURE 4–3   A Voice Evaluation Form
This type of form helps to organize the case history according to each informant. (*The Boone Voice Program for Children*, Austin, Texas. Copyright © 1993 by PRO-ED, Inc.)

Consistently from these descriptions we view a patient who was showing some tension signs when relating to other people. He was hypersensitive during laryngoscopy attempts, his vocal patterns and facial-hand mannerisms suggested tension, and his description of his problem voicing with other people all suggested psychological tension as a possible contributing factor to his dysphonia. Aronson (1990) has written, "If the dysphonia is of greater severity or different in character than warranted by the lesion, a psychogenic component is strongly suspected" (p. 120). The bilateral polyps alone should not have caused the complete voice breakdown the patient experienced while teaching groups at the church. Successful management of this man's problem necessitated a combined voice therapy and psychological counseling approach, similar to what was suggested initially by the speech-language pathologist.

Onset and Duration of the Problem

How long patients believe they have had the voice problem is important. A problem of acute and sudden onset usually poses a severe threat to a patient—that is, it keeps the patient from carrying out his or her customary activities (playing, singing, acting, selling, preaching, teaching, campaigning, or whatever). Sudden onset of aphonia or dysphonia deserves thorough exploration by both the laryngologist and the speech-language pathologist. Some dysphonias develop very gradually. Such gradual, fluctuating dysphonias are often related to varying situations in which patients may find themselves; sometimes they only occur during moments of stress or after fatigue. A history of slow onset sometimes suggest a gradually developing pathology, such as the development of bilateral polypoid degeneration of the vocal folds or dysphonia that is but an early developing symptom of some kind of progressive neurological disease. Long-term chronic dysphonia usually exists for so long because the patient has never been particularly disturbed by the voice problem. Voice therapy, like other forms of remedial therapy, is usually more successful with those patients who are motivated to overcome their problems. Patients with a long history of indifference toward their dysphonia usually present a more unfavorable prognosis than the ones who have recently acquired the disorder, depending, of course, on the type and etiology and relative extent of the pathology involved.

Variability of the Problem

Most voice patients can provide rather accurate timetables of the consistency of their problem. If the severity of a voice problem is variable a clinician may be able to identify those vocal situations in which the patient experiences the best voice and the worst voice. The typical patient with vocal hyperfunction reports a better voice earlier in the day, with increasing dysphonia as the voice is used more. For example, a high school social studies teacher reported a normal-sounding voice at the beginning of the day; toward the end of a day, after 6 hours of lecturing, he reported increasing hoarseness and a feeling of "fullness and dryness in the throat." Voice rest and then dinner at the end of the day usually restored his voice to its normal level. Obviously, such fluctuations in the daily quality of the voice enables the clinician to easily identify the situations contributing to the patient's vocal abuse. Another patient, whose dysphonia was closely related to allergy and postnasal drip experienced during sleep, presented this kind of variation in hoarseness: severity in the morning upon awakening, decrease in severity with usage of the voice, complete disappearance by late afternoon, and severity again the next morning.

The variation of the voice problem can provide even more specific clues as to what situations most aggravate the disorder. A nightclub singer reported that she had no voice problem during the day in conversational situations or while practicing her repertoire. She developed hoarseness only at night and only on those nights she sang. Further investigation of her singing act revealed that the adverse factors were the cigarette smoke around her, to which she was unusually sensitive, and the noise of the crowd, above which she had to increase her volume to be heard. Her singing methods were found to be satisfactory. A change of jobs to a summer tent theater provided her with immediate relief. Variability of situation also affected a housewife allergic to a specific brand of meat tenderizer. This patient lost her voice completely shortly after using the tenderizer during meal preparation. When she discontinued the use of this product, she did not lose her voice; when the product was reintroduced, the aphonia followed. Inhaling only a small amount of this substance rendered her almost completely aphonic for 15 minutes or more.

Description of Vocal Use (Daily Use, Misuse)

Abuse, misuse, and overuse of the voice cause most functional voice problems. It is important for clinicians to determine how voice patients are using their larynges in most life situations. The voice a child or adult exhibits in the speech-language pathologist's office may in no way represent the voice used on the playground, in the classroom, or in other settings. Sometimes patients can re-create some of their aversive laryngeal behaviors as a demonstration for the clinician, but more often a valid search for aversive vocal behaviors requires the clinician to visit the environment where the abuse-misuse occurs. Successful voice clinicians must thus build into their schedules actual visits to playgrounds, theaters, churches, courtroom, or offices. In reducing one child's vocal abuse (and vocal nodules) a major factor was our visiting the school lunchroom and changing his manner of repeating the phrase "Do you want white or chocolate milk?" 300 times each day as he passed out the milk during the noisy lunch period. Similarly, we were able to make major vocal gains with a dysphonic attorney only after attending the courtroom trial where we observed his excessively loud and effortful legal objections and jury addresses and modified them firsthand. Apparently, only a little voice abuse-misuse in whatever setting is all that may be needed to keep a glottal membrane inflamed or a pair of vocal nodules irritated and fibrotic. Case (1991), for instance, has demonstrated the effects of cheerleading on the larynges of teenagers, comparing them with laryngoscopy before and after 2 weeks of attendance at a cheerleading camp. His data strongly suggest that continued cheerleading has a direct aversive effect on the larynges of the majority of the adolescents studied. It is obviously important for the clinician to identify the vocal use pattern of the patient.

Special attention must be given to the identification of playground screaming and yelling in children. One only has to listen to the noise level of the typical primary-school playground to realize that yelling at play appears to be a normal childhood behavior. A child with a voice problem, however, often has a history of yelling a little louder and a bit more often than normal-voiced peers. Sometimes public school clinicians must enlist the help of teachers, friends, and the family to determine the everyday vocalization history of the child. Perhaps the most important part of voice therapy for children is identifying vocal abuse and developing strategies to reduce its occurrence.

Additional Case History Information

It is important to determine at the time of the voice evaluation if the patient has ever had previous voice therapy. If so, what type of past therapy would have obvious relevance to present management? When previous voice therapy attempts have failed to improve the vocal quality or have been unsuccessful in reducing a vocal pathology, the knowledge of previous therapy is important. We must, however, make every effort to present the appearance of a fresh and different approach to the patient who has experienced failure in previous voice therapy (McFarlane and Lavorato, 1983). Even if we use the same goals of therapy as before, we must redirect the new approach to voice therapy in a manner that appears to the patient to be headed down a completely different road.

Determining whether other members of the family have similar voice problems is helpful. We have had particular patients present a certain voice problem, only to interview members of the family and find that all or many of them have the same voicing patterns. Deviations in resonance are often the most commonly observed family patterns.

Voice evaluations should also include some kind of health history, an example of a health history taken from a child evaluation form (Boone 1993) is shown is Figure 4–4. Certainly for adult patients it is important to determine such conditions as allergies, medication or hormone therapy, smoking, use of alcohol, and use of drugs. It is also very important to check the level of hydration by asking about daily fluid intake. Once a patient is comfortable with an examiner, or perhaps after voice therapy has begun, a social history should be taken to provide the clinician with useful information about the patient as a person. One patient spoke with two completely different voices, constantly shifting between one voice and the other. When we asked why she used these two voices she said her first voice was "her voice before she died." Further case-history questioning revealed that she had been a patient in a mental hospital on two occasions. It became clear as the interview progressed that she was still having psychological problems and her voice disorder was a symptom of a more serious unresolved disorder.

THE VOICE EVALUATION AND OBSERVATION OF THE PATIENT

Observations of our patients often tell us more about them than our histories and our test data. Speech-language pathologists must become critical observers, attempting to describe behavior they see rather than merely labeling it. Writing observations about a patient is one of the few ways clinicians can note what they observe (audio and video tape recordings are two other means). Even here, however, it is important for clinicians to minimize any subjectivity by describing only what they see and hear, and not adding interpretation to the observation. For example, an adult laryngectomy patient was seen preoperatively and gave this report:

> I work as a hod carrier. I have done this kind of work for years. A question I have is how will this operation go along with my work? My Mom and I live together and she needs my help and my paycheck. If I have a hole in my neck what about the cement dust. Can I still work? My boss likes my work and I have done it for a long time. And what about my girlfriend, will she be able to understand me? I go to a bar and have a beer and sandwich sometimes and it is loud in there. Will they hear me?

During his interview the patient gave "little cues" about his doubts concerning his skills and his ability to work at other jobs. We asked him if he could read or write. He said "How did you know? Only one other doctor ever knew in all my thirty-eight years." He was fearful that he might never be able to return to work, and without the ability to read and write he was not likely to find another job, and he and his mother would

---

SECTION 2
Health History

*Informant:*_____

Birth History
_____

Feeding Problems
_____

Illnesses and Allergies
_____

Accidents
_____

Surgery
_____

Medications
_____

Voice Change
_____

Family Voice Problems
_____

Previous Voice Therapy
_____

FIGURE 4–4   A Health History Form
This type of form helps to organize a health history. (*The Boone Voice Program for Children*, Austin, Texas.
Copyright © 1993 by PRO-ED, Inc.)

be without an income. He became not only a good alaryngeal speaker using the Tokyo Larynx and somewhat of a celebrity in his community, but he also learned to read and write when we referred him to an adult literacy program. He also went back to his hod-carrying work. It was important to notice clues that gave important information about the patient. He would never have told us that he was unable to read or write. His mother or girlfriend would fill out papers for him. He had picked up our clinic form and brought it in at his visit all completed by his mother.

Because voice difficulties are often symptomatic of the inability to have satisfactory interpersonal relationships, it is imperative that the clinician consider the patient's degree of adequacy as a social being. The patient who exhibits extremely sweaty palms; who avoids eye contact with the person to whom he or she is speaking; who uses excessive postural changes, demonstrates facial tics or sits with a masked, nonaffective facial expression; or who exhibits obvious shortness of breath may be displaying behaviors frequently considered as symptomatic of anxiety. The struggle to maintain a conversational relationship may be accompanied by much struggle to phonate. Such observed behavior in the voice patient may be highly significant to the voice clinician planning a course of voice remediation. The decision about whether to treat a problem symptomatically or by improving the patient's potential for interpersonal adjustment (perhaps by psychotherapy) is often aided by a review of the observations of the patient. A patient who demonstrates friendly, normal affect is telling the clinician, at least superficially, that he or she functions well in a two-person relationship; such information may well have clinical relevance. Such observations are extremely valuable to voice clinicians planning treatment approaches. Note, however, that in our experience very few voice patients require referral for psychotherapy.

THE VOICE EVALUATION AND TESTING OF THE PATIENT

A voice rating scale of some kind aids the clinician in separating the various processes contributing to voice into separate components. A children's voice rating scale is shown in Figure 4–5. This particular scale permits clinicians to observe each of seven parameters: pitch, loudness, quality, nasal resonance, oral resonance, speaking rate, and variability of inflection. This particular scale is basically a seven-point rating scale with normal production checked in the middle. To the left of normal are the rating slots for insufficient performance of the parameter to be rated; for example, a voice pitch that appears too low would be rated on the pitch scale to the left of normal. The individual's pitch level is compared with the pitch levels of age peers. The mild, moderate, and severe boxes are checked according to the clinician's judgment. The rating scale is not a test per se but provides clinicians with a structure for systematizing their observations. Actual measurements of frequency, intensity, quality, and resonance are made separately, and these data can often help clinicians make the summary judgments placed on the voice rating scale. Because rating scales force clinicians to focus their measurements and observations into some kind of summary, many voice clinicians have developed scales and found them useful (Perkins, 1971; Wilson & Rice, 1977). Wilson (1987) describes several equal-interval scales having ratings from 1 to 7, with interjudge reliability in excess of .90. Let us consider some of the measurement instruments used by speech-language pathologists in voice evaluation.

The Oral Evaluation

Careful assessment of the oral mechanisms is part of the voice evaluation. Although we focus on evaluation of the larynx and respiratory systems, some examination of facial structures, mouth,

SECTION 8 ▬▬▬
Voice Rating Scale

	−			N			+
Breathing	1	2	3	4	5	6	7
(words per breath)	too few			normal			too many
	−			N			+
Loudness	1	2	3	4	5	6	7
	soft			natural			too loud
	−			N			+
Pitch	1	2	3	4	5	6	7
	low			natural			high
	−			N			+
Pitch Inflections	1	2	3	4	5	6	7
	none			normal			excessive
	−			N			+
Quality	1	2	3	4	5	6	7
	breathy			normal			harsh
	−			N			+
Horizontal Focus	1	2	3	4	5	6	7
	front			normal			back
	−			N			+
Vertical Focus	1	2	3	4	5	6	7
	throat			normal			nasal
	−			N			+
Nasal Resonance	1	2	3	4	5	6	7
	denasal			normal			hypernasal

FIGURE 4–5   A Voice Rating Scale
This seven-point rating scale allows clinicians to rate various aspects of voice during conversation, play, and
oral reading. (*The Boone Voice Program for Children*, Austin, Texas. Copyright © 1993 by PRO-ED, Inc.)

dentition, tongue, teeth, hard and soft palate, pharynx, and nasal cavities
is required. Incorporated into the voice evaluation may be the peripheral
mechanism forms offered in such evaluation-diagnosis books as Dickson
and Jann (1974) and Nation and Aram (1977). In our evaluation of the
peripheral mechanisms of the voice patient, we must pay particular
attention to possible signs of neural innervation problems. Every now
and then, when we evaluate a patient with "functional dysphonia," we
find some subtle neurological signs of fasciculation and atrophy of the
tongue, or asymmetries of the velum related to neural innervation
changes, and so on. Subsequent medical-neurological evaluations may
find that the early dysphonia is simply the beginning symptomatology of
a serious neurological disease such as multiple sclerosis, muscular
dystrophy, amyotrophic lateral sclerosis, or myasthenia gravis. It is
important to evaluate the voice patient specific to structural and
functional adequacy for all parts of the oral mechanisms. In Chapter 2 we
presented sites of possible hyperfunction where voice patients may have
some difficulty. We now review some of these sites of hyperfunction
closely as part of our total peripheral mechanism evaluation. Beyond

observing obvious problems in breathing, attention should be given to the amount of neck tension. The accessory neck muscles and the supralaryngeal strap muscles in some patients literally stick out like bands as the patient speaks or the untrained singer performs. Often, mandibular restriction is closely associated with neck tension; affected patients speak with clenched teeth, with little or no mandibular movement. Such restricted jaw movement places most of the burden of speech articulation on the tongue, which, to produce the various vowels and diphthongs in connected speech, must make fantastic adjustments if no cavity-shaping assistance from the mandible is forthcoming. Another externally observable hyperfunction of the vocal tract is unusual downward or upward excursion of the larynx during the production of various pitches. Any unusual movement upward while phonating higher pitches or unusual movement downward while phonating lower ones should be noted. The angle of the thyroid cartilage may be felt digitally as the patient sings varying pitches; typically the fingertips will feel little discernible change in thyroid angle as the patient sings up and down the scale. Sometimes, however, the thyroid cartilage can be felt rocking forward slightly in the production of high pitches, as it sweeps upward to a higher position toward the hyoid bone. Any noticeable amount of lifting or lowering of the larynx, as well as the tipping forward of the thyroid cartilage in the production of high pitches, should be noted as possible hyperfunctional behavior. The majority of hyperfunctional behaviors associated with voice problems are probably not directly observable from examination of the peripheral mechanism. For example, to determine the extent of the tongue's impinging on the oral-pharyngeal space we would need to rely on oral or nasal endoscopy or videoendoscopy.

Endoscopy

The endoscope may be introduced intraorally or intranasally; the light at the tip of the scope (which comes fiber-optically from an external light source) illuminates the nasal and oral pharynx that is viewed through a window lens on the other end of the endoscope. Of relevance to voice evaluation is that the tip lens of the oral endoscope can be directed up at the velopharyngeal closure mechanism or down at the larynx below. A nasal endoscopic voice evaluation is pictured in Figure 4–6.

When the oral or nasal endoscope is attached to a small video camera, the examination is termed a videoendoscopic evaluation. It provides a permanent video record of the observations. Using a stop-frame feature of the video recorder and a video printer, we can make a hard copy picture of the observation to include in the patient's file of voice evaluation. When we use a stroboscopic (flashing) light source instead of a steady-state light source, we can produce what appears as a slow motion observation of the vocal physiology (video stroboscopic endoscopy). With such instrumentation we are able to make valuable observations of deviations in both vocal tract anatomy and, more importantly, physiology (McFarlane, Watterson, & Brophy, 1990). The mucosal wave, which is responsible for normal and abnormal voice, can be studied with stroboscopy. With most voice patients, these deviations are subtle, inappropriate vocal adjustments in glottal approximation of the vocal folds, in tongue position, or in pharyngeal constriction, rather than the result of laryngeal lesions. For most observations and measures of intraoral phenomena contributing to normal and faulty voice, we are forced to use various measuring instruments that help quantify aspects of respiratory, phonatory, and resonance function. Videolaryngealstroboscopy is an extremely valuable tool for the speech-language pathologist interested in voice disorders. Many inappropriate laryngeal adjustments produce vibratory abnormalities leading to disordered voice. These adjustments usually cannot be seen without videostroboscopy.

Respiration Testing

Because the vocal folds are activated for phonation by the outflowing airstream passing through the closed glottis, some observation and measurement of respiratory adequacy is a necessary part of the voice evaluation. Early phoniatrists placed emphasis on breathing adequacy, particularly with regard to adequacy for singing; such a view was advocated by singing teachers and frequently cited by Luchsinger and Arnold (1965). Many speech-language pathologists continue to show interest in how well voice patients breathe, and particularly in how well

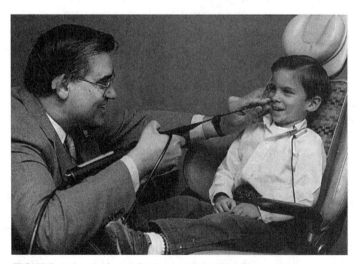

FIGURE 4–6   A Nasal Endoscopic Voice Evaluation
This procedure allows for the study of laryngeal function during typical
phonation (dysphonia) and during clinical stimulation conditions.

patients are able to extend and use their exhalations for phonation. It is commonly recognized, for example, that shortness of breath or speaking after much breath is already expired will noticeably affect phonation. Because lung capacities are generally far greater than the amount of air required for typical speaking situations, patients' *use* of air supply is usually more important than their lung volumes. This is true even for patients who present severe breathing disorders such as emphysema or chronic obstructive pulmonary disease, or even with patients who have only one lung. Large lung volumes are more important for singing than for speaking. We shall consider separately those instruments that can be used for measuring various aspects of respiratory movement and, finally, those observations and tests that we can use to assess patients' use of respiration as it applies to phonation. Specifically, we shall consider separately four types of information: lung volume, air pressure, airflow, and measures and motions of the torso.

Lung Volume   It is important to determine how much of the total lung volume a patient uses in phonation. We can observe the patient speak or sing, and make a judgment about the overall adequacy of respiration while the patient is performing the task. Does she run out of her air supply before finishing the planned utterance? Is he forced to renew air intake more often than is desirable? Part of evaluating respiratory adequacy is measuring the patient's lung volume. Specific measurable dimensions of volume include vital capacity (maximum amount of air that can be expelled from the lungs following a maximum inspiration), tidal volume (amount of air inspired and expired in a normal breathing cycle), inspiratory reserve (maximum amount of additional air inspired after a tidal inhalation is completed), and expiratory reserve (maximum volume of air expired after a tidal expiration). Normal speakers use a small amount of their total vital capacity when speaking. Hixon, Goldman, and Mead (1973) wrote that normal speakers use only about twice the air volume for speech that they use for quiet, normal (or tidal) breaths. Does the typical patient use greater or lesser volumes than this? The capacities and volumes we need to measure can be determined by using wet or dry spirometers. In the wet spirometer, a container floats in water placed in a larger container. As air is introduced to the smaller floating container, it floats higher in proportion to the volume of air introduced. The distance or rise of displacement is measured in cubic centimeters or liters. A 14-year-old boy tested on a wet spirometer was found to have these lung volumes:

Vital capacity	=	3.8 liters
Tidal volume	=	.4 liter (400 cc)
Inspiratory reserve	=	3.3 liters
Expiratory reserve	=	3.4 liters

We see in this example that the normal tidal volume and the maximum amount of air the boy can expire after the tidal breath in several trials approximate his vital capacity or total maximum expiration following maximum inhalation. Some spirometers are of the dry type. A flexible container enlarges on inspiratory tasks and decreases in volume on expiratory tasks, in both instances measuring the volume of displacement. The wet spirometer appears to have greater clinical usage and also to provide greater volume accuracy. Again, we should point out, however, that volume data do not have the same clinical relevance as measures of expiration (pressure and flow) and data specific to neck, thoracic, and abdominal movements.

Airflow Pressures   One can hear the effects of air pressure on the perceived loudness of the voice. Greater vocal intensities require higher airflow volume and pressures passing through the glottis for a shorter time, producing greater excursions of the vibrating vocal folds. We often hear symptoms of inadequate airflow volume and pressure in voice patients who experience varying and inadequate loudness; we may also hear quality disturbances related to inadequate pressure for normal fold vibration.

Relatively inexpensive pressure measuring gauges and manometers are available for the measurement of airflow pressures. In measuring air-pressure adequacy for voice, we are interested in finding an individual's oral pressures. One way of doing this is to ask the patient to produce a series of /pa/ syllables. In the initial production of /pa/ the glottis is open, and the pressure peaks during the production of the /p/ phase of the /pa/. Netsell and Hixon (1978) found that the oral pressures obtained in the /pa/ production or in a blowing task (when the mouthpiece has a small air leak) correspond to the pressures found in the lungs and at the glottis. They concluded that if patients can produce 5 to 10 cm of pressure over a period of 5 seconds in a sustained blowing task, they probably have sufficient expiratory pressures to produce normal voice.

Pressure measurements are used diagnostically more often when attempts are made to measure velopharyngeal adequacy, described in some detail in Chapter 7. Using some kind of manometric device, the patient is asked to produce a consonant such as /p/ or /k/; oral pressure measures are taken and nasal pressures (a nasal olive is inserted in the nares attached to the flow tube) are also determined. Sometimes the oral and nasal measurements are taken sequentially back to back, but such measures are perhaps more meaningful when taken simultaneously. For simultaneous oral-nasal pressures, the patient wears a face mask that is divided into oral and nasal sections, which provides separate oral-nasal pressure ratings (Hixon, Saxman, & McQueen, 1967). Oral speech should have little or no nasal pressure flow; as puffs of air escape through an inadequately closed velopharyngeal port, the sensitivity of the pressure gauge would detect such inappropriate escape.

Airflow Measures An important diagnostic measure in voice evaluation is a measurement of airflow, which indicates the volume of air passed through the glottis in a fixed period of time. For example, the normal production of a vowel requires about 100 cc of air passage through the glottis in 1 second. A patient with large bilateral nodules who cannot effect adequate glottal closure will exhibit much higher airflow rates and perhaps will use 100 cc in far less than a second. His or her voice would be characterized by breathiness, and the leakage of air caused by the lack of normal glottal resistance would be audible. Poor glottal resistance to the airflow, as would be caused by the formation of nodules on the glottal margin, results in elevated airflow measures. Or a patient with unilateral vocal fold paralysis may have an airflow rate as high as 1,000 cc per second. An opposite kind of problem, where the glottis is highly constricted, such as is observed in spasmodic dysphonia, results in markedly reduced flow rates perhaps a low as 50 cc per second.

The rate of flow, particularly when combined with pressure ratings, thus gives much diagnostic information about what is happening to the outgoing air at the level of the glottis. Measurements of airflow are usually substantiated by critical listening to the voice. If a voice appears to be produced by a relatively lax glottal closure as observed in breathiness, the flow rates are high; if the voice appears harsh and sounds constricted, flow rates are often markedly diminished. Not only is flow rate information of diagnostic importance, but it also helps us measure the effects of therapy. For example, as we attempt to move patients into more optimal phonatory behaviors, we see flow rates shift toward normal values (such as 100 cc per second).

An extremely useful instrument is the Phonatory Function Analyzer (see Figure 4–7). We have used this to great advantage in clinical situations (Paynter, 1991). This device makes five simultaneous measures of phonation that demonstrate the efficiency of the larynx during phonation. It also demonstrates the interaction of these five measures (phonation time, frequency, intensity, airflow rate, and total volume of expired air) with one another. When one parameter, such as pitch, is altered during clinical stimulation, the effect on another parameter, such as airflow rate, is easily demonstrated. The tracing (see Figure 4–8) from the Phonatory Function Analyzer demonstrates that a slight elevation in pitch during the production of a vowel can reduce the excessive airflow rate that gives rise to the perception of extreme breathiness in this adult patient with bowed cords. An improved vocal quality, with reduced breathiness, is correlated with the tracing of reduced airflow. The airflow measurement is made in milliliters per second (ml/sec), which is the practical equivalent of cubic centimeters (cc) mentioned earlier.

In the past, the pneumotachometer was used for measuring airflow. The patient produces vowel prolongations with airflow captured in the oral mask, and the flow rate is measured by the pneumotachometer. Much data are available for normal flow rates both in children (Leeper, 1976) and adults (Yanagihara & von Leden, 1967), as are many references examining changes in flow for various voice disorder groups (Gordon, Morton, & Simpson, 1978; Isshiki & von Leden, 1964). Somewhat related to a measure of flow are the various duration studies that determine how long the individual can sustain a voiced or voiceless expiration (Bless & Saxman, 1970; Eckel & Boone, 1981; Ptacek & Sander, 1963; Tait, Michel, & Carpenter, 1980). One measure of differential duration measures that can be used diagnostically in the voice evaluation is the s/z ratio we discussed earlier in this chapter. As mentioned, here the patient is asked first to sustain the /s/ as long as possible, and then to sustain the /z/ The typical s/z ratios of normal subjects approximate 1.0, indicating that the voiceless expiration time (the /s/) closely matches maximum phonation time (the /z/) (Tait et al., 1980). In 95% of their patients with glottal margin pathologies (nodules, polyps, thickening), Eckel and Boone (1981) found elevated s/z ratios in excess of 1.4, indicating marked reduction in voiced duration values. The clinical value of the s/z ratio to pressure and flow measures are illustrated by the application of all three measures in the following clinical case:

A 19-year-old university singer was self-referred to the University Speech and Hearing Clinic for her continuing "breathiness and hoarseness." Initial

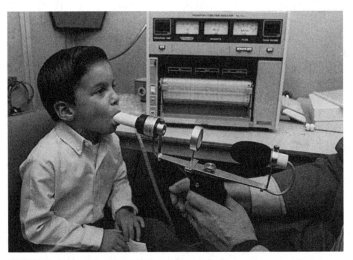

FIGURE 4–7   Phonatory Function Analyzer
The phonatory function analyzer is used here to evaluate phonation time (in seconds), fundamental frequency (Hz), vocal intensity (dB SPL), airflow rate (Ml/sec), and total volume of air (Ml) during each phonation attempt.

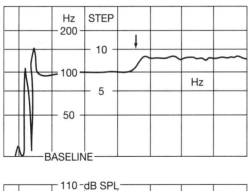

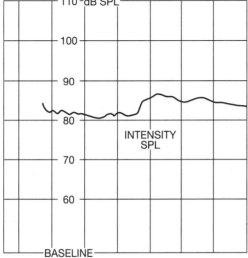

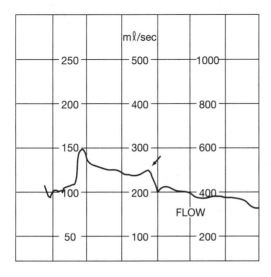

FIGURE 4–8 Tracings from a Phonatory Function Analyzer
These tracings from the phonatory function analyzer demonstrate how a change in one vocal parameter (pitch, for example) can make a significant change in another parameter (such as rate of airflow). As the pitch level is raised from 100 Hz to a level of 130 Hz, the airflow rate is reduced from 260 Ml/sec to a level of 180 Ml/sec. Intensity is also increased from 83 to 88 dB SPL.

voice evaluation techniques included a pneumotachic evaluation, which found airflow measurements of 240 cc/sec with oral pressure readings of 5.5 cm H_2O; her initial /s/ duration was 18, her /z/ duration was 11, and her s/z ratio was computed at 1.64. Initially, she resisted having a medical evaluation that included indirect laryngoscopy. The clinician, however, knowing that her high s/z value may well have been predictive of laryngeal disease, insisted that she have laryngoscopy. A subsequent examination found her to have bilateral vocal nodules that occupied almost a third of her total anterior-posterior glottal length. Following laryngoscopy, she was enrolled in individual voice therapy. Repeated testing after 9 weeks of voice therapy revealed a lower airflow measure of 219 cc/sec and higher oral pressure readings of 7.3 cm H_2O; her s/z ratios had decreased to 1.28.

These improved scores all suggested better laryngeal function. Subsequent laryngeal examination confirmed some decrease in the size of the nodules, although small bilateral nodes were still present. Her voice quality had improved. The s/z ratio as used here provided one additional measure (which requires no instrumentation other than a stopwatch) and observation for the clinician in conducting the overall voice management of the patient.

A simple but useful clinical maneuver for the clinician without instrumentation that can be employed to demonstrate the presence of excessive laryngeal tension is the application of hand pressure to the patient's abdomen during phonation of the sustained /i/ or /u/ vowel. The palm of the hand is placed firmly over the middle of the abdomen just above the level of the belt (Figure 4–9). The hand is pulsed as the phonation is sustained. The more hyperfunction present during the voice production, the less the voice will pulse; conversely, the more relaxed the vocal folds and the larynx are, the more the voice will pulse in response to the hand pressure. When the clinician applies the technique to patients who are producing their typical voice, and then reapplies the technique after using a facilitating approach such as glottal fry, the dramatic difference in vocal pulsing becomes obvious to the patient.

Motions of the Torso   For years students of voice have been able to use the pneumograph to track and record thoracic and abdominal movements during inhalation and exhalation. The pneumograph is usually connected to a recording device, of which there are two main types, the kymograph and the polygraph, both of which provide graphic measurement write outs. The pneumograph provides straps, which are placed around the thorax or abdomen; at the ends of the straps are rubber tubes. As the tubes are stretched, a partial vacuum is created within them, and the amount of vacuum is communicated to the recording instrument. The pneumographic recordings help speech-language pathologists study the frequency of the respiration cycle, focusing on the regularity of the inhalation-exhalation ratio. How well a patient can sustain an exhalation can be determined by using the pneumograph with a kymographic or polygraphic write out. Today, for the study of differential movements of the thorax in inspiration, newer methodologies are favored over the pneumograph. The Respiratrace is now becoming common as a clinical research tool with applications in stuttering and voice as well as with other clinical populations.

To study the relative coordination between abdominal movements and thoracic movements, Hixon et al. (1976) have used magnetometers to examine the relative "anterior-posterior diameters" of both the abdomen and thorax, particularly as the two areas relate to each other. When using the magnetometers, the clinician can determine the synchrony of movements of the rib cage and the abdomen during speech breathing. Some clinical voice disorders related to such problems as cerebral palsy or other motor-speech disorders produce severe problems in this synchrony between the different parts involved in breathing. Small magnets are placed on the back, on the front chest wall, and on the lower back and abdominal wall; the anterior-posterior distance varies between the magnets in each area (chest or abdomen), and this information can be traced either on an oscilloscope or on some kind of graphic printout.

The experimental use of the electromyograph (EMG) in investigating the use of particular muscles in breathing during speech has been explored in several studies reported by Hoshiko (1962), but there has been little regular use of the EMG as a clinical tool for respiration assessment. Which muscle is doing what and when may be determined by the clinical EMG, whereby recordings are made of the variations in electrical potential as detected by needle or surface electrodes inserted into or placed on a

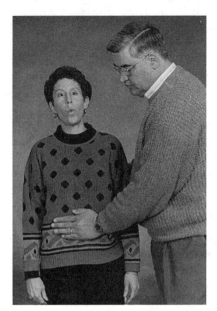

FIGURE 4–9 Demonstrating the Presence of Excessive Laryngeal Tension
A simple but useful clinical maneuver that can be employed to demonstrate the presence of excessive laryngeal tension is the application of hand pressure to the patient's abdomen during phonation of the sustained /i/ vowel.

muscle. Whenever that muscle becomes active (contracts), its electrical activity is displayed on a graphic write out.

Movement of the thorax and the downward excursion of the diaphragm can be identified very well by various X-ray techniques. The degree of inflatability, as seen by thoracic expansion and downward movement of the diaphragm, has been evaluated with convenience by still X-ray. Still X-rays taken at moments of maximum inhalation and exhalation have been helpful in identifying those sites of respiration (apical versus base of lungs) that show the most deflation or inflation and have provided knowledge about the type of breathing the patient employs: abdominal-diaphragmatic, midthoracic, or clavicular. Similar information can be obtained by viewing the respiratory mechanism in action, assessing actual movement by the use of other X-ray techniques—namely, fluoroscopy and videofluorography.

Other Aspects of Respiration Testing

The type of breathing the patient uses can often be accurately determined by careful clinical visual observation. The most inefficient type of breathing, *clavicular*, seems to be the easiest to identify. The patient elevates the shoulders on inhalation, using the neck accessory muscles as the primary muscles of inhalation. This upper chest breathing, characterized by noticeable elevation of the clavicles, is unsatisfactory for good voice for two reasons: First, the upper, apical ends of the lungs, when expanded, do not alone provide an adequate respiration; and second, the strain in using the neck accessory muscles for respiration is often visually apparent, with individual muscles "standing out" (particularly the sternocleidomastoids, as they contract to elevate the upper thorax). Although little research evidence clearly identifies the negative effects on speech of clavicular breathing, no serious singer would waste time developing such a shallow, upper-lung reservoir of air. The excessive muscular tension created has a detrimental effect on voice quality. Clavicular-type breathing requires too much effort for too little breath and contributes to excessive muscle tension.

Diaphragmatic-abdominal breathing may well be the preferred method of respiration, especially if the patient has heavy vocal demands, as in singing, acting, or speaking without electronic amplification, such as on stage in opera. If the patient is employing diaphragmatic-abdominal breathing, this should be noted on the voice evaluation form. This use of lower thoracic breathing is usually identifiable by the presence of abdominal and lower thoracic expansion on inspiration, and a gradual decrease in abdominal/lower thoracic prominence on expiration. When asked to take in a deep breath, such a patient will demonstrate, upon inhaling, relatively active expansion of the lower thorax and little noticeable upper chest movement.

We can perhaps obtain a more accurate assessment of how patients breathe for speech when we ask them to demonstrate various voices, such as a pulpit voice, a calling-the-kids voice, a talking-to-superiors voice, and so on. Most voice patients exhibit breathing patterns that are somewhere in between clavicular and diaphragmatic abdominal breathing, and for these persons we use the somewhat nondescript term *thoracic* on voice evaluation forms. Thoracic breathers exhibit no noticeable upper thoracic or abdominal expansion on inhalation. The general mode of breathing can often be assessed if the clinician observes the patients closely as they speak.

Measurement of Pitch

Observations of voice pitch tell us whether a voice is low or high for the patient's age and sex, but only when we measure pitch can we determine the exact fundamental frequency of a voice. Of the various aspects of voice, frequency as measured in cycles per second (cps) now in Hertz (Hz) is one of the most useful and perhaps the most measurable. As part of a voice evaluation, the patient's total frequency range (lowest to highest note) should be determined as a prelude to finding that person's best pitch level (the patient's easiest and most compatible voice pitch) at which to begin therapy probes. Measurements should be made of the patient's habitual pitch (the most frequently occurring or modal pitch level used by the patient). We first discuss the instruments available for measuring these aspects of frequency and pitch.

The Visi-Pitch (Figure 4–10) is an excellent clinical instrument for measuring different aspects of frequency: frequency range, best pitch (we use the term *best pitch* here, since *optimal pitch* is not a real entity, as has been demonstrated experimentally), and habitual pitch. We are aware for example that if there were an actual optimum pitch the singer would sound best only at that pitch and would be severely limited in range and repertoire. The Visi-Pitch offers both a digital display of frequency and an oscilloscopic display. For determination of range, the patient is asked to say the /i/ vowel (e e e) at a comfortable pitch and loudness level and then repeat the /i/ at decreasing musical steps, down to the lowest "note" the patient can produce. The patient is then asked to produce successively higher notes until reaching the top of his or her range. Even though the clinician will have a digital write out of fundamental frequency for each separate vocalization, the productions can be stored on the scope and frequency values can be determined after the patient has completed the sequence. A cursor feature on the Visi-Pitch allows the clinician to search the stored tracings on the scope to determine the exact frequency of any particular phonation. The lowest and highest frequencies the patient is able to produce represent the patient's range.

The concept of optimal pitch can be challenged (and has been in the literature) for a number of reasons, but there is some clinical utility in the notion of a pitch level that is best for the patient during the period of initial voice retraining. One level of pitch usually sounds better in vocal quality, and thus the facilitating approach of *chant talk* takes advantage of this observation (see Chapter 5). "Best pitch" (the pitch level that produces the least amount of hoarseness or roughness) can be determined by using both the frequency and intensity write outs of the Visi-Pitch at the same time. The best pitch is usually the frequency that is slightly louder and clearer in quality; relative changes in both intensity and quality can be determined by viewing the scope tracings (greater vertical excursion indicates greater intensity, and improved sharpness of tracing line indicates better periodicity or improved quality). One way habitual pitch can be determined is by playing a conversational tape jacked into the Visi-Pitch; for every 8 seconds of conversation, the most commonly occurring frequency level can be spotted in the scope tracings (which can be stored until they are reviewed) and then measured. The patient can also produce live conversation or oral reading directly into the Visi-Pitch microphone for a time period of 8 seconds; the tracings of frequency can be stored on the scope and then measured. The most often occurring frequency can be easily identified. The Visi-Pitch has been designed as a clinical instrument that will easily provide frequency data both at the time of the evaluation and as ongoing feedback information during the course of voice therapy.

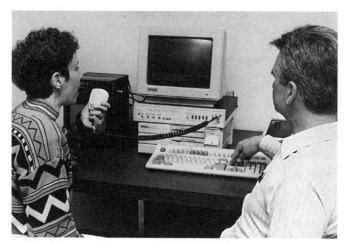

FIGURE 4–10   The Visi-Pitch
The patient is able to use the visual feedback from the Visi-Pitch
screen to modify her pitch and intensity output. Using the split screen
(upper/lower) capability, the patient and clinician can compare typical
performance with performance under clinical stimulation.

The Phonatory Function Analyzer, mentioned in our earlier discussion of flow rate and volume, provides an excellent measure of pitch during sustained vowels. If a face mask is used, the pitch can be measured in connected speech. Of particular value is the fact that this instrument is capable of five simultaneous measures of voice. The instrument provides a hard-copy printout for the patient's chart and also five dials (corresponding to each parameter) that the patient can monitor for feedback during voice production.

Another relatively inexpensive clinical instrument for the measurement of pitch is the Fundamental Frequency Indicator. This device is used by holding a microphone to the larynx or under the nose while producing a sustained vowel or /m/. Repeated syllables such as /mi mi mi/or /bi bi bi/ and voiced phrases such as "Miami millionaire" and "Momma made lemon jam" (see Nasal/Glide Stimulation section in Chapter 5) can be produced and measured. The pitch level can be read from the dial, and the red and green light can be set at levels that will indicate a patient's achievement of a certain level of pitch. The device can be useful in establishing a pitch level to begin facilitating techniques such as chant talk, tongue protrusion /i/, or glottal fry (see Chapter 5). The patient's habitual pitch level, pitch range, and best pitch level can be determined with this device, as Figure 4–11 shows.

Another instrument for measuring both pitch range and habitual pitch is the Tunemaster III. When the tone switch is on, the instrument is capable of generating pitch levels over a one-octave range; for example, the instrument can generate the 12 semitones from C_3 to B_3, and by switching on the octave switch, one can extend the range up another octave to B_4. When the musical frequency is generated in step-by-step semitones, patients are asked to match the tone with their own voices. For adult male subjects whose fundamental frequencies may be well below C_3, (128 cps), clinicians have to convert the matched pitch of the patients to the instrument pitch level by dropping the machine value by one octave. For example, if the instrument is generating an F_3 and a male patient is "matching" the tone with his lowest pitch production, the patient would be producing an F_2 pitch level. The Tunemaster III is useful for establishing a new pitch level, as described in Chapter 5. With the meter switch on, an internal microphone picks up external sounds. If the sound is within a two-semitone range of a target note that has been predetermined and set in the instrument, a "valid reading" light will go on, and a meter pointer will show how sharp or flat the speaker's pitch is specific to the target pitch.

It is possible to measure frequency range and make other measures of frequency without instrumentation other than a piano or pitch pipe. An initial voice recording made at the time of a patient's first clinic visit is a useful tool for analyzing the patient's habitual pitch level. This analysis can be made after the patient has left the clinic. One method we have used is to stop the recorder at random points and attempt to match the voice pitch level with a pitch pipe or a piano. After some experience with a pitch pipe, it is possible to match pitch levels between the pitch-pipe frequency and the patient's voice. This is facilitated by remembering key pitch values for average voices. For example, in cycles per second, the typical adult male voice is somewhere near C_3 (128 cps), and therefore is not very different from the C_3 note on a pitch pipe. Using the pitch pipe, we would start at C_3 and then go by gradations (sharps and flats) until we reached "near" the recorded level of the patient's voice. With an adult female, we might select as our beginning pitch A_3 (213 cps) and go up or down to match her voice. A typical starting place for a prepubertal child would be middle C (256 cps). In a 2- or 3-minute sample from a voice recording, we might select seven or eight voice samples for analysis of pitch level. After we have determined the approximate pitch of the patient's voice samples, we then count the various pitch levels and look for the modal pitch value (the pitch level that occurs most often) and record this as the patient's habitual pitch level. Using the modal pitch probably gives us a more valid habitual pitch than averaging the obtained sample values and using the mean.

A patient's pitch range can also be determined by using voice models. This may be done by asking the patient first to match a pitch level provided by the clinician. It is usually easier for patients to match their own voices with another person's voice than to a generated pitch level from some instrument such as a piano, a pitch pipe, and so on. For this reason, it is most useful to have on hand some recordings of normal voices (adult male, adult female, several children's voices), producing vowels, prolonging each vowel for about 3 seconds. These samples can be recorded on small cassette tapes, discs, or on blank Language Master

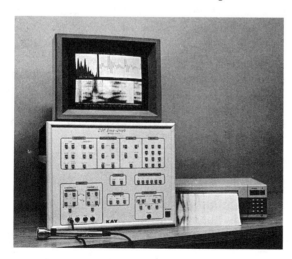

FIGURE 4–11   The Fundamental Frequency Indicator

The spectograph allows for voice analysis, producing spectograms demonstrating acoustic energy associated with various perceptual voice qualities.

cards (1979). On playing the sample voice, which should be close to the patients' observed pitch levels, we ask the patients to say "ah" with the sample voice, matching it as closely as possible. This allows us to provide the patients with a model, showing how we want them to sing down to the lowest note they can make, descending by one full note on the musical scale for each production. In our model sample, we prolong each note for about 3 seconds. Patients' performances should be recorded on tape, whenever possible, and the actual frequency analyses done later in the laboratory. Patients now attempt to sing down to the lowest notes they can produce, then sing up one full note at a time, until reaching the highest notes they can produce including the falsetto, and then sing down, one note at a time, until reaching their lowest notes again. Finally, when the lowest notes are reached, they are asked once again to sing up to the highest note of their ranges. This pitch-range task is usually easiest for patients if they are instructed to sing one note at a time, taking a breath between each 3-second production. Many voice patients, and perhaps the population in general, have real difficulty matching their own voices to a pitch model and producing a range of their lowest to their highest pitch productions. It may be impossible for some patients with vocal fold pathology, such as nodules or polyps, to vary much the pitch of their voice. By providing various models and encouragement at the right times, the experienced voice clinician can usually obtain some pitch-range information.

Each individual seems to have a voice pitch level that can be produced with an economy of physical effort and energy. This relatively effortless voice production has been called optimum pitch and is apparently the pitch level at which the thyroarytenoids and other intrinsic muscles of the larynx can produce vocal fold adduction with only minimal muscular effort. The vibrating frequency emitted from the approximated vocal folds is directly related to the natural length and mass of the thyroarytenoids, without much lengthening or shortening. It is doubtful, however, that optimum pitch represents any exact cycles-per-second value. Optimum pitch, in the literature has been reported to be more often found at two or three notes somewhere at the bottom of the individual's pitch range, several notes higher than the lowest possible pitch production. The classic notion of optimum pitch may not be valid, but a clinical use of best pitch can be helpful. Using the Visi-Pitch, we confirm a note or two toward the bottom of the patient's total range where the periodicity of fold vibration is improved (a sharper line appears on the scope), accompanied by relative increases in intensity. A traditional way of determining optimum pitch, described by Fairbanks (1960), requires individual patients to phonate their entire vocal ranges, including the falsetto, from their lowest productions to their highest. The total range of full-step musical notes is then counted. For adult males, the optimum pitch level is considered to be the one located one-fourth of the way from the bottom of the total pitch range; for female adults, it might be one or two notes lower than the one-fourth level. Although the concept of optimum pitch has been questioned (Thurman, 1958), the concept of an "easy, natural" pitch level (*best pitch*) is useful in voice therapy. Because so many voice patients seem to have problems of vocal hyperfunction, an attempt to have patients produce easy, relatively effortless phonations has obvious diagnostic and therapeutic implications. If a patient can easily produce a good voice, such a voice can become an immediate therapy goal. When a best pitch has been determined, the patient should be asked to produce various other vowels and words at that general pitch level. We have used various different vowels to determine which produce the best vocal quality at different pitch levels. Our experience with voice-disordered patients has revealed that the /i/, /u/, and /o/ vowels almost always produce the best voices, whereas the /a/ and /æ/ always produce the poorest. A qualitative judgment should be made as to how the voice sounds.

Other methods of optimum pitch determination have been described, including these methods described by Murphy (1964):

> (a) the loud-sigh technique: take a deep breath and intone as on expiration; (b) the grunt method: grunt ah or o, gradually prolonging the utterances until a passage is chanted at the original grunt pitch level; (c) the swollen tone technique: stop up the ears, sing ah or hum m up and down the scale until the pitch level at which the tone swells or is loudest is identified; (d) cough sonorously on an ee sound. (p. 95)

We might add to Murphy's list two other brief methods that help to determine best pitch. Ask the patient to yawn and sigh (the relaxed phonation of a sigh is often the optimum speaking pitch) and also to say "uh-huh" (this somewhat automatically produced, affirmative utterance often approximates the best pitch level and was described by Cooper (1973). The six methods—these two and Murphy's four—usually yield pitch levels that are close to one another, even if not the same. Indications from the Visi-Pitch further help the determination of the best vocal quality at a given pitch level. Remember, however, that for clinical purposes we are interested in a particular area of the frequency range (usually a note or two, several notes above the bottom of the total range) that seems to produce the "best" voice with the least amount of effort.

Variations in Pitch as a Diagnostic Aid

An inappropriate pitch level may at times contribute to the development of a voice disorder. Some vocal fold pathologies, on the other hand, produce changes in voice pitch, often because of the weighting or increased mass size of the involved fold(s). Some functionally produced low-pitched voices may be called "the voices of profundity or the voice of authority." A young professional may employ an artificially low voice to assert authority and knowledge; a preacher may try to "hit the low ones" in a sermon; a young woman may think a low-pitched voice is more professional sounding. Conversely, a high-pitched voice is often symptomatic of general tension and difficulties in relaxation. In addition, a postmutational falsetto in a postpubertal male may be the result of serious psychological identity problems, or may serve the patient little or not at all and persist out of habit or set. If a patient's pitch appears incongruous with his or her sex and chronological age, the clinician should first determine if that patient has the functional ability to speak at a pitch level more compatible with his or her overall organism. If pitch variation is impossible, the condition might be the result of cord paralysis, or of certain virilizing drugs that have permanently changed the vocal folds, or of glandular-metabolic changes.

Variations in Loudness

Some patients are observed to speak too loudly or too softly for particular vocal situations. There is no optimal loudness level for any one individual, as voice loudness will vary according to the situation. In an evaluation session a clinician can make a judgment about the loudness of the patient's voice. If it appears to be impossible for the patient to speak in a loud-enough voice, the dysphonia may be related to vocal fold paralysis, or to increases in the mass of the folds (e.g., due to vocal nodules), or to bowed vocal folds worn out from continuous use (*myasthenia larynges*). Soft voices may also be heard in patients who feel relatively inadequate and inferior, and their softness of phonation is consistent with their overall self-image. There are some neurological disorders, such as Parkinson's disease and bulbar palsy, where the patient characteristically speaks in a voice that may be barely audible. At the other end of the spectrum, are patients who speak with voices that may be perceived as uncomfortably loud. Some dysphonic patients, particularly those who speak with hyperfunction, may have inappropriately loud voices as part of their total problem or related to hearing loss. Another intensity variation that may be observed at the time of voice evaluation is a patient who speaks with little or no fluctuation in loudness, and perhaps with no variation in pitch.

Because the loudness of the voice frequently varies according to the setting, the interactions of the speaker-listener, background noise levels, and so forth, it is difficult to measure a representative intensity of someone's speaking voice. One of the best ways we have of measuring loudness is to use a sound-pressure level meter that gives the sound-pressure level of the voice for a particular distance (from speaker's mouth to sound-level microphone). To measure voice intensity, patients are seated so that their mouth is about 1 meter from the microphone. The intensity level of the voice can be read from the sound-level-meter dial in terms of decibels. Remember, however, that this laboratory measure of intensity does not have practical application to the loudness levels the patients may be using in more natural settings. The Visi-Pitch can provide relative measures of intensities.

The Visi-Pitch "screen is divided into a grid, and each vertical division represents 10 dB of sound pressure level" (pp. 2–13). The Visi-Pitch can also provide data for the interaction of frequency and intensity because the instrument allows the simultaneous plotting of both values. Typically, the speaker, or singer for that matter, uses higher-intensity levels for higher-frequency levels. With practice it is possible for speakers to hold their pitch level constant and vary the intensity curve without altering frequency. The Visi-Pitch intensity values are relative values that can be inferred from the oscilloscope display rather than from direct measurements of sound-pressure level.

As mentioned earlier in this chapter, the Phonatory Function Analyzer makes careful intensity measurements in dB SPL as intensity interacts with airflow, frequency, total volume of air, and total phonation time in seconds. This makes the instrument helpful both diagnostically and therapeutically with dysphonic patients. Most measures of voice intensity level should be related to other information specific to airflow and air pressure, frequency, relative opening of the mouth, body position, and so on. If intensity measurements are possible, they are usually supplemented by perceptual rating scale judgments of loudness, as discussed earlier in this chapter.

Measurement of Vocal Quality

One early diagnostic sign of a voice problem is the emergence of some kind of vocal quality disorder, such as hoarseness or breathiness. Usually some form of dysphonia (the term used through this text for all disorders of voice quality) signals to the patient that he or she has a voice problem. At the time of evaluation, the clinician should listen closely to how the patient speaks and attempt to describe what is heard. The verbal description of dysphonia is extremely difficult, however. Until the state of the art improves, clinicians will simply have to find terms to describe the voices they hear. Fairbanks (1960) lists three quality conditions, breathiness, harshness, and hoarseness, that may well be related to difficulties in optimal approximation of the vocal folds on phonation.

In breathiness, we can usually observe an audible escape of air as the approximating edges along the glottis fail to make optimum contact. Breathiness may be related to a patient's functional inability to bring the folds firmly together; the person may have the functional capability of firmer vocal fold approximation, but, for whatever reason, prefers to speak with a breathy voice. Some patients with rheumatoid arthritis or with chronic lower back pain may take various muscle relaxants that produce excessively breathy voice quality as a side effect. Sometimes breathiness is related to growths on the folds, such as nodules or polyps, which prevent optimum adduction; sometimes it results from cord paralysis, which prevents fold adduction. In a voice signal that is characterized as breathy, the periodicity of vocal tone is reduced and aperiodicity or noise is increased. We frequently observe at the beginning of an utterance marked aperiodicity that decreases as the vocal folds begin to vibrate. The breathy voice is often produced by the vocal folds approximating slowly together after the initiation of the outgoing air stream has already begun.

The spectrograph provides a visual display of what we hear. Figure 2–17 showed that the breathy voice produces noise across the sound spectrum with less definition of a periodic sound wave, as seen in the distinct print of the first three formants in the normal voice spectrogram. Other laboratory measures for quantification of breathiness can be made, such as measuring airflow and air pressure and spectral noise levels (Sansone & Emanuel, 1970), and determining jitter (variations or perturbations in frequency) and shimmer (variations in amplitude) as described by Michel and Wendahl (1971). The perceptual judgments of the clinician and other listeners continue, however, to play an important role in the observation and diagnosis of breathiness.

A harsh voice is usually heard by listeners as unpleasant. Ainsworth (1980) described the difficulty of defining harshness:

> Verbal descriptions of harshness are difficult to make without using "impressionistic" terms, i.e., grating, rasping, rough, gutteral, raucous. There often are frequent and "hard" glottal catches, i.e., the initiation of tones with an explosive release of air by the vocal folds, and excessive glottal (vocal) fry which is a low-pitched "popping" sound. (p. 7)

Aperiodicity of laryngeal vibration can be seen in the spectrogram for the harsh voice. Often abrupt initiation of voice is characterized by hard glottal attack. Patients sound as if they are working hard to speak. A harsh voice may be described as strident, metallic, or grating; whatever the description used, the connotation is unpleasant. The Visi-Pitch or any kind of spectrum analyzer like the spectrograph will visualize harshness with increased aperiodicity across the spectrum, a reduction of fundamental frequency, a scatter of resonance across the spectrum, and abrupt glottal attack as observed in sudden initiation of phonation. In our judgments of harshness we often focus on the metallic aspects of resonance, whereby the voice seems to come out of a pharynx and oral cavity that appears to be in a state of hypercontraction. Instead of hearing softness and some absorption of sound waves, we hear a hardness described by Coffin (1981) as a "voice produced by hard, reflective surfaces rather than by soft, absorbing surfaces." It is difficult to describe the harsh voices we sometimes hear.

Hoarseness is the most common laryngeal quality disturbance, although the term is often used in a meaningless manner to label any kind of laryngeal problem in phonation. Anything that interferes with optimum vocal fold adduction can produce hoarseness.

Many patients exhibit it on a purely functional basis—that is, because they approximate the vocal folds too tightly or too loosely

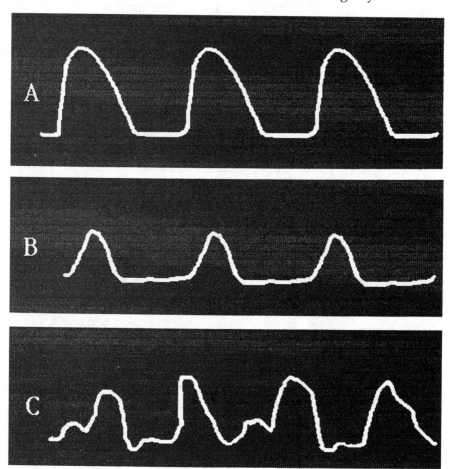

FIGURE 4–12   Glottograms

These three glottograms are productions of the /i/ vowel with (A) normal vocal quality, (B) breathy quality, and (C) hoarse vocal quality. The normal trace (A) demonstrates a sharp vertical rise, a narrow peak, an even return to baseline, and a substantial closed phase. Trace (B), the breathy voice quality, is represented in the sloping voice onset, rather than the vertical rise seen in the normal trace and the long open phase. Trace (C), the hoarse voice, is indicated by the lack of a uniform wave form from one cycle to the next.

together, they produce hoarseness. Darley (1965) wrote that "hoarse voice quality combines the acoustic characteristics of harshness and breathiness and usually results from laryngeal pathology" (p. 57). Typical dysphonic patients display the kind of hoarseness we hear in patients with some form of laryngitis. The hoarse voice heard in patients with bilateral vocal nodules includes a breathy escape of air and is often accompanied by hard glottal attack as patients attempt to compensate for their phonation difficulties. Hoarseness may be related to mucus on the vocal folds, or sometimes to destruction of all or a part of the folds. The spectral printout of the hoarse voice in Figure 2–17 confirms the combination of breathiness and harshness, as we see increased noise across the spectrum with a heavier concentration of acoustic energy in the first formant at the bottom of the spectrogram.

Many patients with hoarseness begin to compensate for their poor voices by driving the mechanism even harder; they may feel, for example, that they must have abrupt initiation of glottal attack to "get their voices started." The Visi-Pitch is easy to use to determine the abruptness of glottal attack combined with hoarseness. Any kind of air-pressure instrument can likewise verify sudden onset of expiration. The visual imprints on the oscilloscope attached to such a monitoring instrument will show sudden and abrupt phonation onsets, characterized by vertical excursions at onset, as opposed to a more gradual sloping rise of the onset curve.

The *electroglottalgram* (EGG) is an excellent device to demonstrate the abruptness of glottal onset or the opposite, a breathy onset, and to depict the ratio of long open phase to closed phase that characterizes the breathy voice on an EGG trace. It also depicts the reverse situation of long closed phase to short open phase as in a hypertense voice. The device also displays aperiodic vocal fold vibration by clearly demonstrating the lack of similarity from wave to wave (McFarlane & Watterson, 1991). The more dissimilar each wave is from the preceding and following waves, the more aperiodicity in the voice. Figure 4–12 shows a glottogram or laryngogram of a prolonged /i/ vowel produced with a very hoarse voice quality. This laryngogram may be contrasted with one of a normal vocal quality and one of a breathy vocal quality during the production of the /i/ vowel.

A clinician's judgment of hoarseness must supplement any instrumental measurements we are able to make. The advantage of some kind of instrument quantification of hoarseness at the time of the initial evaluation is that the measurement data can be compared with data taken subsequently during and at the end of therapy. It has also been our experience that the instruments that provide evaluation data can be used to provide feedback to patients in therapy about particular components of voice. For example, for a patient with hoarseness, it may be advantageous to provide visual feedback on the oscilloscope relative to improvement of periodicity as the voice is heard to be "less hoarse." Like most evaluation data, it should be used not only in the diagnostic-decision process in planning therapy, but also given to patients as a continuing feedback and confirmation of their therapy progress. This can be extremely motivational. When instrumentation is used with clinical stimulation such as the facilitation techniques in Chapter 5, the data obtained help to plan and direct therapy and assist in making a prognostic statement.

Other variations in vocal fold approximation may produce symptoms of glottal fry, register variations, pitch breaks, and phonation breaks. Most voice evaluation forms have checkoff lists that would include these terms. Glottal fry can be detected using the Visi-Pitch. Instead of a single tracing line representing a single fundamental frequency, the voice is represented by two or more broken lines, indicating that the patient is producing two or three simultaneous fundamental frequencies The multiple phonation pulses are usually of low frequency and are usually observed at the bottom of the patient's frequency range. The phenomenon of fry is usually observed as slight hoarseness that comes into the individual's voice toward the bottom of the pitch range. It has been described as sounding like an outboard motorboat, a creaking door, popcorn popping, and so on. Moore and von Leden (1958) termed glottal fry "dicrotic dysphonia." Others have described the vocal folds during the production of fry as thick, with the ventricular bands in close contact with the superior surface of the true vocal folds. It is undoubtedly this thickness of folds that produces the lower fundamental pitch that usually accompanies glottal fry. With some elevation of voice pitch, or slight increase in subglottal air pressure, the fry will usually decrease. We consider glottal fry to be a normal vocal register. Register variations, rarely mentioned in American speech pathology texts, do exist as clinical problems in some voice patients. The concept of vocal register comes from the organ stop, which in German is called "register." Luchsinger and Arnold (1965) wrote:

> In chest voice, the cords vibrate over their entire breadth, whereas the falsetto voice reveals vibration limited to the inner cord margins.
> When phonating low tones, the cords appear rounded, full, and relaxed, while they are sharp-edged, thin, and taut for falsetto tones. These differences may readily be seen on frontal laryngeal tomograms. (p. 97)

Register variation is related to the relative changes in the cross section of the vocal folds, produced by differential contraction of the vocalis section of the thyroarytenoid muscle. In his classic article "The Mechanism of the Larynx," Negus (1957) used the terms *thick* and *thin* to correspond to the cross-sectional differences seen in the production of the chest register and the head register. Sometimes we observe voices that seem incompatible with the resonating bodies of the patient. Certain patients may produce variations by attempting to speak at their lower pitches with vocal folds approximated in the manner typical of high-pitched head register. Conversely, sometimes higher pitches are produced with the folds approximated in their fullest broad dimension, the typical pattern of the low-pitched chest register. Register variation (fold approximation incompatible with the desired pitch level) can best be confirmed by frontal X-ray of the approximating glottal surfaces, as seen in frontal tomograms. Typical tomographic configurations for varying registers were shown in Figure 2–15.

When pitch break is observed, it is usually in a voice that is pitched too low. As the patient is phonating, the pitch level suddenly breaks upward to a falsetto level, often one octave above the pitch level the person was using. Pitch breaks may also be observed in a voice pitched too high, and then the break is downward, usually a full octave below the previous pitch level. In an adult patient, voice breaks can be extremely embarrassing. Sometimes pitch breaks are a patient's primary, and perhaps sole, reason for seeking voice therapy. Pitch breaks in children are much more common but are rarely considered to be clinical problems, although they may be embarrassing for the child. Curry (1949) found in his voice studies of adolescents that although voice breaks can occur in prepubescent males, they are much more common at around the age of 14, when rapid pubertal changes take place. In 18-year-olds, Curry found virtually no pitch breaks. Pitch breaks in children, particularly in males at around the time of puberty, are, in fact, fairly common and usually disappear with continuing physical maturation. In adults, pitch breaks are relatively rare and appear most often to be symptomatic of inappropriate habitual pitch levels—too low a pitch with involuntary pitch breaks upward or too high a pitch with the breaks occurring downward.

The phonation break or abductor spasm (see Chapter 6) is a temporary loss of voice that may occur for only part of a word, a whole word, a phrase, or a sentence. An individual may be phonating with no observable difficulty when a loss of voice or phonation break suddenly occurs. Patients who experience voice breaks usually exhibit some degree of voice hyperfunction as they speak. They *work too hard* at talking. Typical patients with voice breaks (e.g., teachers) may use their voices a lot. After prolonged speaking, they begin to experience vocal fatigue and try to improve the sound of their voices by raising or lowering the voice pitch or speaking through clenched teeth. The result is increased vocal mechanism tension. Finally, while they are phonating, the vocal folds spontaneously abduct and they temporarily lose their voices. By throat clearing, coughing, swallowing water, or whatever, they restore phonation until the next phonation break. Most voice patients, even if they have occasional phonation breaks, will not exhibit such temporary voice loss during evaluation sessions. The two different types of phonation breaks or abductor spasms result from different causes. One, as we have described, is the cessation of phonation that results from the sudden abduction of the vocal folds, or from the loss of sufficient glottal resistance, such as when two opposing nodules meet and allow too much air to escape. Too little subglottal pressure remains to drive the cords, and phonation is lost momentarily. Another type of phonation break occurs when there is a phonatory arrest, as in spasmodic dysphonia, hyperkinetic dysphonia, or ventricular phonation. The vocal folds are simply overadducted, which prevents phonation.

Resonance Testing

Our focus in this chapter is on evaluation is the evaluation of patients with phonation disorders. That is not to say that patients may not have accompanying resonance disorders; phonation and resonance disorders may go hand in hand Many patients, however, have voice problems that are primarily of voice resonance. We discuss the problems of voice resonance, their evaluation, management, and therapy in Chapter 7.

SUMMARY

The voice evaluation is the time when the clinician first meets the voice patient, providing opportunity for observation and testing. The evaluation continues as part of every therapy session, particularly as the clinician continually searches with the patient for new and better vocal behaviors The speech-language pathologist must continue to evaluate and observe the patient's respiratory, phonatory, and resonance functions. Whenever possible, these functions should be quantified with instrumentation. The patient's voice data are used for comparison purposes to quantify vocal changes, in response to clinical probes, between the first visit, subsequent therapy sessions, and the final outcome session. Patient performance, both as observed and as measured, is offered back to the patient as a continuing feedback, helping the patient become aware of voice performance. The evaluation enables the voice clinician to decide on what management steps to take for the patient. If voice therapy is indicated (a decision made by the speech-language pathologist), the evaluation will help the clinician to develop a therapy plan and to predict the patient's outcome prognosis.

Chapter 5

Voice Therapy for Problems of Vocal Hyperfunction

Most voice problems are related to vocal hyperfunction, related to using excessive effort and force while singing or speaking. Effective voice therapy for reducing vocal hyperfunction begins with identifying possible vocal abuse and misuse and then systematically attempting to decrease these aversive behaviors. We then search for the most efficient voice the patient is able to produce by using various voice therapy techniques, called in this text *facilitating approaches*. Those approaches that facilitate easier, better voice are then used in voice therapy with a particular patient. In this chapter, we present 25 approaches, presenting the therapy procedures for each approach followed by discussion on the usefulness of the approach with particular voice disorders.

In voice therapy, patients often must learn to use their vocal mechanisms more optimally. Interference with optimal vocalization can be caused by vocal abuse and misuse, requiring an all-out effort by the clinician to identify such abuse-misuse and to establish a program to reduce their occurrence. An example of vocal abuse would be continuous throat clearing. If throat clearing is extensive enough, it can produce edematous (swelling) changes of the glottal margin, which causes hoarseness and breathiness. Throat clearing may also result from an additive lesion that serves as a glottal margin irritant, so that the patient clears the throat to change the feeling that "something is there." Such a patient may soon begin to clear the throat out of habit. Continuous throat clearing can add irritation to an already irritated site, and the throat clearing itself may thus become part of the production of the irritation. Efforts must be made, if the voice therapy is to be successful, to reduce the occurrence of the throat clearing or of any other form of vocal abuse.

Similarly, voice misuse can add irritation to the glottal margin, which can, in turn, contribute to the beginning and the continuation of a voice problem. An example of vocal misuse could be speaking with excessive hard glottal attack. A typical patient speaks with sudden initiation of voice onset, and the voice sounds forceful and strained. To improve the quality of such a voice, the patient should change from speaking in such an abrupt manner to using an easier phonatory style.

There is little difference in the kind of voice therapy given for the different kinds of dysphonia related to vocal hyperfunction. A 10-year-old boy with a husky voice and a normal larynx would require about the same therapy program as his 10-year-old friend with a husky voice and a larynx with bilateral vocal nodules. The type of facilitating approaches might be different because what helps one person may not help another. Both children would profit, however, from a voice program designed to reduce vocal abuse and misuse, and a voice production program whereby the clinician and the children use various facilitating approaches to find the voice they are able to produce with the least amount of effort. Many adult problems of dysphonia and vocal fatigue demonstrate no structural change of the laryngeal mechanism, either as a cause or as a result. Functional voice problems without pathology usually respond to the same techniques of voice therapy as dysphonias related to cord thickening, vocal nodules, polyps, and so on. A differential therapy approach—that is, a certain method for nodules, a different one for polyps—is not needed for each voice disorder. Rather, therapy might be more effective and relevant if, after analyzing the voice disorder along the dimensions of pitch, loudness, and quality, clinicians then applied a therapy appropriate to those dimensions.

It would be easy, and very wrong, to identify for patients the various things they are doing wrong vocally and then provide them with a series of specific remedial therapy techniques. Rather, voice therapists must continually search for the patients' best and most appropriate voice production. This searching is necessary because so much of vocal behavior is highly automatic, particularly the dimensions of pitch and quality. Patients cannot volitionally break vocalization down into various components and then hope to combine them into some ideal phonation. Therapy techniques are primarily vehicles of facilitation—that is, a clinician tries a particular therapy approach to see if it facilitates the production of a better voice. If it does, then that approach is utilized as therapy practice material. If it does not, it is quickly abandoned. As part of every clinical session, the clinician must probe and search for the patient's best voice. When an acceptable production is achieved, it becomes the patient's target model in therapy.

Note that the best voice is not necessarily the best-sounding one. For example, the voice of someone with vocal nodules may sound "worse" after the individual is instructed to take the "work" out of phonation. Without the excessive loudness or the hard glottal attack, there may not be enough driving airflow and subglottal pressure to produce adequate phonation with the weighted (heavy with vocal nodules) vocal folds. The temporary result may be increased dysphonia; however, the target goal with such a person is to reduce the aversive vocal behaviors. Without the added effort to phonate, the voice may sound increasingly dysphonic. This must be considered a "temporary condition that will exist until the nodules get smaller." Eventually, the voice will also sound better. Meanwhile, the optimal voice is a voicing attempt that is free of unnecessary effort and tension. The patient's own best voice becomes the therapy goal. This requires, of course, the continuous use of feedback to the patient of some aspect of the best voice production. Various kinds of feedback could include the auditory playback of voice productions using a cassette or reel-to-reel audiotape recorder, a looptape recorder, or a videotape recorder, and presenting the patient's production back on a television monitor, or using various kinds of biofeedback equipment so that the patient might monitor a physiological aspect of voice production. Biofeedback might include monitoring some aspect of respiration using a manometer or a pair of magnetometers, or letting a patient watch his or her velopharyngeal closure using an endoscope attached to a video unit. Often a patient can progress in voice therapy with only the feedback of his or her own best voice as the target model; sometimes voice patients need additional feedback provided by other devices.

Voice therapy for problems of vocal hyperfunction might well follow this kind of four-point program:

1. Identify abuse-misuse.
2. Reduce occurrence of identified abuse-misuse.
3. Search for the optimum vocalization by using facilitating approaches.
4. Use the approaches that work as practice techniques.

The following description of the vocal management of a 9-year-old boy with vocal nodules utilized this four-point program. Note that his voice actually sounded better when various facilitating approaches were used (this is not always an immediate result of early therapy attempts).

Eric, age 9, had a 4-year history of hoarseness and occasional loss of voice. In a third-grade school screening program he was found to have a severe dysphonia by the speech-language pathologist, who referred him to an ENT physician for indirect laryngoscopy. The ENT doctor found that Eric had "large bilateral nodules that occupied about one-third of his total glottal length." A voice therapy program was initiated that put beginning focus on identifying his vocal abuses and misuses. Eric was observed to yell continually at play, clear his throat excessively (sometimes twice a minute), and make funny animal sounds as a way of entertaining his family and friends. The reduction of abuse-misuse section of *The Boone Voice Program for Children* (1993) was very successful in providing Eric with the insights he needed to curb his yelling and throat clearing. Various voice therapy approaches were used including chewing, open mouth, and the yawn-sigh. These approaches gave Eric a better-sounding voice, and he subsequently enjoyed using them as therapy techniques. His better-sounding voice was his positive reinforcement. The clinician also found that Eric's intelligence and sensitivity allowed him to profit much from her explanations of his problem. Audio feedback, which confirmed for him the improvement in the way he sounded, was also critical to his progress in voice therapy. The boy saw his public school clinician for individual voice therapy twice weekly for a total of 26 weeks. At the end of that time, repeat laryngoscopy found "only a slight thickening on the right fold with the left fold completely normal." His voice began to sound like the voices of other boys his same age. When he entered fourth grade, no further voice therapy was indicated.

Similar to the excellent progress experienced by Eric, voice therapy for problems of vocal hyperfunction often produces spectacular, positive results. Such therapy gains must, however, be followed by a vocal hygiene program (Andrews, 1986; Cooper, 1977; Wilson, 1987) that is designed to prevent further vocal abuse and misuse. Such a vocal hygiene program is presented in Chapter 6.

ESTABLISHING WHERE TO START IN VOICE THERAPY

Voice therapy must begin where the patient is able to perform. We cannot ask patients to do more than they are capable of doing. In addition, the beginning of voice therapy must relate to the final outcome of the therapy. In applying dismissal criteria to 73 voice patients (Boone, 1974), we found that at the first therapy session we had to determine the size of laryngeal lesion (if there is one), make a voice recording of the patient, and analyze what kind of physical sensations the patient may experience while voicing. We then compared these initial data to data *after* therapy and used them as part of the decision process in terminating therapy. The effect of subsequent voice therapy could never be fully determined without some preliminary data on the presence or absence of a laryngeal lesion. The site and size of the lesion, if one is present, will greatly determine the beginning steps of voice therapy. For example, large fibrotic vocal nodules might well require a surgical approach, followed by voice rest and then voice therapy. Small, beginning thickenings at the anterior-middle third junction of the folds would offer a prompt and convincing signal for the speech pathologist to initiate a voice program to reduce vocal hyperfunction. Some beginning documentation of the lesion is necessary if we are to compare pretreatment and posttreatment effects.

Voice therapy progress can be clearly documented only if it is built upon thorough beginning diagnostic information. Two important early steps must be taken for voice therapy: an initial voice recording, for both immediate analysis and later comparison, and a determination of the patient's somatic feelings of the disorder (dryness, pain). The initial voice recording should include the patient's name, the date, spontaneous conversation, oral reading, and specific vowel and phrase repetitions that best illustrate the disorder. Subsequent and final recordings should always contain basically the same spoken material. Because many voice problems related to vocal hyperfunction create physical discomfort to the patient, sometimes, in the absence of dysphonia, it is important to determine the patient's self-reports of dryness, pain, fullness, and so forth. Eliminating these symptoms often represents a real improvement to the patient. Initial time in therapy should be spent exploring the speaking conditions and situations that precipitate these self-reports of discomfort.

Voice therapy programs for vocal hyperfunction are highly individualized. A particular approach that works for one patient may not be facilitative for another. Clinicians employ various facilitating approaches to determine whether their application allows patients to produce easier voices (which may or may not sound better). If an approach is successful, it is continued; if it does not seem to help, the clinicians try another approach. Sometimes, some of the steps of an approach are facilitative for good voice while others may not be. We determine both the effects of an overall approach and the steps in that approach by marking a form similar to that shown in Figure 5–1.

VOICE THERAPY FOR YOUNG CHILDREN

When preschool children are brought to a voice clinic because of some kind of dysphonia, the emphasis is placed on early diagnosis and identification rather than on voice therapy per se. A sudden hoarseness, perhaps accompanied by laryngeal stridor (noise on inhalation), prompts concern that the child may have a serious laryngeal disease, such as papilloma or laryngeal web. Direct laryngoscopy (which often necessitates a general anesthetic in a preschool child) or endoscopy may identify such a lesion. If the problem is papilloma, the management would be primarily medical-surgical. If the problem appears to be related to vocal fold thickening or nodules, or to some other vocal hyperfunction, the family and the speech-language pathologist can together decide what procedures to follow. The management may be confined to counseling with the parents, or it may also involve direct therapy with the child. The child's hyperfunctional vocal behavior may be part of an overall pattern of hyperactivity, which is sometimes a mode of behavior during the

VOICE IMPROVEMENT RECORDING FORM
The Boone Voice Program for Children

Name_____ Date Therapy Initiated_____ Date Therapy Terminated_____
Check (✓) if Vocal Abuse Program is in effect_____ .

DATE	FACILITATING APPROACH #	STEP NUMBER		NEGATIVE CHANGE	NO CHANGE	SLIGHT IMPROVEMENT	GREAT IMPROVEMENT

CHECK (✓) APPROPRIATE BOX

FIGURE 5–1 The Voice Probe
The clinician measures the effectiveness of various facilitating approaches with the patient. (*The Boone Voice Program for Children*, 2nd ed. Austin, TX: PRO-ED, 1993.)

preschool years. At the preschool level, voice therapy for hyperfunctional voice problems may not always be warranted.

School-age children often demonstrate hyperfunctional voice problems, most of which are remediable with voice therapy. A national speech and hearing survey (Hull, Mielke, Willeford, & Timmons, 1976) found that about 10% of all school-age children (grades 1 through 12) did not have acceptable voices; the prevalence was 25% at first grade and as low as 3% in grades 11 and 12. Most children who have dysphonia exhibit vocal hyperfunction—using too much effort and force as they speak. Most voice programs (Andrews, 1986; Boone, 1993; Case, 1991;

Wilson, 1987) place early emphasis on identifying abuse-misuse and outlining specific steps for reducing the occurrence of such behaviors.

The clinician can probably do nothing more effective than identify those situations in which the child is vocally abusive, such as yelling at a ballgame, screaming in the playground, crying, imitating noises below or above his or her speaking pitch range, and so on. Many children maintain their vocal pathologies simply by engaging in abusive vocal behavior for just brief periods each day. It is usually not possible to identify these vocal abuses through interview methods or by observing the child in the therapy room; rather, the child must be observed in various play settings, in the classroom, and at home. This need for extensive observation requires that clinicians solicit the help of the children themselves to determine where they might be yelling or screaming. Teachers can provide some helpful clues about the child's vocal behavior both on the playground and in the classroom. Meeting with parents will often reveal further situations of vocal abuse, and the parents may be asked to listen over a period of time for abusive vocal behavior in the child's play or interactions with various family members. At times, we have had good luck using the siblings or peers to help us determine what a child does vocally in certain situations.

Once the abusive situations are isolated, clinicians should obtain base-line measurements of the number of times a vocal abuse is observed in a particular time unit (an hour, a recess period, a day, and so on). Figure 5–2 shows a vocal-abuse graph, which plots the number of abuses a child had recorded over a period of two weeks.

Notice that the first plot on the abscissa is the first day's base-line measurement, which tells on the ordinate how many times the child caught himself yelling on that particular day—for this child, 18 separate yells. The overall contour shows a linear decrement in voice yelling, which is a somewhat typical curve for young children. Having to monitor his offensive behavior seems to motivate the child to reduce it. The child may keep a card in his pocket on which to mark down each occurrence; at the end of the day, he tallies that day's occurrences and plots the total figure on the graph. The review of the plotting graph is a vital part of the therapy, and the child's pride in his graph (which usually shows a decrement in the behavior) helps him continue to curb the vocal abuse. Some children require assistance in making this kind of plot, and sometimes we ask teachers, parents, or friends to also keep tally cards to record the number of events they observed in a particular time period. If children are given proper orientation to the task and clearly know why they must reduce their number of vocal abuses, their tally counts seem to be higher, and perhaps more valid, than the counts of external observers.

Another variation of the tally method requires the child to take his tally card for the date and plot his voice abuse-misuse against that reported by another child or the clinician. For example, in *The Boone Voice*

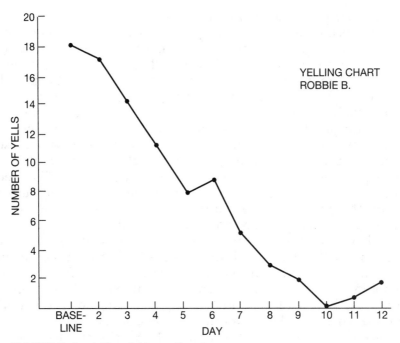

FIGURE 5–2   A Vocal-Abuse Graph

Program for Children (1993) are play materials for a hot-air balloon race in which the clinician "races" the child in plotting changes (in this case abuse-misuse) with hot-air balloons across a sky backdrop. Setting up some kind of reward, such as winning the balloon race, helps the child to become more aware of the desirability of curbing voice abuse-misuse.

An important prelude to the tally method—indeed, to any form of speech therapy, particularly voice therapy—is for the clinician to explain to the child what the problem is, what the child seems to be doing wrong vocally, and what can be done about it. Obviously, a child must first know that there is a voice problem (rarely does a child recognize such a problem independently) before he or she can do anything about it. Such explanations are also especially important because most children with voice problems are not self-referred. Their dysphonias have been discovered by someone else. To the child, there may be no problem.

VOICE THERAPY FOR ADOLESCENTS AND ADULTS

The abusive vocal behaviors of adults are likely to be more difficult to isolate than those of children. It is the relatively rare adult voice patient whose vocal abuses are bound only to particular situations. Preachers or auctioneers whose voice problems appear only on the job may be excellent examples of vocal misuse; however, dysphonic adolescents or adults generally have hyperfunctional sets toward phonation. They work to talk in most situations. Sometimes the exaggerated efforts are related to a generalized feeling of tension that becomes more acute in particular settings, such as when they speak to authority figures or when they try to make favorable impressions on listeners. This common observation—that many people with hyperfunctional voice problems exist in a milieu of tension—has fostered the belief among laryngologists and voice clinicians that the symptomatic treatment of voice disorders should be avoided in favor of a more comprehensive psychological approach. Gray, England, and Mahoney (1965) have described an approach that combines elements of traditional voice therapy with an emphasis on deconditioning patients' anxiety and tensions by using the behavioral approach of reciprocal inhibition. It is our point of view that although unresolved tension and anxiety contribute to the voice problems of some voice patients, most patients are fully capable of producing a good, optimum voice, providing someone (the clinician) will only help them "find" it.

Therefore, the primary task of voice clinicians is to explore with patients the various therapy techniques that might produce that "good" voice. We advocate the same approach with adults as we do with children: using facilitating techniques as therapy probes. The approach that works is then used as a therapy practice approach. Once the patients are able to produce a model of their own best voice, this model, and the techniques used to achieve it, become the primary focus of voice therapy.

Voice clinicians also provide patients with needed psychological support, and together they explore various facilitating techniques to be used in particular situations. Hierarchies of stress can often be identified (Boone, 1982; Wolpe, 1987), and behavioral approaches used at these times of stress may minimize symptoms. Patients are taught to isolate those situations in which they experience poor voice and to substitute at those times more optimum forms of behavior—that is, easier voice.

Voice disorders in adolescents and adults often have a negative impact on their lives because they may interfere with life interactions and employment. Some patients become desperate over their vocal problems, and so seek professional help. The family physician is often the first professional who identifies a voice problem as a disorder that needs the expert help of an otolaryngologist or speech-language pathologist. The physician subsequently refers the patient for a voice evaluation that, more often than not, involves the evaluation-diagnostic procedures described in Chapter 4. Voice therapy is often the recommended step after the diagnostic evaluation.

VOICE THERAPY FACILITATING TECHNIQUES

As described in earlier chapters, a *voice therapy facilitating approach is a therapy technique that seems to produce optimum voice.* Using such an approach generally allows an individual to produce voice with less effort and strain, and perhaps even to sound better. This easy voice may be designated the target voice in therapy. Once a particular approach is found helpful in producing the target voice, the approach is used as a practice focus in therapy. Symptomatic voice therapy requires clinicians to probe continually with various facilitating techniques, using the one that seems to produce the target voice, and avoiding those that seem to have negative or little effect. This kind of therapy requires that clinicians search continually for "can-do" vocal behaviors. What may work (or facilitate the target voice) for one patient may not work for another patient with the same kind of voice problem. The selection of voice facilitating approaches in therapy is thus highly individualized. Although clinicians should be familiar with the application of all therapy techniques, they should apply such techniques selectively. The selection of a particular approach should not be an arbitrary, trial-and-error decision. Rather, the possible effects on the parameters of pitch, loudness, and quality must be considered.

Table 5–1   Twenty-Five Facilitating Approaches in Voice Therapy

Facilitating Approach	Parameter of Voice Affected		
	Pitch	*Loudness*	*Quality*
1. Altering tongue position			x
2. Change of loudness	x	x	x
3. Chant talk		x	x
4. Counseling (explanation of problem)	x	x	x
5. Digital manipulation	x		x
6. Ear training	x	x	x
7. Elimination of abuses		x	x
8. Elimination of hard glottal attack		x	x
9. Establishing a new pitch		x	x
10. Feedback	x	x	x
11. Focus	x		x
12. Glottal fry		x	x
13. Half-swallow, boom		x	x
14. Head positioning	x		x
15. Hierarchy analysis	x	x	x
16. Inhalation phonation	x	x	
17. Masking	x	x	x
18. Nasal/glide stimulation			x
19. Open-mouth approach		x	x
20. Pitch inflections	x		
21. Relaxation	x	x	x
22. Respiration training		x	x
23. Tongue protrusion	x		x
24. Warble	x		x
25. Yawn-sigh	x	x	x

Table 5–1 lists 25 facilitating approaches to be used in voice therapy. Serious students of voice pathology may notice that some approaches listed in previous editions (1971, 1977, 1983, 1988) of this text have been omitted in this edition, and that four new approaches have been added. In applying various therapy approaches over the years, it becomes apparent that certain techniques have only limited usefulness. Extensive feedback from clinicians who tell us what approaches they use and which techniques they never use, have all contributed to our decisions as to what facilitating approaches to use in this edition, as seen in Table 5–1. Dropping a technique does not mean that the approach should no longer be used. For example, in this edition of this book two approaches, chewing and pushing, that have been in all previous four editions appear to be rarely used today by practicing voice clinicians. There may still be occasional cases, however, where the chewing and pushing techniques would be helpful for finding a desirable target voice.

This list of 25 facilitating approaches is used currently by the authors. Each approach is basically a therapy method that can be used in therapy. In addition to knowing these approaches, there are many other voice therapy techniques described in the literature: Andrews (1986), Aronson (1990), Case (1991), Colton and Casper (1990), Cooper (1977), Filter (1982), Greene and Mathieson (1989), and Wilson (1987).

The facilitating approaches in Table 5–1 are listed alphabetically. After each approach a notation (X) is made to indicate the voice parameters that the particular approach has the potential to influence. For example, approach 1, altering tongue position, in most cases has little influence on the pitch or loudness of the voice; its biggest influence is usually on vocal quality. Consequently, for the three columns in Table 5–1—pitch, loudness, quality—only the quality column is marked with an X. Other techniques, such as 25, yawn-sigh, influence all three parameters of pitch, loudness, and quality. Some experienced voice clinicians combine various facilitating approaches in their search with the patient to find the target voice. Each of the 25 facilitating approaches in Table 5–1 is discussed from the following four perspectives: A) Kinds of problems for which the approach is useful; B) Procedural aspects of the approach; C) Typical case history showing utilization of the approach; and D) Evaluation of the approach.

1. ALTERING TONGUE POSITION

A. Kinds of problems for which the approach is useful   The position of the tongue within the oral cavity has a direct influence on both vocal quality and resonance. Laver (1980) describes the lingual "neutral settings" as having the tongue body not too far forward or too far backward within the oral cavity. The distinguishing characteristics of vowels and consonants are produced by tongue positioning, and any group of people speaking the same language will make basically the same tongue movements— that is, if one's vowels or consonants are to be intelligible to one's listeners, he or she must make them in the same way the listeners do. In the faulty positioning of the tongue that contributes to voice disorders, it is not the individual phoneme placement that is in error, but the overall carriage of the tongue. Some patients carry the tongue backward, almost occluding the pharynx, which contributes to a hollow-sounding cul-de-sac resonance; the focus of the voice appears to be pharyngeal. Boone (1966) has pointed out that "deaf boys and girls, regardless of age, have a tendency for a pharyngeal focus in their vocal resonance" (p. 691). Some voice patients retract their tongues into the pharynx during moments of tension, reporting problem voices only at these times. Other patients have the opposite problem, carrying their tongues too far forward, creating a "thin quality." This is the baby-talk voice; lacking the full resonance of back vowels, it sounds immature or pathologically meek and submissive. Both the muffled voice with posterior resonance focus and the weak, thin voice with anterior carriage can sometimes be favorably improved by direct work in modifying tongue position.

B. Procedural aspects of the approach

1. For posterior tongue carriage, the following activities will help promote a more forward tongue positioning:

a. Preface any exercises with a discussion and demonstration of pharyngeal tongue positioning and its effect on voice. Check the posture of the patient and be sure that the chin is neither tucked in toward the chest nor excessively extended.

b. Begin practice with the whispered production of tongue tip— alveolar consonants, such as /t/, /d/, /s/, and /z/. Require that the patient whisper a rapid series of *ta* sounds, perhaps 10 per breath. After several minutes of using *ta*, go on to the next front-of-the-mouth phoneme. Each practice series of several minutes should be followed by some analysis with the patient of what has just been done—for example, "What does the front-of-the-mouth production feel like?" Keep the early practice confined to whispered productions. Other front consonants that lend themselves well to practice are /w/, /wh/, /p/, /b/, /f/, /v/, /θ/, /ɡ/, and /ð/. The following vowels have a relatively high oral focus and lend themselves well to joint practice with the above consonants, /i/, /ɪ/, /e/, /ɛ/, and /æ/.

c. After progress with whispered productions, add voice lightly. Read orally those exercises that are heavily loaded with tongue-tip consonants and front vowels. Practice contrasting this new front resonance with the old posterior resonance. On recorded playback, listen to the difference critically; evaluate the difference in the "feeling" of the two productions.

2. For excessive anterior carriage of the tongue, the following activities will help develop a more normal tongue position:

a. After explaining the problem, determine whether the patient is using an appropriate pitch level (often he or she is not).

b. Instruct the patient that he or she does not have to shape the tongue in any particular way. By saying the back vowels aloud in as full a voice as he or she can, the patient has usually already brought the tongue back to where it should be. These vowels should be practiced first in isolation, with some effort given to sustaining each one for a period of about 5 seconds: /a/, /ɑ/, /o/, /v/, and /u/.

c. Practice reading materials heavy with the back consonants /k/ and /g/, and heavy also with the back vowels. When the patient has achieved some success in posterior productions, ask him or her to contrast the old method of speaking with the new, perhaps using both methods for each word or phrase read aloud. Spend some time listening to the two and discussing the difference in sound and feeling between them.

C. Typical case history showing utilization of the approach

F. D., a 27-year-old male teacher, found himself in situations in which his voice would become muffled and almost inaudible. The voice evaluation found him to have a normal larynx and a "tendency to withdraw his tongue posteriorly into the pharynx during moments of stress." By using the facilitating technique called hierarchy analysis, the patient was able to identify those situations that produced the most stress—situations in which he would almost reflexively draw his tongue back in his pharynx. The patient was taught to alter his tongue carriage to a more anterior position by practicing, in whispers, front-of-the-mouth consonants and vowels. He then practiced using this anterior tongue carriage in various situations in the hierarchy of stress, maintaining optimum tongue position with good voice production in increasingly tense situations. The patient maintained this success in most situations; he reported that only occasional situations, such as speaking up at a teacher's union meeting, were characterized by the old voice.

D. Evaluation of the approach   Many voice patients appear to develop faulty tongue positioning as part of their overall problem of dysphonia. Altering the main carriage of the tongue, whether it be excessively posterior or anterior, can be achieved to some degree by most patients. A slight alteration of position toward a more normal carriage usually has a profound influence in improving the quality and resonance of the voice. Proper positioning of the tongue apparently enables the oral resonance cavities to function more naturally in filtering the laryngeally produced fundamental frequency. The relatively normal positioning of the tongue appears to be an important component of a normal voice.

2. CHANGE OF LOUDNESS

A. Kinds of problems for which the approach is useful   Some patients have voices that are either too soft or too loud. The prolonged use of inappropriate loudness levels can result in pathologies of the vocal folds, such as nodules or polyps. Many of the vocal pathologies of children are related to such excesses of loudness as screaming and yelling. Weak, soft voices may develop as a consequence of the prolonged hyperfunctional use of the vocal mechanism that results in the eventual breakdown of glottal approximation surfaces—for example, a patient with vocal nodules who loses much airflow around the nodules and is unable to produce an intense enough vocal fold vibration to achieve a sufficiently loud voice. Some speaking environments require a loud voice, and untrained speakers or singers may push for loudness at the level of the larynx rather than adjust their respiration. Inappropriate loudness of voice is most often not the primary causative factor of a voice problem, but rather a secondary, if annoying, symptom. Reducing or increasing the loudness of the voice lends itself well to direct symptom modification through exercise and practice, and often, if other facilitating techniques are being used, does not even require the use of loudness techniques per se.

B. Procedural aspects of the approach

1. For a decrease in loudness:

a. See that the patient has a thorough audiometric examination to determine adequacy of hearing before any attempt is made to reduce voice loudness. Once it has been established that the patient has normal hearing, the following steps may be taken.

b. For young children, ages 3 through 10, the change of loudness steps in *The Boone Voice Program for Children* (1993) are useful. Ask the child to develop awareness of five different voices:

i. Voice 1 is presented as a whisper.

ii. Voice 2 is presented as the voice to use when not wanting to awaken a sleeping person, a quiet voice.

iii. Voice 3 is the normal voice to use to talk to family and friends.

iv. Voice 4 is the voice to use to talk to someone across the room.

v. Voice 5 is the yelling voice to call someone outside.

c. With patients over 10 years old, discuss with the patient the observation that he or she has an inappropriately loud voice. The patient may be unaware of the loud voice, and should listen to tape-recorded samples of his or her speech. The best demonstration tape for loudness variations would include both the patient's voice and the clinician's, to provide contrasting levels of loudness. Then ask the patient, "Do you think your voice is louder than mine?"

d. Focus on making the patient aware of the problem. Once the patient becomes aware that his or her voice is too loud, ask, "What does a loud voice in another person tell you about that person?" Loud voices are typically interpreted to mean that the speaker feels "overly confident," or "sure of himself," or that the speaker is putting on a confident front when he or she is really scared, or that he or she is mad at the world, impressed with his or her own voice, trying to intimidate listeners, and so on. Some discussion of these negative interpretations is usually sufficient to motivate the average patient, to learn to speak at normal loudness levels.

e. Practice using a quiet voice (voice 2 in section b). The practice for the quiet voice can be facilitated by using instruments that give feedback specific to intensity, such as the Vocal Loudness Indicator and the Visi-Pitch. The Vocal Loudness Indicator, for example, has a series of lights that are illuminated by increases in voice intensity. Keeping the instrument at a fixed distance, the patient can quickly learn to keep his or her voice at a lower intensity level to prevent the light (all or a few) from coming on.

f. For practice materials, use some of the excellent voice drill books available for controlling loudness of voice, such as Newcombe (1986); Modisett and Luter (1984); Stemple and Holcomb (1988); Glenn, Glenn, and Forman (1989).

2. For an increase in loudness:

a. Determine first that the inappropriate softness of the voice is not related to hearing loss, general physical weakness, or a severe personality problem; for these cases, a symptomatic approach is not indicated. The steps that follow are for voice patients who are physically and emotionally capable of speaking in a louder voice.

b. Discuss with the patient the soft voice. A tape-recorded playback of the patient's and clinician's voices in conversation will usually illustrate for the patient the inadequacy of the loudness. After the patient indicates some awareness of his or her soft voice, ask, "What does a soft, weak voice tell us about a person?" Inadequately loud voices are typically interpreted to mean that the speaker is afraid to speak louder, is timid and shy, is unduly considerate of others, is scared of people, has no self-confidence, and so on. Some discussion of these negative interpretations is usually helpful.

c. By exploring pitch level and fundamental frequency, try to achieve a pitch level at which the patient is able with some ease to produce a louder voice. If the patient habitually speaks near the bottom of his or her pitch range, a slight elevation of pitch level will usually be accompanied by a slight increase in loudness. The Visi-Pitch has been useful in helping patients associate changes in pitch with relative changes in intensity. Certain frequencies produce greater intensities. When the patient finds the "best" pitch level, he or she should practice sustaining an /a/ at that level for 5 seconds, concentrating on good voice quality. He or she should then take a deep breath and repeat the same pitch at a maximum loudness level. After some practice at this "home base" pitch level, ask the patient to sing /a/, up the scale for one octave, at one vocal production per breath; then have him or her go back down the scale, one note per breath, until he or she reaches the starting pitch.

d. Explore with the patient his or her best pitch—that is, the one that produces the best loudness and quality. Auditory feedback devices (such as loop tape recorders) should be employed, so that the patient can hear what he or she is doing. Some counseling may be needed about the practice pitch used, because the patient may be resistant to using a new voice pitch level. Note that the practice pitch level may well be only a temporary one, and not necessarily the pitch level the patient will use permanently. It is important that the work be pursued both in and out of therapy. A change in loudness cannot be achieved simply by talking about it. It requires practice.

e. Sometimes respiration training (which we discuss later in the chapter) is necessary for a patient with a loudness problem. Remember, however, that even though loudness is directly related to the rate of airflow through the approximated vocal folds, little evidence indicates that any particular way of breathing is the best for optimum phonation. Any respiration exercise that produces increased subglottal air pressure may be helpful in increasing voice loudness.

f. Particularly effective in functional voice loudness problems is the pushing approach. When pushing is coordinated with phonation, little air is wasted and vocal fold approximation is firm, both of which result in louder phonation. However, if a patient can achieve adequate loudness through initial counseling, "best" pitch practice, and some help in respiration, the pushing approach and other techniques requiring physical effort can be avoided.

g. For patients who appear to resist increasing the loudness of voice, it might be necessary to introduce loud noise as a competing sound to the feedback of the patient's own voice. The Lombard effect (speaking at louder voice levels during conditions of competing noise) lends itself well therapeutically to the demonstration of greater voice loudness. The clinician may use white noise, a pure tone (such as 125 or 250 Hz), or the patient's own voice amplified on a simultaneous or delayed auditory feedback device. The procedures of the approach are as follows: (a) Ask the patient to read aloud a passage of about 100 words; (b) tape-record the patient's oral reading; (c) at about word 30, introduce the loud competing auditory stimulus; the patient's voice will increase in loudness; (d) at about word 50, shut off the sound stimulus; the patient will immediately use a softer voice; (e) for the balance of the reading, alternately introduce and stop the sound source at about 15-word intervals; (f) complete the procedure by having the patient listen to the recorded playback, noticing the Lombard effect on the loudness of his or her voice. An extension of the approach might be to ask the patient to attempt to match his or her own loudness models.

3. A few patients demonstrate little or no loudness variation. To achieve variation:

a. Have the patient listen to a tape recording of his or her voice. Then, after making appropriate comments, ask the patient how he or she likes his or her voice, and whether he or she thinks it should be changed. People who become aware of the monotony of their voices, and who are concerned about it, can usually develop loudness inflections with practice.

b. Maintaining an unvarying level of loudness seems to require a great deal of energy. Less work is involved in speaking naturally, which means speaking with a mouth well open and with pitch-loudness variations. The rare patient with hyperfunctional voice problems who speaks in a loudness monotone should be encouraged to increase loudness variation. Any good voice and diction book includes useful practice materials for developing such variation.

C. Typical case history showing utilization of the approach

C. T., a 31-year-old teacher, complained for more than a year of symptoms of vocal fatigue—that is, pain in the throat, loss of voice after teaching, and so on. Laryngoscopy revealed a normal larynx, and the voice evaluation found that the man spoke at "a monotonous pitch and low loudness level, with pronounced mandibular restriction, at times barely opening his mouth." Early efforts at therapy included the chewing approach, with special emphasis given to varying pitch level and increasing voice loudness. The patient was highly motivated to improve the efficiency of his phonation; he requested voice therapy three times a week and supplemented the therapy with long practice periods at home. After 9 weeks of therapy, pretherapy and posttherapy recordings were compared, and the patient agreed with the clinician that he sounded "like a new man." Speaking in a louder voice for this patient seemed to have an immediate effect on his overall self-image, resulting in an almost immediate increase in his total communicative effectiveness. Not only did the patient achieve a better-sounding speaking voice, but he reported no further symptoms of vocal fatigue.

D. Evaluation of the approach   Inappropriate loudness of voice penalizes the patient. Happily, many of the facilitating techniques described in this chapter have some influence on voice loudness, and inadequate loudness is also highly modifiable. In fact, more often than not the use of various other facilitating techniques will have an indirect effect on voice loudness, obviating the need for loudness techniques per se.

3. CHANT TALK

A. Kinds of problems for which the approach is useful   Voice problems related to hyperfunction are often helped by the chant approach. The chant in music is characterized by reciting many syllables on one continuous tone, creating in effect a "singing monotone." We hear chanting in some churches and synagogues, performed by clergy and select groups. The words run continuously together without stress or a change in prosody for the individual word segments. In singing, the *legato* is very similar to the chant we use in voice therapy. A common dictionary definition of legato is "smooth and connected with no break between tones." The chant in therapy is characterized by an elevation of pitch, prolongation of vowels, lack of syllable stress, and an obvious softening of glottal attack. Once a patient can produce the chant in its extreme form (such as in a Gregorian chant), it can usually be modified to resemble conversational phonation. We have used chanting with other facilitating approaches, such as chewing, open mouth, and yawn-sigh.

B. Procedural aspects of the approach

1. The chant-talk approach is explained to the patient as a method that reduces the effort in talking. It is important to point out to the patient that the method will only be used temporarily as a practice method and will not become a permanent and different way of talking. Demonstrate chant talk by playing a recording of a religious chant. Then imitate the recording by producing the same voicing style while reading any material aloud.

2. Urge the patient to imitate the same chant voicing pattern. Most patients are able to do this with some degree of initial success. For those who cannot chant in initial trials, present a chant recording again and then follow it with the patient's own chant production. Some lighthearted kidding is useful to tell the patient that the chant is a different way of talking and will only be used briefly as a voice training device. If the patient cannot chant after several attempts, use another facilitating approach. For those patients who can chant, go on to step 3.

3. The patient should now read aloud, alternating the regular voice and the chant voice. Twenty seconds has been found to be a good time for each reading condition. Ask the patient to read aloud first in the normal voice, then in a chant, then back to normal voice, then in a chant, and so on.

4. Record the patient's oral reading. On playback, contrast the different sound of the normal voice with the chanted voice. Discuss the pitch differences, the phonatory prolongations, and the soft glottal attack.

5. Once patients are able to produce chant talk with relative ease, they should try to reduce the chant quality, approximating normal voice production. Slight prolongation and soft glottal attack should be retained as the patient reads aloud in a voice with only slight chant quality remaining.

C. Typical history showing utilization of the approach

C. C. was a 28-year-old woman who sold telephone directory advertising. She began to experience increased dysphonia and "dryness of throat," particularly toward the end of a busy day of calling on customers. On endoscopic examination, she was found to have bilateral vocal nodules with unnecessary supraglottal participation during phonation. She spoke at an inappropriately low pitch, with mandibular restriction and noticeable hard glottal attack. Twice a week she received voice therapy designed to "take the work out of phonation." The chewing approach, coupled with the chant-talk approach, dramatically changed her overall voicing style. She was able early in therapy to incorporate the soft glottal attack of the chant into her everyday speaking voice. Other approaches, such as open mouth and yawn-sigh, were added with various self-practice materials she could practice. The patient reported that she practiced throughout the day in her car, driving between appointments. In about 12 weeks, videoendoscopy revealed that the nodules had disappeared and that her supraglottal larynx stayed open during normal voicing. There was no evidence of hard glottal attack at the time of her clinic discharge.

D. Evaluation of the approach   The chant-talk approach is easy for most patients to use. Initially, it is important to let the patient know that chanting is only a temporary behavior, designed to take the work out of phonation. We have found that the method works well with children, who seem to enjoy the "different" way of talking. For those patients who need to reduce hard glottal attack, the chanting approach seems to produce dramatic results for softening voicing onsets.

4. COUNSELING (EXPLANATION OF PROBLEM)

A. Kinds of problems for which the approach is useful   Counseling the voice patient, including direct explanations of the voice problem, has proved to be one of the most effective techniques in voice therapy. Putting the voice problem in its proper perspective can often free the patient from overwhelming concern. Patients with hyperfunctional voice disorders, in particular, profit from hearing the clinician describe the voice problem in words they can understand. Clinical experience has taught these authors that if they can help individuals know why they have the voice problem, sometimes nothing more is needed to change a phonation style or to curb vocal abuse-misuse. In the case of those dysphonias that are wholly related to functional causes (such as hyperfunction), it is important that clinicians not confront patients with the implication that they "could talk all right if they wanted to." Instead of saying, "You are not using your voice as well as you could," a clinician might say, "Your vocal folds are coming together too tightly." The latter statement absolves the patient of the guilt he or she might experience if the clinician indicated that the patient was doing things "wrong." The patient will be much more receptive to a statement that puts the blame on the vocal folds. For patients with structural changes of the vocal folds, such as nodules or polyps, it may be necessary to explain that the organic pathology may well be the result of prolonged misuse, and that by eliminating the misuse, the patient will eventually experience a reduction of vocal fold pathology.

B. Procedural aspects of the approach   Counseling the patient is highly individualized. One of the most common counseling approaches in voice therapy is helping the patient to put his or her voice problem in its proper perspective. For some patients, the voice problem is the cause of all of their ills, such as poor job performance, social inadequacy, or general unhappiness. The clinician must have some sensitivity to the depth of the patient's overall attitude and self-image. If the clinician senses psychological or social problems well beyond his or her counseling-psychological training to deal with such problems, referral should be made to professional counselors, psychologists, or psychiatrists. More often than not in voice therapy, a direct explanation of the patient's problem proves to be most effective.

In voice problems related to vocal hyperfunction, it is important to identify for the patient those behaviors that maintain the dysphonia. No exact procedure for this can be laid down; each case has its own rules. For problems related to abuse and misuse of the voice, identify the inappropriate behavior and demonstrate to the patient some ways in which it can be eliminated. In the vocal abuse reduction section of our voice program for children (Boone, 1993), we put much focus on having the child cognitively approach the problem of vocal abuse. By using comic pictures with an accompanying story text, we help the child understand the consequences of continued abuse, and emphasize what can be expected (a better voice) if he or she reduces or eliminates such abuses.

For truly organic problems, such as unilateral adductor paralysis, the same explanations must be made, but in terms of inadequate and adequate glottal closure. Most voice patients want to understand what their problems are and what they can do about them. Make use of medical and diagnostic information, but explain things to the patient in language the patient can understand. Such imagery as "your vocal cords are coming together too tightly," or "you seem to place your voice back too far in your throat," may lack scientific validity, but may help the patient understand the problem. Make explanations brief and to the point, but take care not to put the patient psychologically on the defensive during the first visit. If, after the evaluation, it appears that some psychological or psychiatric consultation is necessary, further diagnostic-therapy sessions may have to be held before the patient can agree to find out more about his or her feelings. An explanation of the problem does not have to be completed before voice therapy begins; in fact, Olsen's (1972) data suggest that an explanation of the problem is an important part of every session of voice therapy as practiced by experienced clinicians.

C. Typical case history showing utilization of the approach

Dr. M., a 72-year-old retired professor, developed speech and voice symptoms shortly after retiring. He was diagnosed by a neurologist as having a congenital myotonia (family history revealed that several male relatives had myotonia that began at much earlier ages than the patient's). He came to the hospital speech-voice clinic for "my poor speech." Subsequent evaluations found that Dr. M.'s primary communication problem was a pronounced hypernasality caused by a relatively immobile velum. Because his disease symptoms were relatively static and his overall speech articulation was normal, a palatal lift was recommended. His nasal voice resonance was isolated as his primary symptom; air-pressure flows and a recording playback were provided for the patient, as were detailed explanations about voice resonance and his hypernasality problem in particular. Recordings of several other patients who had been fitted with palatal lifts were played to demonstrate for the patient the before and after vocal resonance. A description of how a palatal lift is constructed and a prediction of the patient's probable outcome were then provided. The explanation of his problem not only suggested what direction the patient should take to improve his voice, but also convinced him that he would experience a good outcome. The patient was subsequently fitted with a palatal lift, attached to his own modified upper denture. Results were excellent, producing normal airflow data and a pronounced reduction in nasal resonance. After the lift was fitted, only one counseling and therapy demonstration session was required.

D. Evaluation of the approach   With a little guidance by the clinician in helping the patient understand his or her voice problem, what causes it, and what can be done about it, the typical voice patient can often make progress in overcoming the voice problem. Both children and adults profit from an explanation of their voice problem and from understanding how particular behaviors, like yelling or clearing one's throat excessively, keeps their voices in trouble. Sometimes an explanation of the problem is the primary treatment with no other facilitating approaches required. For those patients who need much practice with various approaches, they seem to make better progress when they understand the rationale behind what they are practicing.

5. DIGITAL MANIPULATION

A. Kinds of problems for which the approach is useful   There are several ways that voice clinicians can facilitate a target voice by finger manipulation of the patient's larynx. For voice problems related to an inappropriately high pitch level, external digital pressure by the clinician on the patient's thyroid cartilage is often effective in establishing a lower pitch. The external pressure nudges the thyroid cartilage slightly backward and shortens the vocal folds; this increases their mass and produces a lower fundamental frequency. Another form of digital manipulation, described by Case (1991), involves the clinician's or patient's monitoring any vertical movement (often interpreted as symptomatic of too much force while speaking) by placing fingers on the lateral walls of the thyroid cartilage. Perhaps the most active method of laryngeal manipulation is recommended by Aronson (1990) for problems of vocal hyperfunction, where tension is reduced in the laryngeal area by maneuvering the larynx to a lower position by placing the fingers "over the superior borders of the thyroid cartilage" and working "the larynx gently downward, also moving it laterally at times" (p. 341). Phonation produced by the larynx in a lower fixed position with only minimal vertical excursions is often observed in trained, efficient users of voice, such as professional singers.

B. Procedural aspects of the approach   The three digital procedures used in voice therapy are quite distinct from one another. We list the steps separately for each of the three procedures:

1. Digital pressure for lowering pitch.

a. With the exception of some men with falsetto voices, patients will respond to digital pressure by producing a lower voice pitch. Ask the patient to prolong a vowel (/a/ or /i/). As the vowel is prolonged, apply slight finger pressure on the thyroid cartilage. The pitch level will drop immediately.

b. Ask the patient to maintain the lower pitch after the fingers are removed. If the patient can do this, he or she should continue practicing the lower pitch. If the high pitch quickly reverts back, repeat the digital pressure.

c. If the method is used to let the patient hear and feel a lower pitch, the patient should practice producing the lower pitch with and without digital pressure on the thyroid cartilage.

2. Monitoring the vertical movements of the larynx.

a. For a patient with excessive pitch variability and tension related to much vertical movement of the larynx, demonstrate how to place the fingers on the thyroid cartilage and monitor laryngeal vertical movement while phonating.

b. Ask the patient to produce a pitch level several full musical notes off the bottom of his or her lowest note. Keeping the fingers on the thyroid cartilage, ask the patient to lower pitch one note at a time to the lowest note in his or her pitch range. Usually, the larynx will lower its position in the neck at the low end of the pitch range. Then ask the patient to sing one note at a time up to the top of the singing range, exclusive of falsetto. Toward the top of the scale, the patient should feel (through the fingertips) a slight elevation of the larynx. Review both the lowering and rising of the larynx at the extremes of the pitch range.

c. Once the patient has experienced vertical movement in the preceding steps, point out that in production of a speaking voice that is relatively free of strain, no vertical movement of the larynx should be felt during digital monitoring. Oral reading and speaking should be developed with little or no vertical laryngeal movements. Practice in oral reading with encouraged pitch variability can then be monitored by slight digital pressure of the thyroid cartilage with the patient's confirming (hopefully) no vertical movement.

3. Maneuvering the larynx to a lower neck position.

a. Encircle the hyoid bone with the middle finger and thumb.

b. With light finger pressure, place the fingers within the thyrohyoid space, just above the thyroid notch. With the fingers over the superior border of the thyroid cartilage, begin gently to "work" the larynx downward, with downward pressure and slight lateral movements. The larynx will usually move slightly downward with this gentle pressure (provided the patient does not fight the movement by observable tension and resistance).

c. If the technique does not work, repeat steps a and b a few more times. With the larynx in the lower position, ask the patient to prolong vowels and monitor laryngeal positioning using the procedure described in step 2. If the lower position is achieved and maintained, use a number of other voice facilitating techniques.

C. Typical case history showing utilization of the approach

J. F. was a 17-year-old male who had been raised exclusively by his mother until her sudden death about a year before. Since that time he had lived with a maternal uncle who was concerned about the boy's effeminate mannerisms and high-pitched voice. Laryngeal examination revealed a normal adult male larynx. The boy was found to have a habitual pitch level of around 200 cps, well within the adult female range, but below the level of falsetto. The most effective facilitating technique for producing a normal voice pitch was to apply digital pressure on the external thyroid cartilage. The young man was able to prolong the lower pitch levels with good success, but any attempt at conversation would be characterized by an immediate return to the higher pitch. After three therapy sessions, he was able to read aloud using the lower pitch, but was unable to use the lower voice in conversation except with his male clinician. Subsequent psychiatric evaluation and therapy were initiated for "identity confusion and schizoidal tendencies." Voice therapy was discontinued after 2 weeks, when it was clearly demonstrated that the patient could produce a good baritone voice (125 cps) whenever he wanted. Unfortunately, follow-up telephone conversations several months after therapy revealed that he was using his high-pitched, pretherapy voice exclusively.

D. Evaluation of the approach

With some problems of vocal hyperfunction, particularly cord thickening and vocal nodules, it is sometimes necessary to work toward lowering the child's or adult's (but not the adolescent's) pitch level as suggested by Aronson (1990) and Wilson (1987). Digital pressure on the thyroid cartilage is an excellent facilitator for many patients developing lower voice pitch. If the method does not produce a lower pitch level, as it may not do for certain cases of falsetto, the method cannot be used. Even though the method may produce an immediate change of voice to a more desired, lower pitch level, as illustrated in the preceding case history, it may not effect a permanent voice change without some counseling or psychotherapy. Digital pressure, though effective in lowering pitch level, rarely brings about permanent success unless other therapeutic approaches are used as well.

A well-trained singing or speaking voice is produced with a minimum of physical effort and relatively little upward-downward movement of the larynx. Some patients demonstrate excessive pitch variability and unnecessary laryngeal excursion as they speak. An excellent method of pointing this out to a patient, and of helping him or her establish a more optimum phonation with only minimal vertical laryngeal movement, is to have the patient place his or her fingers lightly on the laryngeal thyroid cartilage, feeling the downward movement as the pitch lowers and the upward movement as it rises. Lowering the larynx by external digital pressure or by using the yawn-sigh approach (Boone & McFarlane, 1993) are both effective.

6. EAR TRAINING

A. Kinds of problems for which the approach is useful   Most voice therapy involves the identification and elimination of faulty vocal habits and their replacement by more optimum ones. The basic input modality in developing appropriate phonation is the auditory system, particularly the patient's self-hearing. Individuals do not have much awareness of what they are doing laryngeally, whether they are approximating their folds or shortening or lengthening them, except as they hear their own voices. The surprise nearly always evoked in people hearing their own voices on recordings is one indication of how gross our self-hearing is. This lack of voice feedback has always presented problems to clinicians because patients literally do not know what they are doing when they phonate. Music teachers have historically attempted to circumvent the problem by using imagery in their training attempts, because the voice will often respond appropriately to psychological-anatomical instructions—for example, "Put your voice forcefully down in your chest"—even though the physiology of the described event is in error. In voice therapy, we are concerned with making patients critical listeners. Patients, however, may need practice in learning to listen to their own voices. Davis and Boone (1967) reported that some voice patients, like some people in the normal population, demonstrate difficulty in pitch discrimination and tonal memory as measured by subtests of the Seashore Measures of Musical Aptitude (Seashore, Lewis, & Saetviet, 1980). Such patients may have serious problems in voice therapy in making pitch discriminations and in remembering the sounds of their own target voices. Up to a certain point, gross pitch discrimination and tonal memory can be taught by ear-training practice, wherein the patient learns how to listen critically to his or her own "good" and "bad" voices and to the voices of others. Through auditory feedback devices, such as loop tape recorders, the patient learns to hear and monitor auditorially his or her own phonation. For patients who have defective listening skills, voice training may include instruction in making pitch discriminations, improving tonal memory, and learning to hear one's "good" and "bad" voices. But clinicians should first assess patients' listening skills because many voice patients have no problem in this area; others, just as some people in the normal population, may have surprisingly deficient listening abilities. The latter group may profit from ear training.

B. Procedural aspects of the approach

1. Take a base-line measurement of how well the patient can make pitch discriminations. The ear-training cassette from *The Boone Voice Program for Children* (Boone, 1993) contains 20 pitch-discrimination pairs that were produced with a music synthesizer and 20 singing voice pitch discriminations. The tape provides for easy contrast discrimination. You may also make your own taped or "live" discrimination presentations, or use the Seashore pitch discrimination subtest, a piano, or pitch pipe. Present to the patient a pair of tonal stimuli, asking if the stimuli are the same as each other or different. Follow this by voiced pitch discriminations, either produced by you or prerecorded. If the patient is unable to discriminate between one whole note and its flat or sharp, the indication is that the patient's pitch discrimination is not normal, but not necessarily that pitch discrimination therapy is needed. In gross departures, however, such as the patient's being unable to discriminate between notes that are more than a third apart (say, between a C^4 and an F^4), some discrimination training may be needed if the patient is ever going to match successfully a target model voice.

2. Pitch discrimination training should begin at the patient's base-line "can do" performance. When the patient makes correct discriminations at this level, his or her performance should be positively reinforced. Pitch stimuli can come from a piano, a pitch pipe, or the voice itself; it is often better therapy to mix all three types of pitch stimuli into the practice sequence, rather than to use one type only. Continue this activity for as long as necessary, until the patient is able to discriminate between pitches that are one full musical note apart (e.g., C^4 and D^4). This pitch-discrimination approach can be effectively practiced alone, without the clinician, if the patient listens to prerecorded practice materials and makes "same-different" choices as he or she listens. To learn the correctness of response, the patient can mark choices down on paper and then check them against a master sheet. Simple programming equipment has also been successfully used; here, the patient indicates the "same-different" choice, and a light goes on when the choice is correct.

3. Tonal memory therapy also begins where the patient is. That is, if the patient can remember a two-note sequence (via piano, pitch pipe, or voice), the therapy should begin by presenting two two-note sequences and asking the patient to identify which note varies between the two presentations. The ear-training cassette (Boone, 1993) also contains 20 pairs of contrasting melodies for use in tonal memory practice. It is not necessary for the patient to work beyond remembering a four-note series. When the patient can hear a four-note melody, remember it, and successfully compare it with a second four-note melody (with only one note varying between the first and second presentation), tonal memory is probably good enough for recalling various voice model presentations. Tonal memory therapy is also well suited for self-practice; the patient listens and responds to prerecorded sequences.

4. If a target model voice has been produced by the patient, can he or she discriminate between this good production and a faulty one? It is essential in voice therapy that the patient use his or her own "best" voice as a therapy model whenever possible. The patient may need some practice in learning to listen for his or her own "best" and "bad" voices. Capture the patient's voice productions on recordings, and then edit and splice them into contrasting pairs. The patient should listen discriminatively to these pairings to learn to identify quickly and correctly his or her better phonation. Recordings of other people's voices with similar problems, also paired for discrimination listening, make excellent practice materials. When the patient is consistently able to hear his or her "good" voice, whether or not he or she can produce that voice, there is little need to emphasize ear training. For some patients, just a little listening to their own voices helps; for others, even a great deal of practice is useless. For the rare patient who shows no improvement after trial ear training, further training might as well be abandoned.

C. Typical case history showing utilization of the approach

C. M., a 9-year-old girl with functional hypernasality, was evaluated by a local cleft-palate team and found to have adequate velopharyngeal closure (as demonstrated by cinefluorography), normal manometric pressure ratios, and normal stimulability for producing good oral resonance in isolated words repeated after the examiner. Voice therapy on a twice-weekly basis was recommended. The focus of therapy was on ear training, helping the patient discriminate between her nasal resonance and oral resonance. The first 7 weeks of therapy were spent both in this discrimination listening, which in the beginning was very defective, and in producing contrasting oral and nasal resonations. In the early phases of therapy, orality was stressed only in the therapy and practice sessions, and no attempt was made at any outside carry-over. Eventually, carry-over phrases and sentences were practiced in situations outside the clinic setting. As therapy progressed, the girl showed excellent auditory self-monitoring and was able to develop normal oral voice quality in all situations. Voice therapy was judged a success and terminated after 11 weeks.

D. Evaluation of the approach

In voice therapy, the patient must become a critical listener to his or her own voice. Some voice patients, like some people in the normal population, have real difficulty making pitch discriminations and judgments of tonal memory. Of these patients, some profit from ear training. The patient must learn to hear, if possible, how he or she is phonating. If the patient's listening abilities are poor, ear training should be initiated. If there is no problem in listening, ear training should be avoided.

7. ELIMINATION OF ABUSES

A. Kinds of problems for which the approach is useful   There are many ways that one can abuse or misuse the voice. *Vocal abuse* comprises various behaviors and events that have some kind of deleterious effect on the larynx and the voice, such as:

1. Yelling and screaming
2. Speaking against a background of loud noise
3. Coughing and excessive throat clearing
4. Smoking
5. Excessive talking or singing
6. Excessive talking or singing while having an allergy or upper respiratory infection
7. Excessive crying or laughing

Vocal misuse means improper use of voice, such as:

1. Speaking with hard glottal attack
2. Singing excessively at the lower or upper end of one's range
3. Increasing vocal loudness by squeezing out the voice at the level of the larynx
4. Speaking at excessive intensity levels
5. Cheerleading (Case, 1991)
6. Speaking over time at an inappropriate pitch level
7. Speaking or singing (such as a prolonged show rehearsal) for excessively long periods of time

We could, obviously, add other abuses and misuses to such a list. Identification and reduction of vocal abuse-misuse are primary goals in voice therapy for hyperfunctional disorders such as functional dysphonia with or without such physical changes as vocal nodules, polyps, or contact ulcers. Therapy cannot be successful until contributory vocal abuse-misuse can be drastically reduced. Optimum usage of the voice, such as the vocal hygiene program outlined in Chapter 6, also requires identifying possible abusive voice situations and making deliberate efforts to minimize their occurrence.

B. Procedural aspects of the approach

1. Time must be given early in voice therapy to identifying possible vocal abuse. Once a particular vocal abuse is identified, the patient and clinician should develop a baseline of occurrence. This will often require that the clinician hear and observe the patient in and out of the clinic environment, such as on the playground, at the pulpit, or in a nightclub. The number of times the particular event occurred must be tallied.

2. Children with vocal abuse must become aware of the impact of such abuses on their voices. With children we use the "Vocal Abuse

Reduction Program" (Boone, 1993), which recommends: an explanation of how additive lesions occur, using the story *A Voice Lost and Found*; a review of the child's abuses; and a systematic reduction of the child's abuses, using the Voice Tally Card, the Voice Counting Chart, and the Hot-Air Balloon Race (p. 7). The focus of the reducing abuse program is to make the child cognitively aware of the relationship of vocal abuse-misuse to increasing symptoms of voice. The story in the program is pictorially illustrated with various vocal behaviors related to changes of "the little bumps on the vocal cords."

3. Discuss identified vocal abuses with the patient, emphasizing the need to reduce their daily frequency. Assign to the patient the task of counting the number of times each day he or she engages in a particular abuse. Perhaps a peer or sibling could be brought in, told about the situation, and asked to join in on the daily count. Depending on the age of the patient, a parent or teacher, spouse, or business associate might be asked to keep track of the number of abuses that occur in their presence. At the end of the day, the abuses should be tallied for that day.

4. Ask the patient to plot his or her daily vocal abuses on a graph. Along the vertical axis, the ordinate, the patient should plot the number of times the particular abuse occurred, and, along the base of the graph, the abscissa, the individual days, beginning with the baseline count of the first day. Instruct the patient to bring these graphs to voice therapy sessions. Keeping a graph usually increases the patient's awareness of what he or she has been doing and results in a gradual decrement of the abusive behavior. The typical vocal abuse has a sloping decremental curve, indicating its gradual disappearance. Greet any decrement in the plots of the people observing the patient, but particularly in those compiled by the patient, with obvious approval.

C. Typical case history showing utilization of the approach

Joyce was a 27-year-old secretary who complained of a voice that was often hoarse and that tired easily every day. Subsequent indirect laryngoscopy confirmed a slight bilateral thickening at the anterior-middle third junction. A detailed history and observation of the patient found that she constantly cleared her throat. The throat clearing had become a habit. She rarely felt that she was able "to bring up any mucus" but just cleared her throat in attempt to make her voice clearer. A high-speed motion picture depicting throat clearing was shown to the patient. She was counseled to try to reduce its occurrence. The patient subsequently began to tally her throat clearing and coughing as they occurred, plotting them on a graph at the end of the day. Within 2 weeks, she was able to change her throat-clearing habit. Her vocal quality improved immediately and she never needed formal, long-term voice therapy.

D. Evaluation of the approach
Identifying vocal abuses and attempting to eliminate them by plotting their daily frequency on a graph are effective in helping young children with voice problems. Adolescents are

equally guilty of vocal abuses and profit greatly from keeping track of what they are doing. Typical adult abuses, such as throat clearing, are often eliminated after a week or two of graph plotting by motivated patients. The effectiveness of this approach, in fact, is highly related to the skill of the clinician in motivating the patient to eliminate the abusive behavior. The value of the plotting is more in developing awareness of the frequency of the problem than in the actual count per se. Reduction of vocal abuse has become a primary part of most voice therapy programs for children (Andrews, 1986; Boone, 1993; Wilson, 1987) and for adults (Aronson, 1990; Boone, 1983; Case, 1991).

8. ELIMINATION OF HARD GLOTTAL ATTACK

A. Kinds of problems for which the approach is useful   In the facilitating approach just described "speaking with hard glottal attack" was first on the list of vocal misuses. Speaking with abrupt vocal onsets is extremely taxing on the laryngeal mechanism. Pershall and Boone (1986) found on videoendoscopy that after continuous staccato phonation (abrupt-onset phonation) a normal subject began to show slight edema and redness on the anterior-middle third site of the glottal margin. Hard glottal attack is often heard in the voices of people with posterior lesions, such as contact ulcers. Hard glottal attack is an excellent example of vocal hyperfunction: using too much unnecessary effort and force for voice.

B. Procedural aspects of the approach
    1. Hard glottal attack is a fairly common phenomenon among actors, politicians, and untrained singers. Play recordings of the voices of such people, and of the patient, for the patient, and then demonstrate the contrasting soft, easy glottal attack. The length of the demonstration should depend on the patient's insight.
    2. Demonstrate a child's vocal attack by letting the patient contrast a recording of his or her own voice with the normal voice of a peer. Then practice using words beginning with /h/, taken from various lists, such as those in Fisher (1975), Moncur and Brackett (1974), or Boone (1993). Select monosyllabic words, beginning with the aspirate /h/ for soft attack practice. When the /h/ words are produced correctly, introduce other words beginning with unvoiced consonants for similar practice. Then use words beginning with vowels.
    3. Use the whisper-phonation technique. Choose a few monosyllabic words, each beginning with a vowel. The patient's task is to whisper very lightly the initial vowel, prolonging it by gradually increasing the loudness of the whisper until phonation is introduced and, finally, the whole word is said. The whisper blends into a soft phonation.
    4. The yawn-sigh approach is particularly effective in eliminating hard glottal attack.
    5. By definition the chant approach eliminates hard glottal attack by

its initiating legato into the speaking voice. It can often be successfully combined with the yawn-sigh or the chewing approach.

6. Simultaneous chewing and chanting make abrupt onset of phonation impossible.

7. Once the patient is able to produce easy-onset phonation by chanting, chewing, or yawning-sighing, a good therapy procedure is to have the patient contrast the easy-onset phonation with abrupt-onset phonation. The lack of effort of easy onset and the obvious effort of abrupt onset make a convincing contrast between the two modes of voice onset.

8. Various instruments are useful in providing the patient feedback about the severity of his or her glottal attack or suddenness of initiation of phonation. The display from a spectrograph or the Visi-Pitch can show the relative onset time of phonations; a vertical tracing at the beginning of the word indicates hard, abrupt vocal attack as opposed to a sloping onset tracing that displays a more gradual onset. Using various facilitating approaches, the clinician and the patient can visually confirm the relative suddenness of onset by the slope of the onset curve. The Voice Monitor (1977) has been found useful. The Voice Monitor can be set at various sensitivity levels to alert the patient to sudden initiation of phonation. When the patient initiates a word abruptly, a light goes on. The patient's task is to continue speaking connected speech without abruptness of attack to avoid the warning light. Using the Voice Monitor has the advantage of critically monitoring the patient's voice practice without having a clinician in the room.

C. Typical case history showing utilization of the approach

Louis was a 35-year-old assistant professor of hydrology who came to the voice clinic with the sole complaint of "pain in the throat and hoarseness" after lecturing for more than an hour. A subsequent voice evaluation and visitation to his classes found that Louis was lecturing with a "different voice" from the one he used conversationally. His lecture voice appeared to be at the bottom of his vocal pitch range, and he spoke with excessive glottal attack. He felt (perhaps correctly) that his low-pitched voice and his abrupt way of saying things made him sound a bit more authoritative and "in charge of my subject matter." Although some work in voice therapy involved raising his voice pitch two full steps, focus was on eliminating hard glottal attack. Within a few weeks of starting voice therapy, he reported no discomfort after lecturing, and the dysphonia after prolonged lecturing began to disappear.

D. Evaluation of the approach
Elimination of hard glottal attack is often easily accomplished in voice therapy. When they begin voice therapy, most patients who speak with hard glottal attack are unaware of the amount of unneeded energy they expend by speaking with such abrupt initiation of voice. Once hard attack is pointed out and an easier vocal onset is taught (perhaps by chewing, chanting, or sighing), the typical patient soon prefers the easier way of initiating vocal onsets.

9. ESTABLISHING A NEW PITCH

A. Kinds of problems for which the approach is useful Although it is fairly well established (Bless, 1984; Minifie, 1984) that there is no absolute optimum pitch on which a particular person should speak, some people with voice problems may profit from speaking at a different pitch level. A change of pitch will often have positive effects on voice, such as improving vocal quality and loudness. Speaking at the very bottom of one's pitch range requires too much force and effort. Similarly, speaking habitually toward the top of one's range can be vocally fatiguing. Because a number of instruments available today can portray fundamental frequency in real time (while one is phonating), awareness and feedback of one's ongoing pitch level play prominent roles in establishing new pitches through therapy.

B. Procedural aspects of the approach

1. If pitch needs to be raised or lowered, describe where the patient is and where the target pitch is. The methods for determining habitual and optimum pitches described in Chapter 4 can be applied here. Make a tape recording of the patient producing various pitches, including feedback about the old pitch and the projected target pitch. The playback should always be followed by some discussion comparing the sound and the feeling of the two pitches.

2. Most voice patients can imitate their own pitch models, once they have been produced by the appropriate facilitating technique. Occasionally patients cannot initiate a pitch to match a model, as Filter and Urioste (1981) found in testing college women with normal voices. A useful model can be produced by having the patient extend an /i/ at the target pitch level for about 5 seconds and recording the phonation on a loop tape recorder. If the loop is set for a 5- to 10-second playback, the patient will immediately hear the target production. The loop tape playback will provide the patient with a continuous playback of his or her own voice model of the target pitch. There are many advantages to using the patients' own voices as their voice models, in that they already have voicing experience producing the sounds they are now trying to match. Remain with the loop model /i/ for considerable practice before introducing a new stimulus.

3. Several excellent instruments available today can provide real-time display of fundamental frequency, both with a digital write out and on a display screen on a monitor: PM 100 Pitch Analyzer, Phonatory Function Analyzer, Visi-Pitch, and B & K Real-Time Frequency Analyzer (see reference section at end of book). Usually, these instruments permit the clinician to display patient voice values specific to frequency and intensity. The PM 100 and Visi-Pitch each offer split-screen capabilities, whereby a voice model can be put on an upper screen and the patient's production displayed on a lower screen, permitting comparisons

between model and trial productions. Any instrument that can display fundamental frequency information can provide valuable feedback to a patient attempting to establish a new voice pitch.

4. The Tunemaster III (see reference section at end of book) provides feedback information relative to correctness of patient production. The desired pitch level is set on the Tunemaster III. The display dial can then provide feedback to the patient whether voice production is within 30 cycles (sharp or flat) of the target frequency. Using any of the four instruments previously described in step 3, the patient can receive exact digital feedback about the frequency he or she is producing. Any deviation below or above the target pitch level can be given immediate feedback. Of great therapeutic benefit is that the patient will know immediately when he or she is producing the target frequency.

5. Establishing a new pitch is facilitated by working first on single words, preferably words that begin with vowels. Each word is repeated in a pitch monotone (using the target pitch). Occasionally a patient has more difficulty using the new pitch with certain words. Any such "trouble" words should be avoided as practice material, because what is needed at this stage of therapy is practice in rapidly phonating a series of individuals words at the new pitch level.

6. Once the patient does well at the single-word level, introduce phrases and short sentences. It is usually more productive at this stage to avoid practice in actual conversation because the patient is better able to use the new phonation in such neutral situations as reading single words, phrases, and sentences. When success is achieved at the sentence level, assign the patient reading passages from various voice and diction books. Success in using the new pitch level can be verified by using the instruments described earlier, in step 3.

7. After reading well in a monotone, the patient may try using the new pitch in some real-life conversational situations. In the beginning he or she may have more success talking to strangers, such as store clerks; patients often find it difficult to use the new pitch level with friends and family, because their previous "sets" may prevent them from utilizing their new vocal behavior. Whatever conversational situation works best for the individual should be the one initially used.

8. It is helpful in therapy to tape-record the patient's voice as he or she searches to establish a new and different pitch level. When the patient is able to produce a good voice at the proper pitch level, his or her own "best" voice can then become the therapy model.

C. Typical case history showing utilization of the approach

John, a 10-year-old boy, was referred by his public-school speech clinician for a laryngeal examination because of a 6-month history of hoarseness. The findings included a normal larynx and a "low-pitched dysphonic voice." John could readily demonstrate a higher phonation, which was characterized by an immediate clearing of quality. In the discussion that followed the tape-recorded playback of his "good" and "bad" voice, John stated that he thought he had been trying to speak like his older brother. The clinician pointed out to him that his better voice was more like that of other boys his age, and that the low-pitched voice he had been using was difficult for others to listen to. In subsequent voice therapy with his public-school clinician, John focused on elevating his voice pitch to a more natural level. His success was rapid, and therapy was terminated after 6 weeks.

D. Evaluation of the approach   The pitch of the voice changes constantly, according to the speaker's situation. In some patients, however, the pitch level appears to be too high or too low for the overall capability of the laryngeal mechanism. In other people, an aberrant pitch level is just one manifestation of the total personality. Patients with additive masses to the folds (nodules, papilloma, polyps, and so on) may have lower pitch levels than normal because the thicker vocal folds vibrate more slowly, emitting a lower fundamental frequency. As the lesion is reduced or eliminated, the frequency of the voice becomes higher, perhaps approaching normal limits. For patients with additive laryngeal lesions due to vocal hyperfunction, it is often best to work slowly toward increasing pitch level to approximate levels of the patient's age and sex peers. Some patients use aberrant pitch levels because of personality factors. Counseling such patients and helping them want to change pitch levels might well have to precede actual symptomatic therapy to alter pitch. Typically, however, voice patients who may need to change pitch levels can do so rather quickly, after experiencing marked improvement in overall voice quality because of pitch change.

10. FEEDBACK

A. Kinds of problems for which the approach is useful   Once the patient can produce a model voice—his or her own or one that matches some external model—it is important that he or she attempt to study what the voice feels like and how it sounds. Tactual and proprioceptive feedback are common modalities through which we get some information about our voices as we speak, but we primarily use the auditory feedback system to monitor our own phonation. We have little awareness of what our muscles are doing in the larynx, throat, palate, or tongue, which is why voice therapy relies heavily on the auditory feedback mechanism.

With modern instrumentation, we can provide needed feedback specific to the physiology of respiration, phonation, and resonance. Much of the evaluation instrumentation described in Chapter 4 can be used as effective feedback devices because they permit the patient to view various ongoing speaking-voicing events as they are occurring. It is sometimes helpful to provide the voice patient with information specific to what he or she may be doing in respiration while producing voice. The physiology of respiration can be studied by placing a pair of magnetometers on the chest wall and another pair on the abdomen; Hixon and his associates have studied relative chest wall-abdominal movements during singing (Watson & Hixon, 1985) and in dramatic performances (Hixon, Watson, & Maher, 1987). This use of magnetometers can provide valuable feedback to the patient attempting to develop more optimal breathing patterns.

Nasoendoscopy, as described in Chapter 4, permits direct observation of the actual physiology of various oral, pharyngeal, and laryngeal events while phonating. Supraglottal participation in vocal quality and resonance can be directly observed; the patient can watch himself or herself using various therapy techniques that produce changes in voice. Patients who have marginal velopharyngeal (VP) closure can watch the closure of the VP mechanism on a television monitor and use the experience as direct feedback in therapy (Shelton, Paesani, McClelland, & Bradfield, 1975). For patients with problems of nasal resonance, the Kay Nasometer is a useful feedback device that provides an ongoing ratio of the relative oral-nasal resonance in the patient's voice. By applying a particular therapeutic technique or attempting to match a particular resonance model, the patient and the clinician can get immediate feedback on the patient's production.

Feedback specific to voice frequency and quality can be provided by many electronic instruments, some of which we present later, when we describe some of the procedures using feedback. As the patient is presented various target vocal behaviors to produce or match, instrumentation can provide real-time or delayed feedback specific to the correctness of the response. If the patient is off target in production, he or she can alter the vocalization to more closely match the target model.

Biofeedback specific to the patient's relaxation state can be helpful in voice therapy. The patient is introduced to some kind of biofeedback instrumentation that quantifies physiological changes, such as galvanic response or blood pressure, which are believed to be correlates of anxiety or systemic tension. As the patient becomes more relaxed, the physiological tension data go down; increased tension is characterized by increased data values. The patient in effect learns what it feels like to be more relaxed, and the relaxed state is confirmed by lower tension scores as portrayed on biofeedback instrumentation. Once relaxation behaviors are learned (Stroebel, 1983), the biofeedback confirmation of the relaxed state is often no longer needed.

B. Procedural aspects of the approach

1. Discuss with the patient the general concept of feedback. Tactual feedback might be illustrated by moving the fingertips lightly over the surface of a coin. Proprioception can be demonstrated by having the patient close the eyes, extend an arm, and slowly raise the arm, bending it at the elbow joint. Muscle and joint proprioceptors tell us where our

arm is in space and that it is moving. In the larynx, however, such proprioceptive feedback is essentially lacking; we must rely on hearing our voices as we phonate to monitor what we are doing laryngeally.

2. The conventional tape recorder has never been particularly useful as a training device for auditory feedback. All it can do, essentially, is serve as an amplifying system. By the time you rewind the tape and find the precise recording segment, the patient has already lost his or her focus on that particular stimulus. Many auditory tape devices are available— Language Master, Echorder, Artik (see reference section). You can make your own loop tapes for either reel-to-reel recorders or cassettes by following simple procedures (Boone, 1982). The loop playback provides valuable auditory feedback. A loop recording device, for example, set on a 3-second delay, will give the patient an immediate playback of what he or she has just said. By using such a device, patients can immediately match what they thought they sounded like with the actual playback of what they sounded like externally. Vowel prolongations, single words, and phrases are used as the stimuli in this delayed-feedback practice. Remember that such practice in self-listening is much more effective if coupled with commentary and questions about what was heard, and what was different between the old voice and the new.

3. Introduce the patient to the feedback instruments that will provide the needed feedback. In respiration, any of the measuring devices for air volume and pressures described in Chapter 4 may be useful. Duration measurements, such as how long one can prolong an /s/, can be used for feedback. The magnetometers can provide ongoing information about respiratory physiology. Videoendoscopy can provide excellent feedback for the physiology of VP closure, pharyngeal and supraglottal laryngeal participation in voicing, and vocal fold movements. Information about pitch and quality—for example, digital and graphic data about the patient's ongoing phonation—can be provided by the PM 100 Pitch Analyzer, the Kay Visi-Pitch, and B & K Frequency Analyzers (see reference section at end of book).

4. Once the patient develops an awareness of what he or she is doing with the help of feedback devices, remove the feedback and see if the patient can then maintain the target production. For example, when the patient no longer can see on a scope the normal coordination of abdomen and thorax in breathing for speech, can the optimum pattern be maintained? Both biofeedback of some physiological system and ongoing auditory feedback eventually need to be phased out of the therapy session to facilitate generalization of improved production outside the therapy.

C. Typical case history showing utilization of the approach

Cheryl was a 22-year-old college student with vocal nodules and a severe dysphonia. Her voice evaluation showed that she spoke at the very bottom of her limited pitch range. When she spoke one or two full musical notes higher than the bottom of her pitch range, her voice sounded near normal. We spent time in therapy giving her auditory feedback of her new voice at a higher pitch level, utilizing a 4-second tape loop cartridge. This provided Cheryl with immediate feedback about how she sounded. We then coupled the auditory feedback with the visual feedback of a Visi-Pitch scope, where she could witness the increased periodicity of her voice, indicated by a sharper tracing line on the scope. Not only did she sound better to herself, but she could also see that voicing one or two notes higher than she had been produced a smoother, better-sounding voice. The voice therapy used the auditory and visual feedback, coupled with some practice reducing excessive glottal attack, opening her mouth more, and so forth. At the end of 15 weeks of twice-weekly voice therapy, Cheryl's nodules were gone and we (including the patient) judged her voice as normal.

D. Evaluation of the approach   As instrumentation is developed that can portray various aspects (respiration-phonation-resonance) of voice, it can play an important role in providing feedback to patients. Once a target behavior has been isolated for a patient, such instrumentation can provide ongoing feedback on the appropriateness of patient production. Feedback presents various visual portrayals (values of frequency, jitter, shimmer, and so forth) of what the patient is hearing. Various facilitating efforts in therapy often produce changes in the sound of voice that are confirmed by different feedback devices. Once an optimal voicing pattern has been established, the use of feedback devices is no longer necessary.

11. FOCUS

A. Kinds of problems for which the approach is useful   Good focus of the voice is characterized by the voice coming "from the middle of the mouth, just above the surface of the tongue" (Boone, 1991, p. 71). Problems in "horizontal" voice focus occur when the tongue is too far forward or too far backward within the mouth. The "thin" or baby-sounding voice is produced by carrying the tongue high and forward. The back focused voice, sounding like the country bumpkin voice or the voice of the television character Alf, is produced by carrying the tongue elevated in the back of the mouth. Both anterior and posterior tongue problems are corrected by using approach 1, altering tongue position.

The most common focus problem we see in patients with voice disorders is the voice sounding as if it were deep in the throat. Many patients focus on their throats as the anatomical site of their problem. Such patients profit from this approach, focus, because it shifts their mental imagery from the throat to the upper vocal tract.

Perkins (1981) has written that "voice that feels focused high in the head" is a more efficient voice, and it can survive extensive vocalization. The clinician helps the patient focus on the area of his or her face under the cheeks and across the bridge of the nose. Most patients with chronic dysphonia experience both difficulty finding their voices and continued expectancy of vocal failure. They clear their throats continually, they make phonation rehearsals, and they worry about the poor vocal quality they are likely to have the next time they attempt to speak. For these patients successful voice clinicians often employ two techniques, respiration training and placing the voice in the facial mask, for two reasons: (a) to improve respiratory control and resonance; (b) to transfer the patient's mental focus away from the larynx and place it with the activator (respiration) and the resonator (supraglottal vocal tract).

B. Procedural aspects of the approach

1. The horizontal problems of focus—the front, thin voice or the back voice—are corrected by using facilitating approach 1, altering tongue position.

2. In working with children, we use the pictures shown in the facial mask in Figure 5–3. As described in *The Boone Voice Program for Children* (1993), we follow these steps: "Give the following explanation to the child, pointing to the appropriate places on the picture. (Point to the shaded area on the boy in the picture.) 'A good sounding voice is made right here. We'll do some things today that will put your voice right here.' (Point to the bridge of the nose in the picture, then touch the child in the same place.) 'Then we'll put some voice right here.' (Point to the cheeks in the picture, then touch the child in the same place.)" (p. 118)

3. With adults we use a similar procedure.

4. Demonstrate the method by saying "me" and "one" in an exaggerated manner, which will create sufficient nasal resonance to produce some vibration on the bridge of the nose and above the maxillary sinuses.

5. Request that the patient produce the "me" and the "one" in the same manner. Ask the patient if he or she can feel the vibration on his or her nose and high cheeks.

6. If the patient confirms feeling the vibration produced by the nasal consonant, add a few more words that permit the exaggeration of the nasal consonant. Words like *man, mean, many, went* lend themselves well to this beginning work. If this is done correctly, improvement in vocal quality should be audible. The nasal consonants are used not to increase nasal resonance, but to focus the voice higher in the vocal tract than the patient had been previously.

7. If there is an audible improvement in the sound of the voice using the words with nasal consonants, then introduce other words, such as *baby, beach, take,* and so on, emphasizing the resonance in the facial mask area. Any words may be used at this point.

8. After the patient has had some success in placing the voice "higher," discuss with the patient the imagery of what you are doing. Discuss how this is similar to the singing teacher's using such imagery (we cannot really "place" our voices anywhere), knowing that a singer

who has the imagery of "putting his or her voice somewhere" often shows audible, measurable improvement. This is a good place to use some kind of feedback device, such as a spectrograph or the Visi-Pitch, to confirm any changes in voice quality using the approach.

9. Oral reading and conversation in the voice clinic setting, focusing on the feeling and the "set" for focus are important requisites for generalization of this approach outside the clinic.

C. Typical case history showing utilization of the approach

Richard was a 44-year-old lawyer who developed a functional dysphonia while still maintaining "a normal larynx." At times he experienced a normal voice, but at meetings or on the telephone, he often experienced severe hoarseness, pain in the laryngeal area, and the feeling that talking at all required much effort. The focus technique worked better for him than all the other facilitating approaches we used. He found that the imagery of placing his voice "in his face" seemed to free the tightness he experienced in his throat. Increased periodicity of laryngeal vibration and improvement in overall laryngeal function appeared directly related to shifting his voice concern away from his larynx. From our explanation of phonation, he began to understand that the vocal folds come together "slightly," that the real activator of voice is the outgoing airflow, and that the real sound and quality of the voice are formed in the vocal tract above the larynx. The explanations and the practice placing the voice in the facial mask had lasting effects. Focus, used with respiration training and explanations of the vocal physiology, appeared to restore normal voice in this professional man. A one-year follow up quickly confirmed that he had maintained his normal voice.

D. Evaluation of the approach

The goal in using this approach is to transfer the patient's focus from the larynx to the upper vocal tract. The approach is not used to increase nasal resonance; the heavy utilization of nasal resonance in the beginning steps of the approach is used only to

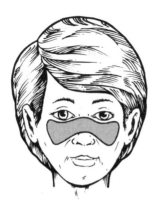 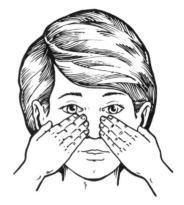

FIGURE 5–3
The imagery of "placing" the voice in the middle of the face is helped by using these two pictures. (*The Boone Voice Program for Children*, 2nd ed. Austin, TX: PRO-ED, 1993.)

develop focus on the area of the nose and face. Singing teachers have successfully used such imagery approaches (Coffin, 1981) as the *um-hum* technique, in which the patient experiences a "tingle or buzz" near the lips or the bridge of the nose. Improvement in vocal quality, using nasal consonants as a method of focusing the voice out of the throat, is part of therapy procedures developed by Wilson (1987) and McClosky (1977, p. 143). Once the patient experiences the nasal vibration of production, the clinician shifts to oral productions, keeping, however, focus on the same somatic site. Our experience has been that the approach is helpful to most voice patients except those whose problems have a hypernasality component.

12. GLOTTAL FRY

A. Kinds of problems for which the approach is useful True glottal fry is produced in a relaxed manner with very little airflow and very little subglottic air pressure (Zemlin, 1981). Glottal fry, considered a normal voice register, is valuable for patients with vocal nodules as well as for patients with other hyperfunctional problems such as polyps, cord thickening, functional dysphonia, and even spasmodic dysphonia and ventricular phonation. Although glottal fry can be an extremely powerful facilitating technique to improve voice in the dysphonic patient and is a useful diagnostic vocal probe, it has a second use, as well: It can be an index of vocal fold relaxation. In order to produce a glottal fry of 65 to 75 Hz, which is desirable, the vocal folds must be relaxed. A patient may not always be able to achieve this fry in the first session, but the accomplishment of a "good fry" of about 70 or 75 Hz is an index that the larynx has been relaxed. The glottal fry can be produced on either inhalation or exhalation. After producing glottal fry phonation for 5 to 10 seconds and then being asked to say a phrase such as "easy does it," a patient with nodules often experiences normal or near-normal vocal quality for the first time in months.

B. Procedural aspects of the approach

1. A common pencil eraser or very dry hard raisin can represent a vocal nodule. When placed between the pages of a hardback book, the eraser keeps the pages apart with a gap on either side of the eraser; likewise, nodules produce a gap between the vocal cords, as was shown in Figure 3–2. If the eraser is placed between two marshmallows instead of between the pages of a book, the marshmallows "wrap around" the mass of the eraser. In glottal fry, the compliant vocal cords can "wrap around" the nodules and improve approximation. A clinician can see this with stroboscopic videoendoscopy and demonstrate it to the patient.

2. Ask the patient to let out half of his or her breath and then say /i/ softly, holding it until it dies away slowly. Encourage the patient to stretch the /i/ as long as possible.

3. Once the patient has a well-sustained /i/ in the glottal fry mode, have him or her open the mouth medium wide and protrude the tongue. Then have the patient make the tone "larger" by "opening the throat." The desired tone is a deep, resonant, slow series of individual pops, which we describe as sounding "like dragging a stick along a picket fence."

4. Have the patient attempt to produce the same tone on inhalation as on exhalation. Some people are better able to produce the glottal fry on inhalation. Also have the patient alternately reverse the tone—first on exhalation, then on inhalation. Next, have the patient say words such as *on* and *off* and *in* and *out* in the glottal fry mode. Suggest that the patient slightly prolong these words and say them on both inhalation ("on," "in") and exhalation ("off," "out"), alternately back and forth between ingressive and egressive airflow. Tape-record the glottal fry so the patient has a model or target.

5. When the patient is able to produce these words well and can produce the sustained /i/ or /a/ in glottal fry, ask him or her to say "easy does it," "squeeze the peach," or "see the eagle." These are almost always produced with greatly improved or normal vocal quality. The patient will generally be able to say only a few words with the improved quality and will then need to go back to the glottal fry mode. Tape-record these phrases and contrast them with the patient's typical voice. Also ask the patient to judge the two.

6. When the correct glottal fry is learned, instruct the patient to practice for a few minutes several (10 or more) times each day. To assist the patient in practice, suggest that he or she tie practice to the environment—for example, by producing the fry each time he or she sees a bus or a red car, or during the last 2 minutes of each hour. The patient must be producing the fry appropriately before you allow practice.

C. Typical case history showing utilization of the approach
Mark, a 10-year-old boy, and Brian, an 11-year-old boy, were referred for voice evaluation by an otolaryngologist who had diagnosed bilateral vocal nodules. Both boys had low-pitched, hoarse voices with frequent phonation breaks during connected speech. They had had these voices for nearly 1 year. After teaching glottal fry as just described, we had "contests" to see who could fry the longest and at the slowest rate. We had the boys say words in the fry mode back and forth to each other. We saw each boy twice a week, once together and once individually, for 45-minute sessions. In 3 months, their voices were normal, and the nodules were completely gone. We should note that with one boy, we reduced vocal abuses during his soccer activity, as well.

D. Evaluating the approach   The approach appears to work because very little subglottic pressure and very little airflow are required to produce the glottal fry. Therefore, there is little stress on the folds. The compliant folds seem to reduce the amount of friction as they meet during phonation. This allows the nodules to be reduced or reabsorbed even though the patient continues to talk. The new talking is done with little fold tension.

13. HALF-SWALLOW, BOOM

A. Kinds of problems for which the approach is useful   This technique is most useful with patients who have unilateral vocal fold paralysis, severe bowing of the cords, or falsetto voice. All of these patients have low loudness levels and air wastage.

B. Procedural aspects of the approach
   1. The instruction to swallow and to *immediately* say a loud "boom" right "on top of the swallow" is critical. We use the term *half-swallow* to stress that the patient is not to swallow and then say "boom" but to say "boom" *during* the swallow. We also ask the patient to say "boom" with a low pitch, which we model first.
   2. Frequently, after only two or three attempts, the "boom" is said in a louder and less breathy (often nearly normal) voice. Record these attempts and play them back to demonstrate the dramatic improvement. Ask the patient to contrast this "boom" with his or her typical voice.
   3. We often use this approach with the head turned to one side and then the other. Also, we try it with the chin lowered and "tucked" in as well. When the best "boom" is produced, ask the patient to say "boom /i/", "boom one," and "boom /i/ boom" right on top of the swallow.
   4. Gradually increase the length of the phrase after the "boom" and finally phase out the "boom." Next, phase out the swallow; by this time, move the head back to the midline, and raise the chin to the normal position.

C. Typical case history showing utilization of the approach
Tom, a 64-year-old retired lecturer for the United States government, was referred by an otolaryngologist who had diagnosed right unilateral adductor vocal cord paralysis. He had a weak, breathy, high-pitched voice (185 Hz) that often failed him in a noisy environment and at the end of the day. Tom experienced frequent phonation breaks and complained of being perceived as a woman when talking over the phone. The half-swallow, boom technique was used exclusively with Tom after the pushing/pulling technique produced a louder but very hoarse voice. He produced a normal voice on "boom" after the fourth or fifth attempt. After 25 sessions, the voice was essentially normal and no longer failed him. After dismissal from therapy, Tom was able to resume speaking assignments to groups. His voice was no longer perceived as that of a female, and his pitch was 135 to 140 Hz. This patient, like many others, developed normal or near-normal voice in the presence of a continuing unilateral adductor paralysis.

D. Evaluating the approach   The swallow produces as much closure of the larynx as is physiologically possible. *Boom* is a brief word composed of voiced sounds that can all be produced as the air is released from the physiologically constricted larynx and the oral opening is minimal, which produces some "back pressure on the larynx." The head turning likely also assists, in a mechanical sense, with laryngeal closure.

14. HEAD POSITIONING

A. Kinds of problems for which the approach is useful   The production of easy, normal voice is sometimes facilitated by changing the position of the head. Head positioning has been found most useful for facilitating both chewing and swallowing in patients with various neurological disorders. For such patients, better oral-pharyngeal competence may result with the head in certain positions. The symptoms of dysarthria, such as in articulation and voice problems, may also be minimized by the relative position of the head during speaking attempts. Occasionally, patients with hyperfunctional voice disorders can experience a marked improvement in voice quality by placing the head in a different position. Several distinct head positions can be tried in therapy in an attempt to find one that facilitates better voice:

1. Normal straight ahead
2. Neck extended forward with head tilted down, face looking up
3. Neck flexed downward with head tilted down, face looking down
4. Neck flexed unilaterally with head tilted to either the left or right, with tilted face looking forward
5. Head upright and rotated toward left or right, face looking in either direction

Any one head position may change pharyngeal-oral resonating structures in such a way that a change in vocal quality (either better or worse) may occur.

B. Procedural aspects of the approach
   1. Introduce the approach by demonstrating various head positions, either by photograph, video, or live demonstration. A simple explanation of the technique should accompany the demonstration: "Sometimes changing the positions of our heads can improve the sound of our voices. The head can either be tilted down or back, or to the left or right. Sometimes we can improve the sound of our voices simply by turning our heads to one side or the other. No one head position seems to help everyone. Let us try a few and listen to any changes in voice we hear."
   2. The best voicing task to use to search for head position influence is the prolongation of vowels, such as /i/, /ɪ/, /ɛ/, /æ/, /o/, or /u/. Once a helpful position is discovered, any kind of voice practice material can be used.
   3. Many gradations in positioning are possible between the normal head position and one of the extreme head positions described previously. For example, when flexing the neck and bringing the head

down in a gradual movement, perhaps at the beginning of the movement, a voice change can be noted. As soon as change can be noted, if it is to occur, the head should be kept at that position without going to the full range of the movement.

4. Neurologically impaired patients may experience some oral-pharyngeal asymmetry from their disease—that is, one side of the neck or oral cavity may function better than the other side. A particular lateral movement of the head may make a sudden and noticeable improvement in voice in such patients. If so, then ask the patient to practice voice material with the head in the lateral position.

5. Patients with vocal hyperfunction—that is, patients who use too much effort to talk—often profit most from neck flexion with the chin tucked down toward the chest. Such downward carriage of the head seems to promote greater vocal tract relaxation. If an easy, target voice is achieved with neck flexion, this head-down position should be held during voice practice attempts.

C. Typical case history showing utilization of the approach

Mary was a 55-year-old housewife who had vocal difficulties for the past 5 years. A subsequent voice evaluation found that she had a moderately severe functional dysphonia accompanied by neck tension with severe mandibular restriction, hard glottal attack, and an inappropriately high voice pitch. Voice therapy was scheduled twice weekly with therapy focus on increasing her mouth opening, developing an easy glottal attack with "a legato phonatory style." The chewing and open-mouth approaches were unsuccessful until changing head position was added to the therapy. Mary was instructed to "tuck in her chin," flexing the anterior neck muscles with her face looking downward. Keeping her chin down, she was able to reduce neck tensions; she experienced immediate improvement in vocal quality. In subsequent therapy sessions, she developed an awareness that much of her past vocal strain was related to her tendency to hyperextend her neck; by using the opposite head position with anterior neck flexion, she was able to produce voice with relatively little strain. This change of head position, coupled with other therapy techniques designed to promote greater oral openness and ease of vocal production, helped Mary reestablish a normal voice.

D. Evaluation of the approach   Using another head position by flexing or extending the neck can have an immediate effect on voice quality. Such an approach is usually used in combination with other voice therapy facilitating approaches. Whereas patients with severe functional tensions often profit from anterior neck flexion—as did Mary, as just described—patients with neurogenic voice problems often profit from using some of the other head positions described earlier, in A. Changing head positions to facilitate better voice requires much trial and error. If a particular head position works, use it; if not, try another position.

15. HIERARCHY ANALYSIS

A. Kinds of problems for which the approach is useful   In hierarchy analysis, the patient lists various situations in his or her life that ordinarily produce some anxiety and arranges those situations in a sequential order from the least to the most anxiety provoking. Individual patients may instead prepare a hierarchy of situations, ranging from those in which they find their voices best to those in which they find them worst. This technique is borrowed from Wolpe's (1987) method of reciprocal inhibition, which teaches the patient relaxed responses to anxiety-evoking situations. After identifying a hierarchy of anxiety-evoking situations, the patient begins by employing the relaxed responses in the least anxious of them and, in therapy, works his or her way up the hierarchy, thereby eventually deconditioning his or her previously established anxious responses. The identification of hierarchical situations (less anxiety–more anxiety; worst voice–best voice) is a useful therapeutic device for most patients with hyperfunctional voice problems, which by definition imply excessive overreacting. Patients with functional dysphonia, or with dysphonias accompanied by nodules, polyps, and vocal fold thickening, frequently report that their degrees of dysphonia vary with the situation. Such patients may profit from hierarchy analysis.

B. Procedural aspects of the approach

1. Begin by developing in the patient a general awareness of the hierarchical behavior to be studied. If, for example, the patient is to be asked to identify those situations in which he or she feels most uncomfortable, discuss with the patient the symptoms of being uncomfortable. Or if the patient is going to develop a hierarchy of situations in which he or she experiences variation of voice, discuss and give examples of what is a good voice or a bad voice. Explain that the patient must develop a relative ordering of situations, sequencing them from "good" to "bad." Some patients are initially resistant to this sort of ordering, perhaps because they never realized that there are relative gradations to their feelings of anxiety or relative changes in their quality of voice. They may not be aware that the degree of their anxiety or hoarseness is not constant.

2. Although the majority of voice patients are soon able to arrange situations into a hierarchy, a few require practice sequencing some neutral stimuli. On one occasion, a woman was taught the idea of sequential order by arranging five shades of red tiles from left to right, in the order of the lightest pink to the darkest red. Having done this, she was then able to sequence her voice situations, proceeding gradually from those in which her voice was normal to those in which it was extremely dysphonic.

3. As a home assignment, have the patient develop several hierarchies with regard to his or her voice. One hierarchy might center on how the patient's voice holds up with the family, another on how it is related to the work situation, and a third on what happens to it in varying situations with friends. An excellent example of hierarchical situations developed by a woman with vocal nodules is discussed in an article by Gray et al. (1965). After these hierarchies have been developed by the patient at home, review them in therapy.

4. In therapy, use the "good" end of the hierarchical sequence first. That is, begin by asking the patient to recapture, if possible, the good situation. The goal of therapy is to duplicate the feeling of well-being or the good voice that the patient experienced in the situation rated as best. Efforts should be made in therapy to recall the good factors surrounding the more optimum phonation. If the patient is successful in re-creating the optimum situation, his or her phonation will sound relaxed and appropriate. The re-created optimum situation thus serves as an excellent facilitator for producing good voice. After some success in re-creating the first situation on the hierarchy, capturing completely his or her optimum response (whether this is relaxation or phonation or both), the patient will then be able to move on to the second situation. Again the goal is to maintain optimum response. The rate of movement up the hierarchy will depend entirely on how successfully the patient can re-create the situations and maintain optimum response. By using the relaxed response in increasingly more tense situations, the patient is conditioning himself or herself to a more favorable, optimum behavior.

5. Although some patients can re-create situations outside the clinic with relative ease, some cannot. As soon as possible, have the patient practice the optimum response outside the clinic under good conditions, so that he or she will eventually be able to use it in the real world in more adverse situations. The patient must not lose sight of the goal of maintaining the good response in varying situations outside clinic.

6. Some patients succeed in going just so far up the hierarchy, only to reach a situation in which they continuously have a maladaptive response. When this occurs, the patient should drop back to a lower hierarchical level and attempt once more to capture the optimum response under more favorable conditions. When a good response is again maintained, efforts at the next level should be resumed.

C. Typical case history showing utilization of the approach

Laurie was a 24-year-old forest conservationist who worked in an office with 10 male conservationists. For 6 months she had experienced recurring dysphonia, particularly when on the telephone at work. Laryngoscopic examination found that she had an "early nodule formation on her left vocal cord"; during the voice evaluation she demonstrated a relatively normal voice. The patient's dysphonia appeared to fluctuate, and it became particularly severe, she reported, in certain anxiety-provoking situations. As part of her 3 months of voice therapy, Laurie was asked to develop several hierarchical scales, listing the situations in order, from those in which she experienced a normal voice to those in which she became all but aphonic. Following is the hierarchy Laurie developed for her vocal responses at the office:

Best Voice
1. Calling mother on the phone every day from the office.
2. The female secretary at the office is easy to talk with, particularly when the older men in the office are not around.
3. Dictating on the dictaphone and talking to the secretary are about the same.
4. Bill W. talks to me a lot at the office and on dates.
5. The younger men kid me about going out with them on field trips.
6. The older conservationists at the office keep reminding me that I have only school and no field experience, which always makes me clear my throat.
7. Talking about forestry projects on the phone is hard.
8. I lose my voice entirely when talking to our regional manager, and if I can't get over this, I will lose my job.
Worst Voice

By rank ordering the situations in which she experienced best voice and worst voice, Laurie developed insight about the role of interpersonal relationships and their direct impact on her voice. Symptomatic therapy coupled with hierarchy analysis in her case did not improve the sound of her voice or reduce the additive lesion on the left vocal fold. Voice therapy was terminated after 3 months in favor of psychotherapy.

D. Evaluation of the approach   Most voice patients report great variability in voice quality, depending on how much they have been using the voice, the time of day, and the psychodynamics of the speaking situations. Hierarchy analysis is often helpful for dealing with vocal inconsistencies experienced while talking with different people in various situations. By analyzing the hierarchical situations in which voice deteriorates or improves, the patient develops an awareness of those situational cues that are causing voice changes. Perhaps for the first time, the patient realizes that voice quality is not a constant; typical of the normal speaker, vocal quality fluctuations are somewhat dependent on how relaxed one feels, how comfortable one is with his or her listeners. Therapy then focuses on using the best voice found low on the hierarchy. The patient attempts to use that optimum voice in those situations in which he or she has previously experienced difficulty. Hierarchy analysis is consistently useful in voice therapy.

16. INHALATION PHONATION

A. Kinds of problems for which the approach is useful   The high-pitched vocalization produced on inhalation is always produced by true vocal fold vibration (Lehmann, 1965). The technique is useful, therefore, for helping patients who are aphonic or who have developed an odd form of phonation, such as ventricular phonation, find true fold vibration. Williams, Farquharson, and Anthony (1975) have written that reverse phonation viewed by fiber-optic endoscopy shows the vibrating folds well. Inhalation phonation is also an excellent method of eliciting true phonation in patients who are experiencing functional aphonia. Greene and Mathieson (1989) write that inhalation phonation can be effectively used as a therapy approach with the occasional patient who exclusively uses "the ventricular band voice." The method is also useful with the occasional patient who is experiencing a functional *puberphonia*—that is, maintaining an inappropriately high pitched voice despite a vocal mechanism that has matured beyond puberty. The ease with which most patients produce the high-pitched inhalation voice makes the method useful in establishing or reestablishing true vocal fold vibration.

B. Procedural aspects of the approach

1. This particular approach, which is similar to masking, is perhaps better demonstrated than explained. Demonstrate inhalation phonation by phonating a high-pitched hum while elevating the shoulders. It is important to time the initiation of the inhalation with shoulder elevation. Elevate the shoulder so you can mark for the patient the contrast between inhalation (shoulders raised) and exhalation (shoulders lowered).

2. After demonstrating several separate inhalations with simultaneous shoulder elevation and phonation, say, "Now, I'll match the high-pitched inhalation voice with an expiration voice." Inhale, raising the shoulders and simultaneously humming in a high pitch, then dropping the shoulders on exhalation and producing the same voice. Repeat the inhalation-exhalation matched phonations several times.

3. Ask the patient to make an inhalation phonation. He or she should repeat the inhalation phonation several times. Now again repeat the inhalation-exhalation matched phonation, taking care to make the associated shoulder movements. Then tell the patient, "Now drop your shoulders on expiration, making the same high-pitched voice as you do it." With a little practice, most patients are able to do it.

4. After the patient has produced the matching hum, say, "Now, let us extend the expiration like this." Demonstrate a continuation of the high pitch, sweeping down from your falsetto register to your regular chest register on one long, continuous expiration. Repeat this several times. Then say to the patient, "Once I've brought my vocal cords together at the high pitch, I then sweep down, keeping them together, down to the pitch level of my regular speaking voice."

5. If the patient is unable to produce this shift from high to low, repeat the first four steps. If the patients can make the shift down to the regular speaking register, say, "Now you're getting your vocal cords together for a good-sounding voice." Take care at this point not to rush the patient into using the "new" voice functionally. Rather, have the patient practice some similar hum phonations. After some practice just phonating the hum, give the patient a word list containing simple monosyllabic words for "true" voice practice.

6. Once the patient is able to produce inspiration-expiration without difficulty, he or she should be instructed to no longer use the pronounced shoulder movements. Elevating and dropping the shoulders are only necessary to mark the difference between inspiration and expiration.

7. Stay at the single-word practice level until normal voicing is established. We often spend several therapy periods practicing the new phonation as a motor practice drill without attempting to make the voice conversationally functional. You might say, "Now we're getting the vocal folds together the way we want them." This places the previous aphonia or ventricular phonation "blame" on the mechanism rather than on the patient. Counseling with the patient at this time is important. The motor practice gives the patient time to adjust to the more optimum way of phonating.

C. Typical case history showing utilization of the approach

Derek, a 5-year-old boy, was found to have small bilateral vocal nodules. His speech clinician placed him on complete voice rest, which unfortunately was enforced for 5 continuous months. At the end of 5 months, the nodules had disappeared, and Derek was instructed by both the physician and the speech pathologist to resume normal phonation. Despite all his efforts, Derek could only whisper. He became completely aphonic, but whispered easily to all people with much animation and relative comfort. This functional aphonia remained for 2 months, after which he was instructed, "Go back and talk the normal way." Derek gestured that he wanted to use his voice but he could not "find it." Therapy efforts for restoring phonation were begun about 7 months after Derek's phonations had ceased. Inhalation phonation was initiated, and at the first therapy session Derek was able to produce a high-pitched inhalation sound and to follow his clinician well by matching the inhalation with an expiration sound. He was able to use an expiration phonation, appropriate in both quality and pitch, by the end of the first therapy session. He was scheduled for two other appointments within a 24-hour period, during which he practiced producing his regained normal voice. He was counseled that his "voice is working now and you'll never have to lose it again." The boy has had normal phonation since his voice was restored using the inhalation phonation technique. Counseling to curb yelling and other vocal abuses appeared to be successful, as Derek has experienced no return of the bilateral vocal nodules.

D. Evaluation of the approach
Some patients who experience either aphonia or ventricular phonation for any length of time lose their ability to initiate normal true fold phonation. The longer the aphonia or dysphonia persists, the harder it might be to use normal voice. Inhalation phonation is a simple way to produce true cord approximation and voicing. The high-pitched voice on inhalation probably results from the vocal folds being longer in their inhalation posture, and even though

they may adduct on command, they remain in their longer configuration. This elongated posture thins them, resulting in the higher-pitched phonation. The patient is able to match the inspiration sound with an expiration sound.

17. MASKING

A. Kinds of problems for which the approach is useful Patients with functional aphonia are often able to produce normal phonation under conditions of auditory masking. Some patients with functional dysphonia produce faulty voices because of poor auditory monitoring of what they are doing. The masking facilitating approach uses a voicing-reflex test, used by audiologists as the Lombard test (Newby, 1972). In fact, the Lombard test was first introduced as a method of finding voice in patients with functional aphonia. When asked to phonate in a loud-noise background, patients with functional aphonia sometimes used light voice. In the voice-reflex situation, the patient wears earphones and is asked to read a passage aloud. As the patient is reading, a masking noise is fed into the earphones. The louder the masking, the louder the patient's voice. At loud masking levels the patient cannot monitor well either the loudness or the clearness of his or her voice. Some patients with functional dysphonias actually experience clearer voices when they cannot monitor their productions because of loud masking. The clinician may make a tape recording of all the patient's oral reading, with and without masking, and then play back the results to the patient. The patient may well experience the "proper" set for more optimal phonation during the masking conditions and be able to maintain this improved production without continued masking.

B. Procedural aspects of the approach
    1. The masking approach is best used without any prior explanation. Because increased voice loudness comes about with increased intensities of masking on a reflexive, nonvolitional basis, there is no need to discuss the method in advance. In fact, there is evidence that some patients can override the voice reflex and maintain constancy of voice loudness despite fluctuations in masking intensity.
    2. The patient is seated next to an audiometer. He or she then puts on headphones and listens to a bilateral presentation of masking at a low level, roughly 40 dB SPL. Once the patient acknowledges hearing the masking, the masking stimulus is discontinued. The patient is then instructed to read aloud and to keep reading, no matter what kind of interruption he or she may hear in the headphones. Typically, the patient is asked to read aloud for a total period of about 2 minutes, with the masking fluctuating off and on throughout the reading. On playback variations in loudness of the patient's voice usually signal when the masking noise was introduced and when it ceased.

3. An audiocassette recording should be made as the patient reads aloud. An aphonic patient's whisper may change to voice under conditions of masking. It is important to have recorded the emergence of voice, which the patient can use in step 5. The dysphonic patient (functional, ventricular, or puberphonic) should also be recorded while using the masking approach. Marked differences in voice quality between the absence or presence of masking conditions will probably be evident.

4. Five- or ten-second exposures to masking are introduced to the patient bilaterally. The intensity levels should be in excess of 90 dB SPL, which is sufficiently loud to mask out the patient's own voicing attempts. Whenever an aphonic patient hears the loud masking, he or she may attempt some feeble vocalization. Under masking a dysphonic patient will produce a louder voice and often a voice with more normal vocal quality, as well.

5. Do not use the masking method beyond the trial stage with those few voice patients who do not demonstrate the voice-reflex effect. If it works well, and produces voice improvement, the method may be used as part of every therapy period. You might then experiment by having the patient listen to tapes of himself or herself, to see whether the patient can match volitionally his or her voice under masking conditions. Recordings can then be made contrasting the voice without masking (attempting to re-create the same voice as heard under masking) and the voice with masking. Try to have the voices sound alike.

6. A patient may profit from reading aloud under masking conditions, and then having the masking abruptly ended to see if he or she can maintain the better voice. Many other variations using the masking noise can be initiated by inventive clinicians.

C. Typical case history showing utilization of the approach

Lillian was a 9-year-old girl who had a history of vocal nodules that had been previously treated successfully with voice therapy. Several months after therapy had been terminated as successful (no nodules, normal voice), Lillian developed a severe influenza that left her with no voice. She was completely aphonic, and could communicate only by whispering and using good facial expressions and gestures. The aphonia continued for 1 month (over the December holiday break) before she returned to the voice clinic. The masking approach was used with Lillian after attempts at modeling and request for voice failed. Lillian was asked to read aloud under conditions of 90 dB masking. Her reading attempts were recorded on a 20-second loop tape. As soon as masking was introduced, light phonation was heard and recorded on the loop cassette. The masking and oral reading were stopped, and Lillian was asked to hear her good voice on the tape. The child clapped her hands in joy that she now had a returned voice. Further masking followed by ear training was used as her voice became stronger. After two follow-up therapy sessions, Lillian was discharged with a normal voice. The pushing approach—producing the word *patch* with sudden extension of arms—

was then demonstrated for Lillian to use "if you ever lose your voice again." Hopefully, her "believing" in pushing as a protection against future voice loss will function as a placebo effect and prevent any recurrence of aphonia. Lillian has had no voice problem in the 2 years since the 1 month of aphonia.

D. Evaluation of the approach The masking approach is most helpful with aphonic patients. It is also helpful for patients with some form of functional dysphonia or young men with puberphonia. If the masking noise is loud enough, in excess of 90 dB SPL, patients cannot hear their voices to monitor phonation. If required to continue speaking by reading aloud under conditions of masking, patients will often produce relatively normal voices under the masking condition. Clinicians should use some care in confronting the patients on audiotape playback with their "good" voices. Improved voices under conditions of masking should be used as the patients' models for their own imitation phonations. Clinicians should use the masking approach with some degree of eclecticism—that is, if the approach works, use it; if it does not, quickly abandon it.

18. NASAL/GLIDE STIMULATION

A. Kinds of problems for which the approach is useful Clinicians frequently note that in voice therapy certain stimulus sounds seem to facilitate an easier-produced, often better-sounding voice. This is particularly true working with children and adults with problems of vocal hyperfunction. Watterson, McFarlane, and Diamond (1993) have found in studying 15 adult voice patients with vocal hyperfunction and 15 matched control subjects that nasal and glide consonants facilitated better voicing patterns and were judged by the hyperfunctional subjects as "easier" to produce. The concept of differences in vocal effort have been also investigated by Bickley and Stevens (1987) and Baken and Orlikoff (1988), generally finding that supraglottal resonance-articulatory postures have a direct relationship to laryngeal physiology and function. Using words that contain many nasal and glide consonants, usually coupled with other therapy techniques, often helps the patient produce desired "target" vocalizations. Using nasal/glide consonants as therapy stimuli is particularly useful for patients with functional dysphonia, spasmodic dysphonia, and dysphonias related to fold thickening, nodules, and polyps.

B. Procedural aspects of the approach
   1. Most therapy techniques require the patient to say something. For example, in the open-mouth approach or in practicing focus, the patient is given a few stimulus words to say. Words that contain nasal or glide consonants will often produce the best-sounding voice or the voice that appears made with the least amount of effort (as compared to words containing other consonants).

2. The clinician can find a number of monosyllabic and polysyllabic words containing nasal consonants for the patient to practice saying as the response when using various facilitating approaches. Here are a few examples: *man, moon, many, morning, many men, moon man, manual lawnmower, Miami millionaire, morning singing.*

3. A variation of the technique is to use nasal monosyllabic words and introduce an /a/ between each word. Ask the patient to say three words in a row with the neutral /a/ between each word. For example, "man a man a man" or "wing a wing a wing."

4. We use the same procedure for words containing glide consonants. It has been found, however, that nasal consonants combine very well with the /l/ and /r/ phonemes and many of our glide words contain nasal consonants: *loll, lil, rare, rah, lilly, arrow, marrow, married, married women, one lonely memory, Laura ran around, remember many lawmen.*

5. Using monosyllabic /l/ and /r/ words with an /a/ between them seems to produce good voice, such as "lee a lee a lee" or "rah a rah a rah."

C. Typical case history showing utilization of the approach

Louise was a 66-year-old housewife who was forced to divorce her husband of some 42 years. She experienced a number of somatic symptoms following the divorce, including a severe functional dysphonia. Endoscopic-stroboscopic examination revealed a high carriage of the larynx with moderate vocal fold compression. The yawn-sigh approach was found to be effective in lowering her larynx and encouraging a more optimal vocal fold approximation. Under the sigh condition, she was asked to say various words. It was found that words with many nasal and glide consonants facilitated the easiest-produced and best-sounding voice. Intensive self-practice and twice-weekly voice therapy for 9 weeks, supplemented by concurrent psychological counseling, resulted in a good functional return of normal voice.

D. Evaluation of the approach

Clinicians are always looking for voicing tasks that facilitate good voice production. Recent research has validated that certain sounds, particularly nasal and glide consonants, facilitate voice production. Among patients with vocal hyperfunction, nasal/glide consonant words are perceived by patients as producing voice with less effort (Watterson, McFarlane, & Diamond, 1993). Word stimuli containing many nasal/glide consonants appear to facilitate in voice therapy a voice that sounds better and is produced (according to patient self-evaluation) with less effort.

19. OPEN-MOUTH APPROACH

A. Kinds of problems for which the approach is useful

Encouraging the patient to develop more oral openness often reduces generalized vocal hyperfunction. Opening the mouth more while speaking and learning to listen with a slightly open mouth allow the patient to use his or her vocal mechanisms more optimally. The open-mouth approach promotes more natural size-mass adjustments and more optimum approximation of the vocal folds, and this helps correct problems of loudness, pitch, and quality. Opening the mouth more is also recommended to increase oral resonance and to improve overall voice quality. The voice also sounds louder. Developing greater openness should be part of any voice therapy program wherein the patient is attempting to use the vocal mechanisms with less effort and strain.

B. Procedural aspects of the approach

1. Have the patient view himself or herself in a mirror (or on a videotape playback, if possible) to observe the presence and absence of open-mouth behavior. Identify any lip tightness, mandibular restriction, or excessive neck muscle movement for the patient.

2. Children seem to understand quickly the benefits of opening the mouth more to produce better-sounding voices. In our voice program for children (Boone, 1993), we use a brief story that illustrates two boys, one who talks with his mouth closed and one who speaks with his mouth open. We then introduce a hand puppet and ask the child if he or she has ever been a ventriloquist. The ventriloquist is described as someone who does not open the mouth, in contrast to the puppet, who makes exaggerated, wide-mouth openings.

3. The ventriloquist-puppet analogy also works well with adults. Let the patient observe the marked contrast between talking with a closed mouth and talking with an open one. Ask the patient to watch himself or herself speak the two different ways in a mirror. Instruct the patient that what he or she is attempting will at first feel foreign and inappropriate. The initial stages of letting the jaw relax are frequently anything but relaxed.

4. To establish further this oral openness, ask the patient to drop the head toward the chest and let the lips part and the jaw drop open. Once the patient can do this, have him or her practice some relaxed /a/ sounds. When the head is tilted down and the jaw is slightly open, a more relaxed phonation can often be achieved.

5. In order for patients to develop a feeling of openness when listening, and as a preset to speaking, they must first develop a conscious awareness of how often they find themselves with tight, closed mouths. One way to develop this awareness is to have patients mark down, on cards they carry with them, each time they become aware that their mouths are closed unnecessarily. The marking task itself is often enough to increase a patient's awareness, and over a period of a week the number of mouth closings will decrease notably. Another way of developing an awareness of greater orality is to have patients place in their living environments (on a dressing table, desk, or car dashboard) a little sign that says "OPEN," or perhaps has a double arrow (↕), or any other code that might serve as a reminder.

6. A patient who wants to achieve greater oral openness must practice a lot. Steps 3 and 4 facilitate greater mouth opening and are thus good practice tasks. In addition, many voice and diction texts have good oral openness tasks (see Modisett and Luter, 1984; Newcombe, 1986). Practice procedures for developing greater oral opening may also be found in voice therapy practice kits (Boone, 1982, 1993) and in voice therapy texts, such as Andrews (1986), Wilson (1987), or Case (1991).

C. Typical case history showing utilization of the approach
J. J., a 17-year-old high-school girl, was examined by a laryngologist about 1 year after an automobile accident in which she had suffered some injuries to the head and neck. Laryngoscopic examination found all visible laryngeal structures normal in appearance and function, despite the fact that since the accident the girl's voice had been only barely audible. The speech pathologist was impressed "with her relatively closed mouth while speaking, which seemed to result in extremely poor voice resonance." Voice therapy combined both the chewing and the open-mouth facilitating approaches. It was discovered in therapy that for 3 months after the automobile accident the girl had worn an orthopedic collar that seemed to inhibit her head and jaw movements. It appeared that much of her closed-mouth, mandibularly restricted speech was related to the constraints imposed upon her by the orthopedic collar. When using the open-mouth approach with her head tilted down toward her chest, she was immediately able to produce a louder, more resonant voice. The open-mouth approach was initiated before beginning chewing exercises, and both achieved excellent results. Therapy was terminated after 6 weeks, with much voice improvement in both loudness and quality.

D. Evaluation of the approach   The voice, both normal and dysphonic, improves in quality with greater mouth opening. Upon opening the mouth a bit more, the voice usually improves immediately. Besides opening the mouth more while speaking, the approach also encourages slight mouth opening while listening. In a previous description of a vocal hygiene approach, Boone (1980) wrote, "A gentle opening of less than one finger wide between the central incisors keeps the teeth apart and generally fosters a relaxed oral posture" (p. 40). The open-mouth approach has been particularly effective with performers who often open their mouths well during performance (acting, singing) but may forget the importance of opening their mouths during conversation.

20. PITCH INFLECTIONS

A. Kinds of problems for which the approach is useful   The prosodic and stress patterns of the normal speaking voice are characterized by changes in pitch, loudness, and duration. In some individuals, the lack of pitch variation is noticeable because the resulting voice is monotonous and boring to listeners. Speaking on the same pitch level with little variation, which for the average speaker is impossible to maintain, requires the inhibition of natural inflection. It is usually observed in overcontrolled persons who display very little overt affect. Fairbanks (1960), who describes pitch variation as a vital part of normal phonation, defines inflection and shift: "An *inflection* is a modulation of pitch during phonation. A *shift* is a change of pitch from the end of one phonation to the beginning of the next" (p. 132). Voice therapy for patients with monotonic pitch seeks not only to establish more optimum pitch levels, but also to increase the amount of pitch variability. Any voice patient with a dull, monotonous pitch level will profit from attempting to increase pitch inflections.

B. Procedural aspects of the approach

1. The patient must first become aware of his or her monotonous voice by listening to playback samples of voices. Play the patient's voice first, and follow it with samples of voices with excellent pitch variability. Follow the listening with evaluative comments. Have the patient self-evaluate, as well.

2. Begin working on downward and upward inflectional shifts of the same word, exaggerating, in the beginning, the extent of pitch change. Voice and articulation books, such as Fairbanks (1960), Modisett and Luter (1984), Newcombe (1986), or Boone (1991), contain good practice materials for improving pitch variability.

3. Using the same practice materials, have the patient practice introducing inflectional shifts within specific words.

4. Pitch inflections can be graphically displayed on many instruments, such as the Visi-Pitch or PM 100 Pitch Analyzer. Set target inflections for the patient, to see if the patient can make his or her pitch level reach the same excursions or movement as the target model on the scope .

5. Record and playback for the patient various oral reading and conversational samples, critically analyzing the productions for degree of pitch variability.

C. Typical case history showing utilization of the approach

Dr. T., a 51-year-old economics professor, received severe course evaluations from his students, who complained of his "monotonous" voice. On a subsequent voice evaluation, during both conversation and oral reading, he used "the same fundamental frequency with only minimal excursion of frequency." His voice was indeed monotonous, not only in pitch, but in loudness, as well. He also used the same duration characteristics for most vowels. Dr. T. was highly motivated to improve his speaking voice and manner of speaking. Subsequent therapy focus was on increasing pitch inflections and improving loudness variations. He was provided with audiocassette tapes, which he practiced daily, matching the target model productions with his own voicing attempts. After 6 weeks of voice therapy and intensive self-practice, Dr. T. demonstrated improvement in both his conversational and lecture voices. Unfortunately, his lack of overall animation and boring affect still resulted in poor course evaluations. However, his conversational voice with increasing pitch inflections appeared to make a much more favorable impression on those around him.

21. RELAXATION

A. Kinds of problems for which the approach is useful   It may well be that most dysphonic voices and laryngeal pathologies are related to continuous and prolonged vocal hyperfunction. Accordingly, a frequent goal in voice therapy is to attempt to take the "work" out of phonation. Using such therapy techniques as the open mouth and the yawn-sigh approaches, it is possible to increase the relaxation of muscles contributing to vocal function. Such symptomatic relaxation methods might well relax the vocal tract but not necessarily lead to overall systemic relaxation. It is usually useless in voice therapy to imply to tense patients that if they would "just relax," then all would be well. If patients could relax, many of them would; if their tension did not, in fact, serve them in some way, they would get rid of it. A certain amount of psychic tension and muscle tonus is normal and healthy, of course, but some individuals do overreact to their environmental stresses; instead of "running at a slow idle," they are like "fast-idle engines," expending far more energy and effort than a situation requires. By relaxation, therefore, we mean a realistic responsiveness to the environment with a minimum of needless energy expended. Some, but certainly not all, voice patients profit from a therapy program designed to reduce unnecessary tension by using relaxation techniques. Relaxation programs (Jacobson, 1957; Wolpe, 1987) and various stress-reducing programs (Staats, 1968; Stroebel, 1983) have been effective in developing greater relaxation and reducing stress in patients with dysphonia. Such relaxation measures might well be combined, however, with voice relaxation techniques such as described by Aronson (1990), Case (1991), or Greene and Mathieson (1989).

B. Procedural aspects of the approach
    1. The classical method of differential relaxation might be explained to the patient and applied. Under differential relaxation, the patient concentrates on a particular site of the body, deliberately relaxing and tensing certain muscles, discriminating between muscle contraction and relaxation. The typical procedure here is to have the patient begin distally, away from the body, with the fingers or the toes. Once the patient feels the tightness of contraction and the heaviness of relaxation at the beginning site, he or she moves "up" the limb (on to the feet or hands, and thence to the legs or arms), repeating at each site the tightness-heaviness discrimination. Once the torso is reached, the voice patient should include the chest, neck, "voice box," throat, and on through the mouth and parts of the face. With some patients, we start the

distal analysis with the head, beginning with the scalp and then going to the forehead, eyes, facial muscles, lips, jaw, tongue, palate, throat, larynx, neck, and so on. Some practice in this progressive relaxation technique can produce remarkably relaxed states in very tense patients.

2. Various biofeedback devices can help the patient develop a feeling of relaxation. Such feedback as galvanic skin response, pulse rate, blood pressure, or muscle responsiveness through electromyographic tracings all seem to correlate well with patients' feelings of anxiety and tension. By performing a particular relaxed behavior, such as yawning, a patient can confirm his or her particular arousal state by the biofeedback data. Using such biofeedback devices, the patient can soon learn what it "feels" like to be relaxed or free of tension.

3. Wolpe (1987) combines relaxation with hierarchy analysis. The patient responds to particular tension-producing cues with a relaxed response, such as feeling a heaviness or warmth at a particular body site, and maintains a relaxed response in the tension situation. The patient may instead develop a situational hierarchy specific to tension and voice by attempting to use a relaxed voice at increasingly tense levels of the hierarchy, as outlined in the adult voice program by Boone (1982).

4. Head rotation might be introduced as a technique for relaxing components of the vocal tract. The approach is used in this way: The patient sits in a backless chair, dropping the head forward to the chest; the patient then "flops" his or her head across to the right shoulder, then lifts it, then again flops it (the neck is here extended) along the back and across to the left shoulder; he or she then returns to the anterior head-down-on-chest position and repeats the cycle, rolling the head in a circular fashion. A few patients will not find head rotation relaxing, but most will feel the heaviness of the movement and experience definite relaxation in the neck. Once a patient in this latter group reports neck relaxation, he or she should be asked to phonate an "ah" as the head is rolled. The relaxed phonation might be recorded and then analyzed in terms of how it sounds in comparison to the patient's other phonations.

5. Open-throat relaxation can also be used. Have the patient lower the head slightly toward the chest and make an easy, open, prolonged yawn, concentrating on what the yawn feels like in the throat. The yawn should yield conscious sensations of an open throat during the prolonged inhalation. If the patient reports that he or she can feel this open-throat sensation, ask him or her to prolong an "ah," capturing and maintaining the same feeling experienced during the yawn. Any relaxed phonations produced under these conditions should be recorded and used as target voice models for the patient. Encourage the patient to comment on and think about the relaxed throat sensations experienced during the yawn.

6. Wilson's *Voice Problems of Children* (1987) includes an excellent presentation on various relaxation procedures for use with children,

developed by Wilson and other authors, which seem to have equal applicability to adults. Most of the procedures described can immediately increase relaxation and reduce tension associated with speaking.

7. Ask the patient to think of a setting he or she has experienced, or perhaps imagined as the ultimate in relaxation. Different patients use different kinds of imagery here. For example, one patient thought of lying in a hammock, but another person reacted to lying in a hammock with a set of anxious responses. Settings typically considered relaxing are lying on a rug at night in front of a blazing fire, floating on a lake, fishing while lying in a rowboat, lying down in bed, and so on. The setting the patient thinks of should be studied and analyzed; eventually, the patient should try to capture the relaxed feelings he or she imagines might result from, or may actually have been experienced in, such a setting. With some practice—and some tolerance for initial failure in recapturing the relaxed mood—the average patient can find a setting or two that he or she can re-create in his or her imagination to use in future tense situations.

C. Typical case history showing utilization of the approach

M. Y., a 34-year-old missile engineer, developed transient periods of severe dysphonia when talking to certain people. At other times, particularly in his professional work, he experienced normal voice. Mirror laryngoscopy revealed a normal larynx. During the voice interview, the speech pathologist was impressed by the man's general nervousness and apparently poor self-concept. In exploring the area of interpersonal relationships, the patient confided that in the past year he had seen two psychiatrists periodically, but had experienced no relief from his tension. Further exploration of the settings in which his voice was most dysphonic revealed that his biggest problem was talking to store clerks, garage mechanics, and persons who did physical labor; some of his more relaxed experiences included giving speeches and giving work instructions to his colleagues. Subsequent voice therapy included progressive relaxation. Once relaxed behavior was achieved, the patient developed a hierarchy of situations, beginning with those in which he felt most relaxed (giving instructions to colleagues) and proceeding to those in which he experienced the most tension (talking with car mechanics). After some practice, the patient was able to recognize various cues that signaled increasing tension. Once such a cue occurred, he employed a relaxation response, which more often than not enabled him to maintain normal phonation in situations that had previously induced dysphonia. As this consciously induced response continued to be successful, the patient reported greater confidence in approaching the previously tense situations, knowing he would experience little or no voice difficulty. Voice therapy was terminated after 11 weeks, when the patient reported only occasional difficulty phonating in isolated situations and increased self-confidence in all situations.

D. Evaluation of the approach   The popularity of many relaxation and stress-reduction programs today is probably due in part to their offering

people with excessive tensions some relief from their agonies. Symptomatic voice therapy focuses on faulty voices and sometimes the tensions associated with (if not the cause of) the vocal problems. A growing number of voice clinicians feel that direct symptom modification, such as teaching relaxed responses to replace previously tense responses, breaks up the circular kind of response that often keeps maladaptive vocal behaviors "alive." In effect, we talk the same way today that we talked yesterday until we learn a better way to respond. Using the voice in a more relaxed manner with less competitive tension is a "better way to respond."

22. RESPIRATION TRAINING

A. Kinds of problems for which the approach is useful   In the first part of the 20th century, some of the articles about voice therapy supported the view that most voice disorders were related to poor breathing patterns—and singing teachers and dramatic coaches to this day include breathing exercises and breathing technique as part of their instruction. The modern-day voice clinician, whether a laryngologist or a speech pathologist, places far less emphasis on faulty respiration than his or her predecessors did. Nonetheless, some voice patients, described in earlier chapters, do profit from improving their control of respiration, especially their control of the expiratory phase of the breathing cycle. Although general improvement in total respiration, such as an improvement in vital capacity, has little effect on the voice, any marked departure in the inspiratory-expiratory cycle may produce noticeable voice alterations.

Among voice and articulation books that have excellent practical exercises for breathing for speech are *Voice and Diction* (Newcombe, 1986), *Your Voice and Articulation* (Glenn, Glenn, & Forman, 1989), and *Effective Voice and Articulation* (Stemple & Holcomb, 1988). Perhaps the most helpful respiration exercises and suggestions in voice textbooks can be found in *The Voice and Its Disorders* (Greene & Mathieson, 1989).

B. Procedural aspects of the approach
   1. Most voice patients profit from a simple explanation of phonatory physiology—a description of the transglottal pressure and flow of outgoing air that sets the approximated vocal folds in vibration. If the patient demonstrates a problem in this area (and work on respiration should be avoided if no problem exists), describe the problem and what can be done about it.
   2. Demonstrate a slightly exaggerated breath, as used in sighing. The sigh is characterized by a slightly larger-than-usual inhalation followed by a prolonged open-mouth exhalation. Describe the type of breath used to produce the sigh as the "breath of well-being," the kind of easy breath one might take when comfortable or happy—the sigh of contentment.
   3. Demonstrate the quick inhalation and prolonged exhalation

needed for a normal speaking task. Take a normal breath and count slowly from one to five on one exhalation. See if the patient can do this; if he or she can, extend the count by one number each time, at the rate of approximately one number per half-second. This activity can be continued until the patient is able to use his or her "best" phonation during the number counts. Any sacrifice of vocal quality should be avoided, and the number count should never extend beyond the point at which good quality can be maintained.

4. Various duration tasks, such as prolonging vowels, provide excellent practice in expiratory control. Prolonging an /s/, /z/, /a/, /ɑ/, /æ/, or /i/ for as long as possible provides an expiratory measure that can be used for comparison. Take a base-line measurement in the beginning, such as number of seconds a particular phonation can be maintained, and see whether this can be extended with practice. Avoid asking the patient to "take in a big breath"; rather, ask him or her to take in a normal breath of well-being, initiating a lightly phonated sigh on exhalation. See if the patient can extend this for 5 seconds. If so, progressively increase the extension to 8, 12, 15, and finally 20 seconds. The voice patient who can hold on to an extended phonation of a vowel for 20 seconds has certainly exhibited good breath control for purposes of voice. Such a patient would not have to work on breath control per se, but he or she might want to combine work on exhalation control with such approaches as hierarchy analysis (to see if he or she can maintain such good breath control under varying moments of stress).

5. Select from various voice and articulation books reading materials designed to help develop breath control. Give special attention to the patient's beginning phonation as soon after inhalation as possible, so as not to waste a lot of the outgoing airstream before phonating. Encourage the patient to practice quick inhalations between phrases and sentences, taking care not to take "a big breath."

6. With young children who need breathing work, begin with nonverbal exhalations. One way to work on breathing exhalation with little children is to use a pinwheel, which lends itself naturally to the game "How long can you keep the pinwheel spinning?" With practice, a child will be able to extend the length of his or her exhalations (the length of time the pinwheel spins). Another method of enhancing exhalation control is to place a piece of tissue paper against a wall, begin blowing on it to keep it in place when the fingers are removed, and keep blowing on it to see how long it can be kept in place. Both the pinwheel and tissue-paper exercises lend themselves to timing measurements; these measurements should be made and plotted graphically for the child; when a certain target length of time is reached, the activity can be stopped.

7. When working with a singer, actor, or lecturer who needs some formal respiration training, you might take the following steps:

a. Discuss the importance of good posture, because normal posture is one of the best facilitators of normal breathing. Any real departure from good posture, such as leaning forward with the head (kyphosis), may contribute to faulty breathing.

b. Demonstrate abdominal-diaphragmatic breathing. First, have the subject lie supine, with his or her hands on the abdomen, directly under the rib cage. In this position, distention of the abdomen upon inspiration will be observable. The downward excursion of the diaphragm, which increases the vertical dimension of the chest, cannot be viewed directly (because the diaphragm attachments are behind and inside the ribs); its effect can be viewed only by the outward displacement of the abdomen. On expiration, as the diaphragm ascends, the abdominal distention lessens. In this form of breathing, then, the patient should deliberately try to relax the abdominal muscles during inspiration and contract them during exhalation. If this can be done successfully in the supine position, the patient should try to duplicate the procedure while standing with the back flat against a wall. Continuing to clasp his or her hands on the abdomen will help the patient develop some initial awareness of the difference between abdominal relaxation-distention and abdominal contraction-flattening. As soon as the subject learns to breathe by this relaxation—contraction of the abdominal muscles—introduce some phonation activities to be done on expiration. The voice patient who has been speaking "from the level of his or her throat," without adequate breath support, will often "feel" the difference that a bigger breath makes only when phonation is added. The voice patient who needed respiration training in the first place must have respiration and phonation combined into practice activities as soon as possible.

8. For serious problems in respiration, which are often related to such illnesses as emphysema or bronchial asthma, the clinician should enlist the help of other specialists to help the patient improve respiratory efficiency. Physical therapists, inhalation therapists, and pulmonary medical specialists may have the expertise required to assist the patient. The voice clinician can often offer the patient ways of phrasing and using expiratory control to better match what the patient is trying to say and thus can supplement the respiration therapy of these other specialists. For example, we have coordinated a breathing-for-speech program for quadriplegic patients, in which the speech pathologist and the physical therapist work closely with the patient to improve both general respiration and expiratory control for speech phrasing and better voice.

C. Typical case history showing utilization of the approach

Libby was a 45-year-old special-education teacher who complained of vocal fatigue as a regular part of her teaching day. She felt that when she was not working, her voice was not a problem. Observation of Libby during her voice evaluation revealed that conversationally she often began to speak without an adequate inspiration. After five or six consecutive spoken words, her voice would become dysphonic and strained. Her voice problems seemed to occur when her air volumes were low and she was experiencing inadequate transglottal airflow. Subsequent voice therapy, designed to reduce the amount of work she was putting into vocalization, gave some priority to increasing her inspiratory volumes, reducing the number of words she attempted to speak on one breath, and teaching her to take "catch-up" breaths when she needed them. Loop tape recordings were used in therapy to monitor her breath support; she would read a 10-word sentence aloud and then immediately listen to a loop playback of the utterance, judging it for respiratory adequacy and lack of strain. After 5 weeks of twice-weekly voice therapy working on better respiratory control, Libby developed an easy phonatory style and a voice that served her well in her various life situations, including her teaching.

D. Evaluation of the approach   A number of voice patients may profit from some kind of respiration training. At the time of the initial voice evaluation, such patients may have done poorly on air-volume and pressure tests, or exhibited poor expiratory control. Vocal attempts, by such patients are often strained and involve too much effort; symptoms of vocal hyperfunction are common. A slight increase of inspiratory volume may produce an immediate effect of reducing vocal strain and improving overall vocal quality.

23. TONGUE PROTRUSION

A. Kinds of problems for which the approach is useful   Many hyperfunctional voice problems are improved by the tongue-protrusion approach. This approach is especially helpful for patients with ventricular phonation (dysphonia plica ventricularis) or "tightness" in the voice, such as when the laryngeal aditus (laryngeal collar) is held in a somewhat closed position. When the tongue is held in a posterior position or the pharyngeal constrictor muscles are contracted to constrict the pharynx, the voice will sound strained or "tight." A patient with such symptoms is asked to produce /i/ with the tongue extended outside of the mouth (but not far enough to cause discomfort). This works to offset the squeezing of the pharynx. The tongue must not protrude so far outside of the mouth that it causes muscle strain in the area under the chin. The /i/ is produced in a high pitch either at the upper end of the patient's normal pitch range or at the lower end of the falsetto register. This approach can be used simultaneously with the glottal fry or the yawn-sigh.

B. Procedural aspects of the approach
    1. Demonstrate to the patient what is expected by opening the mouth and protruding the tongue while producing a high-pitched, sustained /i/. Stress that the jaw is to "drop open" comfortably and that

the tongue is to be extended comfortably. Many patients are reluctant, at first, to stick out the tongue in the presence of a stranger, so demonstrate and reassure them that this is just what you want. You may touch the patient's chin with the index finger to encourage a little wider jaw opening and say, "Roll the tongue out a little farther."

   2. Patient should go up and down in pitch while sustaining the /i/ vowel, with the mouth open and the tongue out. Listen for improved vocal quality. When this is achieved, ask the patient to sustain the tone.

   3. Have the patient chant /mimimimi/ at this level with the tongue still out of the mouth. Then instruct the patient to slowly "slip" the tongue back into the mouth while continuing to produce the /mimimimi/.

   4. At this point, the pitch is usually still high. Demonstrate a sustained /i/ that is lowered by three steps from the pitch that the patient was producing. This often produces a good quality on the first step or the first two steps, but a return to the poor voice may occur on the third step. Repeat the procedure, but only go down two steps. Sustain the second step. Repeat until the tone is established. You may need to return to the original open mouth and tongue protrusion if the target tone is lost.

   5. When the new tone is established, gradually add words to the sustained /i/—e.g., "be, pea, me," "see the peach," and "easy does it."

C. Typical case history showing utilization of the approach

Tammy, a 15-year-old girl, was referred with ventricular phonation of more than 18 months' duration. Her voice, which was consistently hoarse, rough, and low in pitch, was effortful to produce and made her sound like an older male speaker. Tammy had undergone a prolonged bout of flu prior to the onset of the ventricular voice, and she frequently coughed and cleared her throat violently. Strong glottal valving could be heard at times during connected speech. After seven sessions of individual voice therapy using the tongue-protrusion approach just described, Tammy's voice was normal in all situations at home, in school, and at work for the first time in more than 18 months.

D. Evaluation of the approach

This approach appears to work because the tongue, when protruded, pulls its root out of the pharynx and opens the laryngeal aditus. Also, the high pitch is made with a light, breathy approximation of only the true vocal cords. The production of voice with the tongue outside of the mouth is sufficiently novel so as not to trigger the typical pattern of phonation that may have become habituated.

24. WARBLE

A. Kinds of problems for which the approach is useful

When patients have habituated a dysphonia over a long period of time, it is sometimes difficult to break up or interrupt the habitual (almost automatic) mode of phonation producing the hoarse, rough, or breathy voice. In an attempt to break the strongly established pattern, we have used the warble tone phonation. If one has a "muscle set" strongly associated with the onset of phonation, this can be offset by changing the phonatory adjustments of the larynx. This is what happens in the warble approach. Patients constantly change pitch and loudness (to a lesser degree) until they are instructed to extend the tone at a particular level of pitch and loudness. With warble, the pitch is constantly shifted up and down until the phonatory or prephonatory set is disrupted and new vocal tone can be produced free from excessive laryngeal muscle tension and free of the undesirable vocal quality. An instrument that displays the pitch for the patient as well as displays the vocal roughness can greatly aid the patient in his or her use of this technique. The instrument's trace of the frequency and jitter (pitch perturbation) will display the warble tone visually. The "scatter" (produced by jitter in the voice) or departure of the trace from a tight single line trace can easily be seen by the patient as a target for pitch and quality. The Visi-Pitch display works well to display the success of this technique for the patient. Any patient who has a hoarse, rough, strained, or breathy voice may be a candidate for this approach regardless if the voice is secondary to functional adjustments or related to nodules or other cord pathology such as cord thickening and polyps.

B. Procedural aspects of the approach

1. Ask the patient to listen to the clinician produce a tone that is varied up and down in pitch. At the same time, the loudness will usually vary, increasing as pitch is raised and decreasing in loudness with pitch lowering. The patient is instructed to watch the trace on the scope and imitate the clinician.

2. The patient produces the tone with an /i/ vowel for a comfortable duration at a mid-loudness level, constantly shifting the tone up and down. The clinician watches the trace on the screen and listens to the tone. When the tone sounds best the trace will be less scattered or more of a solid line. When the best sound tone and most compact trace are achieved, the tone is extended at that level. It is important that the tone not be interrupted or broken but extended at a desired pitch and loudness level.

3. When the patient has successfully produced a warble tone two or three times and has seen these on the screen display, the next task is to make the warble portion shorter and the steady-state vowel portion longer in duration. For example, if the warble is 2 seconds, extend the steady-state portion for 5 or 6 seconds. This is repeated several times.

4. Next the extended portion is produced without the warble. At this point, usually, the inappropriate muscle set is interrupted. If the patient loses the new mode of phonation initiation, the clinician returns to step 1 above. The new phonatory set or mode of phonation is then transferred into vowel-initiated words and all voiced short phrases such as "even now," "easy days," etc.

C. Typical case history showing utilization of the approach

Margaret, a 39-year-old female with a 4-year history of a rough, very hoarse voice (perturbation, jitter level of 20) was referred by an ENT physician following recurring bouts of throat infection. There were no instances of clearer voice at any time in her speech. Both the ENT exam and the videostroboscopy demonstrated normal laryngeal structure; however, the stroboscopy study revealed a very lax adjustment of the cords. The mucosal wave was extremely exaggerated. Other facilitating techniques failed to produce an improvement in the voice. Using the warble technique at a very high pitch broke up her phonatory set, which had persisted for 4 years. The improved quality of voice production was first extended at 400 Hz and in the same session worked down to 220 Hz. This voice was transferred to the phrase level at 220 Hz with a perturbation level of .4 (which is within the normal range) in the same initial treatment session. In subsequent therapy sessions, the voice was stabilized in conversation and appeared normal in every measure.

D. Evaluation of the approach   The effect of this approach appears to be that the warble fluctuations of pitch and loudness are sufficiently novel to interrupt the inappropriate laryngeal muscle set adopted by the dysphonic patient and used subsequently whenever the patient phonates. It also allows the clinician to use a glide of pitch and loudness adjustments, sliding into a new, more appropriate mode of phonation without the patient being aware of the "slide" into normal or near-normal voice.

25. YAWN-SIGH

A. Kinds of problems for which the approach is useful   The yawn-sigh is one of the most effective therapy techniques for minimizing the tension effects of vocal hyperfunction. Characteristically, in vocal hyperfunction, we see the larynx rise, the tongue lifted high and forward, the vocal folds tightly compressed, and the pharynx constricted (Boone & McFarlane, 1993). The yawn-sigh provides a dramatic contrast: The larynx drops to a low position, the tongue is more back, there is a slight opening between the vocal folds, and the pharynx is usually dilated, as seen in Figure 5–4. The yawn-sigh is frequently combined with other therapy approaches for such problems as functional dysphonia, spasmodic dysphonia, and dysphonias related to thickening, vocal fold nodules, and polyps.

B. Procedural aspects of the approach
   1. With children explain this approach using the pictures and narrative from *The Voice Program for Children* (Boone, 1993). Showing a child the appropriate pictures, we read:
   This girl usually has a tight mouth. She uses too much effort when she speaks. Her voice does not sound good. (Demonstrate) This girl is opening her mouth wide and yawning. She is very relaxed. When she sighs at the end of the yawn, it will be her best voice. (p. 141)
   2. With teenagers and adults explain generally the physiology of a yawn—that is, that a yawn represents a prolonged inspiration with maximum widening of the supraglottal airways (characterized by a wide, stretching, opening of the mouth). You may show the photograph in Figure

5–4 and contrast it with other CT scans of the pharynx taken while subjects were doing other vocal tasks, as displayed by Pershall and Boone (1986). Then demonstrate a yawn and talk about what the yawn feels like.

3. After the patient yawns, following your example, ask the patient to yawn again and then to exhale gently with a light phonation. In doing this, many patients are able to feel an easy phonation, often for the first time.

4. Once the yawn-phonation is easily achieved, instruct the patient to say words beginning with /h/ or with open-mouthed vowels, one word per yawn in the beginning, eventually four or five words on one exhalation.

5. With teenage and adult clients, there are yawn-sigh exercises available, with explanations that the patient can read, in *Is Your Voice Telling on You?* (Boone, 1991, pp. 122–126).

6. Demonstrate for the patient the sigh phase of the exercise—that is, the prolonged, easy, open-mouthed exhalation after the yawn. Then, omitting the yawn entirely, demonstrate a quick, normal, open-mouthed inhalation followed by the prolonged open-mouthed sigh.

7. As soon as the patient can produce a relaxed sigh, have him or her say the word *hah* after beginning the sigh. Follow this with a series of

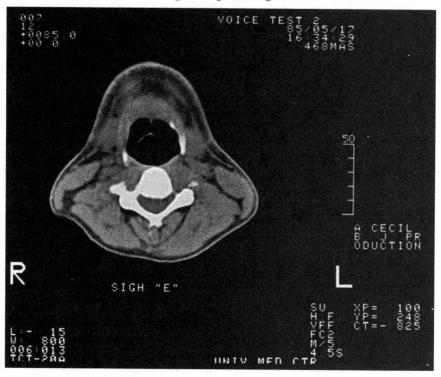

FIGURE 5–4   A CT Scan
A CT scan depicting the dilated pharynx of a normal subject producing a prolonged /i/ vowel on an expiratory sigh. This CT scan was taken near the apex of the arytenoids, showing the horizontal cross section of the neck and mandible. Vertebral bone is shown in white; the open airway (with a slice of epiglottis across it) is represented in black (absence of tissue).

words beginning with the glottal /h/. Additional words for practice after the sigh should begin with middle and low vowels. Take care to blend in, toward the middle of the sigh, an easy, relaxed, relatively soft phonation. This blending of the phonation into the sigh is often difficult for the patient initially, but it is the most vital part of the approach for the elimination of hard glottal contacts.

8. Once the yawn-sigh approach is well developed, have the patient think of the relaxed oral feeling it provides. Eventually, he or she will be able to maintain a relaxed phonation simply by imagining the approach.

C. Typical case history showing utilization of the approach

Jerry, a 47-year-old manufacturer's representative, had a 2-year history of vocal fatigue. He often lost his voice toward the end of the work day. After a 2-week period of increasing dysphonia and slight pain on the left side of the neck, a consulting laryngologist found that Jerry had "slight redness and edema on both vocal processes." The subsequent voice evaluation also found that he spoke with pronounced hard glottal attack in an attempt to "force out his voice over his dysphonia." Using the yawn-sigh approach, Jerry was able to demonstrate a clear phonation with relatively good resonance. His yawn-sigh phonations were recorded on loop tape and fed back to him as the voice model he should imitate. Because Jerry reported some stress in certain work situations, the hierarchy analysis approach was used to isolate those situations in which he felt relaxed and those in which he experienced tension. Thereafter, whenever he was aware of tense situational cues, he employed the yawn-sigh method to maintain relaxed phonation. Combining yawn-sigh with hierarchy analysis proved to be an excellent symptomatic approach for this patient, because his voice cleared markedly, and no recurrence of the periodic aphonia was evident. Twice-weekly therapy was terminated after 22 weeks, and the patient demonstrated a normal voice and a normal laryngeal mechanism.

D. Evaluation of the approach

The yawn-sigh is a powerful voice therapy technique for patients with vocal hyperfunction. During the yawn-sigh, the pharynx is dilated and relaxed. When the patient is asked to sigh an /i/ or an /a/, the voice comes out with little effort and sounds relaxed. For some patients with continued vocal hyperfunction, the voice produced on the sigh will feel relaxed, in dramatic contrast to the patient's normally tense voice.

SUMMARY

Successful voice therapy requires that the clinician identify the patient's aversive vocal behaviors and subsequently reduce the occurrence of such abuses-misuses. Voice therapy for most voice problems requires continuous assessment of what the patient is able to do vocally. By using various therapy approaches as diagnostic probes, the clinician searches for the best voice the patient is able to produce. Twenty-five facilitating approaches were presented; each has detailed specific procedures of application and an illustrative case history showing its particular effects.

Chapter 6

Voice Therapy
for Special Problems

The 25 facilitating approaches in Chapter 5 are broadly used in voice therapy. In this chapter, we look at how these approaches and other management strategies may be used for 12 special problems of voice. Most of these special problems were first described in Chapter 4.

Rather than presenting 12 special problems of voice in alphabetical order, we have made an attempt to group these problems into three overall categories: Special Problems Where There Is No Voice, Special Problems Using a Poor Mode of Phonation, and Special Problems Related to Certain Conditions. While there is some commonality of disorder under each topic heading, as seen in Table 6–1, there is much overlapping and lack of distinct boundaries.

SPECIAL VOICE PROBLEMS WHERE THERE IS NO VOICE

Abductor Spasms

Abductor spasms of the vocal folds produce temporary phonation breaks. A patient may be speaking with a normal voice (or a dysphonic one) when the vocal folds suddenly separate, and produce a fleeting aphonia. In previous editions of this text, the term *phonation breaks* has aptly labeled these annoying and continuing aphonic breaks. Shipp, Mueller, and Zwitman (1980) introduced the term *intermittent abductory dysphonia* to label these sudden phonatory breaks, which seems to indicate that the patient experiences a sudden change of voice, rather than a sudden loss of voice. Aronson (1985) continues to use the term *abductor spastic dysphonia to* describe these "brief moments of breathy or whispered

Table 6–1. Special Voice Problems

Special Voice Problems Where There Is No Voice

Abductor spasms
Functional aphonia
Laryngectomy
Paralytic aphonia

Special Voice Problems Using a Poor Mode of Phonation

Diplophonia
Pitch breaks
Puberphonia
Spasmodic dysphonia
Ventricular phonation

Special Voice Problems Related to Certain Conditions

The aging voice
Dysarthria
Hard of hearing or deaf

(unphonated) segments" (p. 187). Davis et al. (1987) questioned the wisdom of including a patient labeled as having "abductor spastic dysphonia" in their study of 25 patients with spasmodic dysphonia, because airflow, otolaryngologic, and neurologic data demonstrated clear differences between "adductory" and "abductory" spasmodic dysphonia.

Watterson and McFarlane (1992) question the continued use of the terminology *abductor spasmodic dysphonia*, feeling that these abductor spasms have an entirely different etiology and an opposite set of symptoms. The intermittent aspect of abductory spasms appears somewhat related to the degree of vocal hyperfunction in which the speaker is engaged. The greater the amount of tense phonation, the greater amount of abductor spasms.

Therefore, the best management of the problem seems to come from reducing overall vocal hyperfunction. If hyperfunctional behaviors can be identified and reduced, the phonation breaks are usually minimized. For example, a local hard-rock disc jockey suffered from phonation breaks when he was attempting to give the news "straight" for 5 minutes on the hour. It was soon discovered that his broadcasting style away from the news was extremely "hyper" and false and thus produced obvious strain on his vocal mechanism. Voice therapy was directed toward producing a disc-jockey style that was less aversive. The happy result was that he was able to read the news copy free of phonation breaks. Such intermittent losses of voice during voicing are usually the result of prolonged vocal hyperfunction. Once the hyperfunction can be reduced, the phonation breaks usually disappear. Facilitating approaches described in Chapter 5 that have been found useful for eliminating abductory spasms might include counseling, ear training, elimination of hard glottal attack, the open-mouth approach, relaxation, developing greater respiratory efficiency, and the yawn-sigh.

Functional Aphonia

The diagnosis of functional aphonia is made when a patient is examined by endoscopy or laryngoscopy while asked to produce and prolong an "ee" (/i/). Instead of the folds adducting into the midline position when the patient phonates, they simply do not vibrate. The patient's laryngeal muscle function is normal, unlike that of a paralytic aphonic, whose folds (one or both) are paralyzed in a fixed position. In aphonia, patients lose their voice completely and speak in a whisper. Despite the inability to use voice, most patients with functional aphonia maintain excellent communicative pragmatics—for example, looking at the other person, using appropriate social affect and gestures, and, in general, seeking out communication rather than retreating from it.

Our use of the term *functional aphonia* to describe vocal mutism is at variance with two other authors (Aronson, 1990; Case, 1991) who use the term *conversion aphonia* to highlight the psychological origins of lack of voice in patients with normal larynges. Aronson distinguishes between muteness (no articulatory movements, no whisper) and aphonia (an articulated, whispered airstream), although he does not offer a distinct and differential treatment regimen for each voiceless condition. Case views conversion aphonia as "a somatoform" disorder whose symptoms have no organic or physiologic basis, so that the patient often presents evidence of a "strong presumption to psychological disturbance or conflict" (p. 194). Despite the psychiatric focus given by the label "conversion aphonia," both Aronson and Case describe good success in treating the disorder symptomatically.

We recommend using the term *functional aphonia,* which implies that there is no physical cause for the voicelessness, and, more often than not, that the patient is ready to "release" the symptom and experience an immediate return of normal voice. In fact, functional aphonic patients as a group present excellent prognoses. A typical functional aphonic patient experiences complete return of voice within one to three therapy sessions. As stated in Chapter 3, functional aphonic patients are easily conditioned to continue to speak without voice. Whatever the original cause, the behavior is maintained by the reactions of the people around the patient. Such patients soon develop a *no voice* set toward speaking, and they establish habitual responses; they speak this way today because they spoke this way yesterday. Most patients with functional aphonia express a strong desire to regain their normal voice. (A few patients are served well by their aphonia, and they resist all therapeutic attempts at voice restoration.) The bias of the writers, developed from following aphonic patients over time, is that symptomatic voice therapy is usually effective in restoring normal voices in these patients. Once phonation is reestablished, it remains, and the patient does not develop substitute symptoms to take the place of the previous aphonia.

Successful voice therapy for functional aphonia must begin with the clinician's explaining and discussing the problem with the patient. In the physiological description of the aphonia, the clinician must avoid implying that the patient could phonate normally if he or she wanted. Rather, a description of what the patient is doing ("keeping the vocal cords apart") will make it clear that the clinician knows what the problem is. Following the physiological description, the clinician should say something like, "We will do things in therapy that will bring the cords together again to produce normal voice." The clinician should not (at the first session, at least) ask or show undue interest in *why the* patient is not phonating. After the explanation and discussion of the problem, the clinician should evaluate whatever nonverbal phonations the patient may have in his or her coughing, grunting, laughing, and crying repertoire, and then describe them to the patient as normal phonatory activities "in which the vocal cords are getting together well to produce these sounds." These nonverbal phonations should then gradually be shaped into use for speech, at first confining any speech attempts to nonsense syllables, and then moving on to single words, but with no early attempts at phonating during real communication. Attempts at phonating in conversational situations (i.e., in the real world of talking) should be deferred until good, consistent phonation has been reestablished under laboratory, practice conditions.

Steps to be followed in a symptomatic voice therapy program for functional aphonia might include the following:

1. *Counseling.* Point out to the patient that even though the vocal folds are normal, the problem appears to be an inability to "get them started producing voice." Focus the explanation on the *vocal folds* and not on the *patient.* Perhaps show a brief videotape depicting normal phonation.
2. *Coughing.* Ask the patient to cough. By definition, patients with functional aphonia are able to use the laryngeal mechanism for coughing. Take care to ask the patient to cough, not to ask, "Are you able to cough?" Most aphonic patients can cough. If the patient coughs, then ask him or her to prolong the cough with an extended vowel. If this phonatory prolongation can be done, then ask the patient to make a series of cough-initiated phonations, using the vowel /i/. If the patient cannot immediately extend the phonation, go to step 3 after the cough.
3. *Inhalation phonation.* This facilitating approach (see Chapter 5) uses true vocal fold phonation. The high-pitched phonation is always produced by true folds. If a patient can match the high-pitched inhalation with the same sound on expiration, ask him or her to prolong the phonation, as in step 2. Once the expiratory high-pitched phonation is established, introduce monosyllabic words beginning with vowels and /h/ for voice practice.
4. *Masking.* This approach is designed to reestablish phonation in patients with functional aphonia. Ask the patient to read a passage aloud in his or her whispered aphonic voice while wearing headphones attached to some kind of noise generator (such as white noise on an audiometer). As the

patient reads, introduce loud masking at selected intervals. The patient will often reflexively use voice under the masking conditions. Then play back a recording of the patient's reading attempts, which can often reveal true phonation for the patient. (See procedural details of the masking approach in Chapter 5.)

5. *Pacing*. Patients with aphonia should not be pushed too fast. Once normal voice is achieved, often by following one or more of the preceding steps, practice should stay at a single-word (using word lists) level. Making such statements as "Your vocal folds are coming together now" is helpful because they put the "blame" on the folds rather than the patient (Boone, 1966b).

6. *Progression*. Once voice is established by using single words beginning with vowels or /h/, single-word lists using any consonants or vowels can be used. Then progress to polysyllabic words, phrases, and sentences, but defer interactive conversation with the patient until voicing appears consistently.

In functional aphonia, voice can often be reestablished in one therapy session, perhaps followed by several sessions that permit more time for supervised voice practice and counseling. In the last session Case (1991) recommends that the clinician "continue the conversation mode until convinced of vocal stability, then make an appointment for a checkup in a few days" (p. 203). Once voice is reestablished after aphonia, patients rarely experience recurrences of the same symptom.

If the voice clinician has any doubt about the patient's general emotional stability, as indicated perhaps by the patient's continued inability to produce some phonation, he or she should refer the patient for psychological or psychiatric consultation. Sometimes the aphonic patient profits most from symptomatic voice therapy concurrent with psychotherapy. If psychotherapy is needed, however, the typical case involves a fairly rapid recovery of voice with relatively brief voice therapy and a much longer period of psychotherapy.

Laryngectomy

Carcinoma of the larynx continues to be the most serious of all laryngeal diseases. Fortunately, with microsurgery, radiation therapy, and/or chemotherapy, more patients with laryngeal cancers are able to preserve their larynges than ever before. Total laryngectomies used to be performed for smaller lesions than they are today. Unfortunately, however, the prevalence of laryngeal cancer is rising (Myers & Suen, 1989), resulting in a continuing number of new laryngectomy patients (laryngectomees). These patients generally represent one of two kinds of surgical approaches: (a) a total laryngectomy with continued anatomical separation between the trachea and the esophagus or (b) the laryngectomy followed by a surgically created tracheoesophageal shunt, which permits air to flow via the shunt from the trachea into the esophagus. These patients postoperatively require very different speech-voice training.

Both types of laryngectomies (conventional and tracheoesophageal) face problems of adjustment before and after the operation. Preoperative counseling by the speech-language pathologist, sometimes accompanied by a rehabilitated laryngectomee, is usually requested by the surgeon.

A brief preoperative visit by a speech pathologist and a laryngectomee is perhaps the best way to provide the most relevant information about the patient and also to give the patient some psychological support. It is important for the speech pathologist to assess how the patient speaks *before* the operation. Through conversation, the speech pathologist should roughly evaluate the patient's articulatory proficiency and overall speech intelligibility, and, because the long-term goal is to help the patient achieve intelligible speech, he or she should evaluate the patient's performance (independent of obvious voicing problems) in terms of rate of speech, dialect or accent, articulation errors, degree of mouth opening when speaking, eye contact, and so on. In the brief preoperative contact with the patient and his or her family, the speech pathologist should convey confidence that the "patient *will* talk again." In assuring the patient that a method will be found that he or she will be able to use, the speech pathologist should describe several methods of therapy and give a brief demonstration of the artificial larynx. He or she might tell the patient that as soon as the surgeon gives the "go ahead," the patient will be provided temporarily with an artificial larynx, so that he or she will be able to talk to people instead of writing out messages (as many laryngectomees have been instructed to do, as if using the artificial larynx would "contaminate" their chances of learning esophageal speech). As soon as the patient is physically ready postoperatively, as a prelude to receiving voice therapy, the patient is visited again by the speech pathologist and perhaps a lay laryngectomee.

The first postoperative visit should have a certain amount of flexibility, so that the visitors can respond to whatever questions the patient may have about these physical and psychological changes, and perhaps alleviate some of the patient's concerns about talking again. There is some advantage to bringing along some printed material, such as a few of the pamphlets about laryngectomy problems provided by the American Cancer Society. These materials offer the patient and family answers to many problems they may be facing. Selected laryngectomees from local laryngectomy clubs are often effective in relating their firsthand experiences with some of the postoperative problems the patient may have; for example, the physical problem of mucus in the stoma is often an early complaint, and it should be pointed out to the patient that successful control of excessive mucus at the stoma site is usually developed early. Just as with the preoperative visit, the combination team of the speech pathologist and the lay laryngectomee is most appropriate for the first visit after surgery.

Some patients are bothered by the physical disfigurement they begin to become aware of postoperatively. The open stoma in the neck is often the first anatomical disfigurement of which the patient becomes aware. The patient who has additional radical neck surgery for the removal of cancerous lymph nodes experiences additional disfigurement and large vertical scarring in the lateral neck area in addition to the laryngectomy. In the immediate postoperative period, the patient's surgical sites are well covered with bandages. As dressings are removed during the days that follow surgery, some patients experience violent feelings toward the dramatic alterations in their appearance. Both the patient and the family may need some guidance by the physician and nursing staff to help them accept the physical changes in appearance as well as in function of respiration and phonation.

Postoperative Medical Care and Problems of the Laryngectomee   As important as voice restoration may be, and as important as the speech pathologist's role may become, the primary consideration during and immediately after surgery is the preservation of life. Control of bleeding, preservation of the airway, prevention of infection, and nourishment of the patient are of primary concern to the medical team caring for the patient. In a conventional laryngectomy, the entire laryngeal mechanism is removed, including the hyoid bone. The hypopharyngeal opening into the esophagus and the esophagus itself are usually well preserved, although some of their sphincteral functions may be somewhat diminished by the removal of their attachments (hyoid bone, thyroid and cricoid cartilages). The trachea, which loses its connection with the pharynx and mouth, is brought to the skin surface and is attached directly superior to the suprasternal notch at this level. A permanent opening (tracheostomy) is constructed, through which the patient will forever breathe. After surgery an L-shaped plastic tube (cannula) is placed in the stoma (opening) to keep the stoma open and to prevent natural healing. The stoma must be kept open to permit unobstructed breathing. The inverted L-shaped cannula is used in this way: The tube is placed through the opening with the down shaft of the cannula going below the stoma into the trachea and the horizontal shaft remaining within the stoma opening. Some patients wear the cannula tube only for a few weeks after surgery; some laryngectomees prefer to wear the cannula all the time. If there were known or suspected cancerous nodes in the neck, the patient may have had, in addition to the laryngectomy, a radical neck dissection. This procedure involves the removal of the cervical lymph nodes as well as many of the normal-appearing nodes adjacent to the suspected cancer site. The dissection is usually done initially on one side only, and is sometimes followed later by the same procedure on the other side. Radical neck dissection greatly increases the site of surgical alteration, and the postsurgical medical and nursing care required is usually more intensive.

The new laryngectomee usually requires a day or two of absolute bedrest following surgery. The head of the bed should be slightly elevated so that the patient's head will be slightly flexed toward the chest, thus avoiding any tension on the sutures. Ambulation is started as soon as the patient's condition permits, frequently on the second or third day. The patient's fluid and caloric intake require constant monitoring, and attention must be given to his or her vital cardiac, pulmonary, and urinary functions. The patient will receive various antibiotics and analgesics (pain killers) as required. To prevent the patient from swallowing, and thus give the pharyngeal and esophageal structures time to heal, the patient is fitted with a feeding tube inserted through the nose and going directly through the pharynx into the esophagus and hence into the stomach. The feeding tube is usually removed on the 8th to the 10th postoperative day, if there is no unhealed fistula (small opening) between the esophagus and trachea or between the pharynx and the outer skin. About the time that fistulas are healed the surgeon gives approval to start voice-speech instruction. The referral to the speech pathologist and the beginning of voice instruction should be started, if possible, before the patient leaves the hospital.

Some patients fail to learn esophageal speech after a conventional laryngectomy and come back for a modification of the stoma and esophagus, known as a tracheoesophageal shunt. Other patients with their surgeons elect to have the tracheoesophageal shunt put in as the final procedure of the total laryngectomy. Through the open stoma in the neck, the surgeon creates a small surgical opening, or shunt, high on the exposed trachea-esophagus wall. A small prosthesis is then inserted through the shunt opening, two of which are shown in Figure 6–1. Outgoing pulmonary air coming up the trachea is then able to be diverted into the prosthesis and introduced through the shunt directly into the esophagus. The mechanics of using such a Blom-Singer prosthesis are described a bit later.

Voice Training of Laryngectomees The primary goal of speech pathologists working with laryngectomees is to help the patient develop adequate voice to permit functional communication. Many patients begin their training by using an artificial larynx, either a pneumatic type or an electronic artificial larynx. Some patients elect to use the artificial larynx exclusively, while some use it as an adjunctive aid, a device to help in communication. The majority of patients are able to use good esophageal voice, both those with conventional laryngectomies and those who have experienced the added procedure of the tracheoesophageal shunt.

Using the Artificial Larynx   The artificial larynx can be an aid to learning esophageal speech. Postoperatively, the artificial larynx allows the patient to communicate immediately with others. The speech-language pathologist can usually teach the patient quickly to use this new sound source for voice. There has yet to be invented a totally satisfactory instrument that produces a pseudovoice for the laryngectomy patient, although many good instruments are available today, as shown in Figure 6–2.

The steps listed below are good ways for the speech-language pathologist to introduce a new laryngectomee to an artificial larynx:

1. In telling the patient that efforts will now begin to help him or her learn to talk again, point out that he or she faces two problems—first, learning to articulate (pronounce) words again and, second, finding a new source of voice—and that the articulation will be tackled first. Next, demonstrate that the patient has basically the same capability of articulation that he or she had before the operation, but that he or she may have to make some sounds a bit differently, by employing intraoral pressure for some plosive and sibilant sounds instead of the usual pulmonary airstream. If possible, demonstrate the intraoral whisper, articulating to produce a "sound" with no pulmonary airstream. Then ask the patient to imitate these intraoral productions (which are, in fact, easier for a laryngectomee to produce than for the normal person with a larynx). Warn the patient not to try to push the sounds out by using pulmonary air (the use of pulmonary air will be indicated by excessive stoma noises). You must decide the appropriate level of complexity of the discussion and the

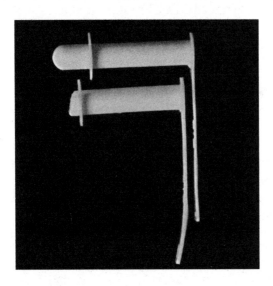

FIGURE 6–1   Two Blom-Singer Prostheses.
The top larger prosthesis is a modification of the original "duckbill" prostheses inserted via a shunt through the trachea into the esophagus. The lower, slightly smaller prosthesis is the newer low-pressure voice prosthesis. (*Photograph is used with permission of Eric D. Blom, Ph.D*).

amount of positive reinforcement to provide each individual patient. Remember, however, that the simpler the explanation and the more focus given to the actual demonstration, the easier the learning task will be.

2. When the patient can produce an intraoral whisper, introduce an orderly presentation of consonants, perhaps having him or her whisper each one 5 to 10 times. The best presentation seems to be along the general order of acquisition of consonants (/p/, /b/, and so on), first practicing the phonemes that are easiest to produce, and then going on to more difficult ones. For some patients the nasals /m/, /n/, and /ng/ may be difficult to produce and may require special attention that deviates from the developmental order. The patient should produce these sounds with as little effort as possible. The "trick," we say, is to go at this type of speech with an "easy does it" attitude and approach, even though the natural tendency is to work hard at learning to talk again. The patient should work for clarity of articulation. Point out to the patient his or her relative lip, tongue, and palatal competencies, as demonstrated by accurate whispering of the consonants. Then go back to the first point made in the therapy, that learning to talk again is a twofold process: articulation and voice. Tell the patient that success in practicing the whispered productions means that he or she is doing very well in the first area. The whispering practice will vary in length, depending on the intelligibility and motivation of the patient.

3. Now introduce the artificial larynx, either the pneumatic or

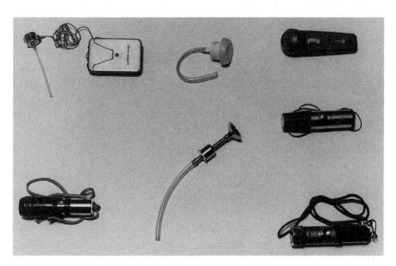

FIGURE 6–2   Seven Artificial Prostheses
Top left: Cooper-Rand intraoral electric larynx; *Top center:* Memacon artificial larynx DSP8 pneumatic; *Top right:* Western Electric neck device; *Bottom left:* Park Jed-Com electrolarynx; *Bottom center:* Tokyo reed type pneumatic artificial larynx; *Center right:* Servox neck device; *Bottom right:* Aurex neck held electrolarynx neovax.

electronic type. We limit our suggested procedures to the two types of electronic larynx. For the neck type, place the vibrating surface of the instrument tightly on your own neck at a site where you have previously determined your best voice to be. You might well repeat some monosyllabic words that include some of the phonemes the patient has just finished using in articulation practice. To these articulations, you should explain, the artificial larynx will introduce the second phase of speech, voicing. You might also use the artificial larynx to demonstrate some connected speech. For the oral-type larynx, take care to show that the intraoral tube does not interfere with the movement of the tongue. We have found that introducing the tube toward the corner of the mouth with the tube angled high toward the palate and about halfway back in the mouth seems to provide the best placement. The phrase "How are you?" is good because the vocal tract is open, and thus the end of the tube is not occluded by the tongue. The success of this production is due largely to resonance (vowels and diphthongs) and has a high probability of working for the patient.

4. Next, in offering the instrument to the patient, take a great deal of care to achieve a good seal between the neck skin of the patient and the surface of the neck vibrator. The vibrator head must be firmly buried against the neck, or the sound source will escape free field and not be directed into the oral cavity. This optimum site of contact, such as just above the site of the laryngeal excision in the midline, is found best by trial and error. The patient should say the same monosyllabic word repeatedly as he or she searches for the site of contact where the intraoral speech or voice sounds best. Much time should be given to achieving this optimum contact of vibrator and neck, because a great deal of early disillusionment with the artificial larynx can come from improper positioning of the instrument. Patients with extensive scarring, such as those who have had radical neck dissections or radiation, may experience real difficulties at first in finding the optimum site of contact. No practice in using the instrument should begin, however, until this critical contact point has been found. Also, once a good sound has been established, the patient will require some practice in working the on-off switch to match his or her articulations. Most patients can learn to do this rather quickly. For the oral instrument, care must be exercised to have the patient place the tube optimally within the mouth and ensure that it not interfere with tongue movement. We first use the phrase "How are you?" because it can be made with relatively little tongue interference. Following this phrase, we generally use number counting as the practice words to find the optimal oral placement of the tube. Trial and error can usually locate the best place to introduce the tube (again, we find that toward the side of the mouth with the tube angled high toward the palate and about halfway back in the mouth seems to provide the best placement).

5. The patient should then practice saying single monosyllabic words in a series, and after that go on to phrases and short sentences. At this point, remind the patient that he or she is now practicing speech. The sharper and clearer one can articulate, the more intelligible the speech will be. The patient should be instructed to discard his or writing pad and begin talking to everyone. The tremendous advantage afforded by the artificial larynx is that it permits the patient to talk shortly after the operation, which provides valuable articulation practice. The more one talks using the artificial larynx, the better his or her speech will usually become. Point out to the patient that the artificial larynx is providing him or her with a voice source while he or she practices improving articulation. After a few days of practice using the instrument, the patient will start learning how to supply his or her own voice by using some form of esophageal voice. Make it very clear to the patient that the artificial larynx and esophageal speech are not competitive forms of voice, but compatible methods that help to achieve good functional speech whenever there is a need to talk.

Teaching Esophageal Speech after Conventional Laryngectomy   Two methods of teaching esophageal speech may be employed: injection and inhalation. We usually begin with the injection method, which is the easiest to teach and is quite compatible with the articulation practice the patient may have used with the artificial larynx.

Both methods, however, employ the same basic principle of compressing air within the oropharynx and injecting this denser air into the more rarefied (less dense) space of the esophagus. Denser air within a body moves in the direction of the less dense body of air whenever the two bodies are coupled together. Some of the compressed air within the oral cavity undoubtedly escapes through the lips, some through the nasopharyngeal port, and some (particularly if the opening of the esophagus is open) into the esophagus. Both methods for esophageal voice bring compressed air into the esophagus; once the air is in the esophagus, external forces compress the air within it and expel it. Hopefully, the esophageal expulsion sets up a vibration of the pharyngo-esophageal (P-E) segment and the patient experiences an eructation or "voice." We consider separately the procedures for teaching the injection method and the inhalation method (sometimes we combine this method with injection).

The Injection Method   Certain consonants appear to have a facilitating effect in producing good esophageal voice. Individual patients may have their own favorite facilitating sounds, but more often than not these are plosive consonants (/p/, /b/, /t/, /d/, /k/, and /g/) or affricatives containing plosives (/tl/ or /d₃/). Stetson (1937) reported many years ago that /p/, /t/, and /k/ were the easiest sounds for the new laryngectomee to use; Moolenaar-Bijl (1953) reported that the same phonemes produced esophageal speech faster in most patients than the traditional swallow method of teaching. Diedrich and Youngstrom (1966) recommended the voiceless /p/, /t/, /k/, /s/, /l/, and /tl/ phonemes as good sounds to employ in the injection method of air intake. The injection of air is best accomplished by using speech that employs some of the consonants just identified. As the patient whispers monosyllabic words with a facilitating consonant before and after the vowel, he or she will sometimes spontaneously inject air into the esophagus and produce an "unplanned" esophageal voice. The production of the consonant facilitates the transfer of air into the esophagus (Shanks, 1986). The injection method is preferred for teaching esophageal voice. Specific steps for teaching injection might include the following:

1. Discuss with the patient the dynamics of air flow, explaining that compressed, dense air will always flow in the direction of less dense, rarefied air. Explain also how the movements of the tongue in the injection method increase the density of the air within the mouth, enabling the air to move into the esophagus. Then demonstrate how the whispered articulation of a phoneme, such as a /t/ or a /k/, is the kind of tongue movement that produces the injection of air into the esophagus. After producing the whispered /t/, demonstrate for the patient an esophageal voice for the word *tot* or *talk*.

2. Now ask the patient to produce the phoneme /p/ by intraoral whisper. Care must be taken that the sound is made by good firm compression of the lips, with no need for stoma noise. Make sure that the patient avoids pushing out the pulmonary exhalation or using tongue and palatal-pharyngeal contact as the noise source. The intraoral whisper can be effectively taught by having the patient hold his or her breath and then attempt to "bite off" a /p/ by compressing the air caught between his or her abruptly closed lips. The patient should continue practicing this until true intraoral articulation is clearly grasped. This is demonstrated when he or she is consistently able to produce a precise /p/. Once the patient can do this, he or she should move to the next voiceless plosive, /t/. Here, the tongue tip against the upper central alveolar process is the site of contact, and practice should be continued until the patient can produce a precise, clear /t/. The same procedure should be repeated for /k/, again first demonstrating for the patient the different site of contact.

3. When good intraoral voiceless plosives have been produced, the patient is ready to add the vowel /a/ to each plosive. With /p/, for instance, he or she makes the plosive, and then immediately attempts to produce an esophageal phonation of /a/, producing in effect the word *pa*. If this is successful, the patient may combine the /p/ with a few other vowel combinations before going on to the /t/ and /k/. If the patient fails to produce the esophageal voice at this point, he or she should go back and work for even crisper articulation of the plosive sounds. If the patient

is still unsuccessful after increased practice in articulation, he or she should attempt the inhalation method as the primary means of air intake.

4. The average laryngectomee experiences some success with the injection method when using the /p/, /t/, and /k/ phonemes. Therefore, he or she might be provided with about five monosyllabic words for each of the phonemes—for example, for /p/, the words *pat, pip, pack, pot,* and *pop.* The task is now to say each word, one at a time, renewing the esophageal air supply *as he or she speaks,* which is an obvious advantage of using the injection method. It is through the mere process of articulation that the patient takes in air. After the patient has demonstrated success with these phonemes, introduce their voiced cognates, /b/, /d/, and /g/. The same procedure should be repeated, ending with about five practice words for each new phoneme.

5. Additional phonemes, such as /s/, /z/, /ʟ/, /tʟ/, /ʒ/, and /dʒ/, may be introduced for practice. As the patient gains phonatory skill with each new consonant, he or she must spend extra time learning to improve both the quickness and the quality of production. Too many patients err in trying to develop functional conversation too early. Considerable practice should be spent at the monosyllabic word level, practicing one word at a time and making constant efforts to produce sharp articulation and a good-sounding voice.

6. Practice with basic control techniques is essential for developing successful and fluent esophageal speech. Therefore, we have the patient practice several skills directly in each speech session. These skills are:

a. Rapid production (one-half second or less) of esophageal phonation on command from the clinician with 100% success in response. If we call for 10 productions of the /a/ vowel, the patient must respond with 10.

b. Ability to sustain a tone for 2 1/2 to 3 seconds or longer.

c. Ability to interrupt the tone into three or four segments.

d. Ability to stress the first or second syllable on command (such as in the word *upper* for first-syllable stress, and *above* for second syllable stress).

e. Ability to make a soft or loud tone on command.

Each of these skills is practiced for a part of each speech session, much as a serious golfer practices on the putting green and driving range as well as playing in a real game. Patients who are too anxious to achieve connected speech and ignore practice may carry bad habits into speech that will detract from their developing good esophageal speech, and that are more difficult to correct at a later date.

7. At this point, if the patient has been successful, the inhalation method can be introduced to further improve air intake and esophageal phonation. The patient should produce a normal inhalation and, at the initial moment of exhalation, produce the consonant and say the word.

Beyond the single words alone, we often couple the words together in phrases, such as "bake a cake, stop at church, park the black cart," and so on. Once plosive-laden phrases are mastered, we then use the oral reading materials from voice and diction books, including, when possible, the facilitative consonants we have been using.

The Inhalation Method   The flow of air in normal respiration is achieved by the transfer of air from one source to another because of the relative disparity of air pressure between the two sources. For example, when the thorax enlarges because of muscle movement, the air reservoir within the lung increases in size, rarefying (decreasing) the air pressure within the lung. Because the outside atmospheric air pressure is now greater, the air rushes in until the pressure within equals the outside pressure. The flow of air is always from the more dense to the less dense air body, and the flow continues until the two bodies are equal in pressure. By this same airflow mechanism the esophagus inflates in the inhalation method of air intake. The patient experiences a thoracic enlargement during pulmonary inhalation, which reduces the compression on all thoracic structures, including the esophagus. If the cricopharyngeus opening into the esophagus is slightly open at the time of the slight increase in the size of the esophagus, air from the hypopharynx will flow into the esophagus. During the exhalation phase of pulmonary respiration, when there is a general compression of thoracic structures, the esophagus also experiences some compression, which aids in the expulsion of the entrapped air. As this air passes through the approximated structures of the lower pharynx-upper esophagus (P-E segment), a vibration is set up, producing esophageal phonation. The advantage of the inhalation method of esophageal air intake is that it follows the patient's natural inclination or pulmonary inhalation followed by exhalation-phonation. Simply to take a breath and then talk is the most natural way of speaking, and for this reason the inhalation method offers the patient learning esophageal speech some early advantages.

In proceeding to the following steps for teaching the inhalation method, remember that the approach is best used in combination with the injection method.

1. Explain and demonstrate to the patient some aspects of normal respiration. Many normal speakers, for example, have never thought much about normal respiration, and many do not know that their voicing has always been an exhalation event. Explain to the patient that when the chest is enlarged by muscle action, the air flows into the lungs, and that, in the laryngectomee's case, the air comes through the stoma opening in the trachea and down into the lungs. Point out that the chest enlarges by muscle action, not by air inflation; thus, the air comes in as the chest enlarges. When the laryngectomee's chest enlarges, a concomitant

enlargement of the esophagus usually takes place; when the esophagus is enlarged, there is a greater chance for air to come into it. When the chest becomes smaller, the pulmonary air is forced out, and the air within the esophagus is also more likely to be forced out. If possible, demonstrate esophageal voice using this method.

2. Before attempting to produce voice, the patient should practice conscious relaxation and correct breathing methods. He or she should become aware of thoracic expansion and abdominal distention on inhalation and of thoracic contraction on exhalation. Respiration practice should only be long enough to permit the patient to develop this kind of breathing awareness, because patients do not seem to benefit much from extended breathing exercises per se.

3. Now the patient should attempt to add air into the esophagus during his or her pulmonary inhalation. Diedrich and Youngstrom (1966) recommended that "the patient be told to close his mouth, imagine that he is sniffing through his nose, and to do so in a fairly rapid manner" (p. 112). Even though the sniff is basically a constricted inhalation, it is frequently accompanied by esophageal dilation (the normal person often swallows what he or she sniffs). As an extension of the sniff, the patient should be asked to take a fairly large pulmonary breath (through the stoma, of course). When his or her lungs appear to be about half inflated, the patient should say "up" on exhalation. This procedure can be repeated until the patient experiences some phonatory success.

4. For the patient who does not experience success in step 3, the following variation of the inhalation method sometimes produces good esophageal air: Ask the patient to take a deep breath, and, as he or she begins the inhalation, to cover the stoma. While the muscular enlargement of the thorax continues (despite the patient's lack of continuing inhalation), there will be a corresponding enlargement of the esophagus, perhaps permitting air to flow into the esophagus. For the patient who can get air into the esophagus but cannot produce the air escape necessary for phonation, the same mechanism applies in reverse. Here, the patient takes a deep inhalation and, as he or she begins to exhale, occludes the stoma; as the thorax begins to decrease in size, there will be increased pressure on the esophagus, which might well result in expulsion of esophageal air (and phonation).

5. If esophageal phonation is achieved by either of the last two steps, the patient should proceed from his or her "up" response to single monosyllabic words beginning and ending with /p/, /b/, /t/, /d/, /k/, and /g/. Time should be spent practicing at this single-word level, until the technique is mastered in terms of loudness, quality of sound, and articulation. The patient who masters the basic techniques of air intake and phonation at the single-word level may become the best esophageal speaker.

6. At this level, use steps 4 to 7 from the injection method.

Teaching Esophageal Voice with a Tracheoesophageal Shunt The patient who has a tracheoesophageal shunt or puncture will generally be able to develop good esophageal voice more quickly than the patient with a conventional laryngectomy. On expiration, by shutting off the open stoma with a finger or by using a one-way stoma valve, the patient is able to divert outgoing tracheal air into the Singer-Blom prosthesis, introducing air directly into the esophagus. Being able to do this negates the need for teaching the patient to trap air in the esophagus by either the injection or inhalation methods.

The decision must first be made whether the patient wishes to wear a one-way valve fastened on the stoma. This valve permits air to come in from the outside on inspiration, but shuts off on expiration, allowing air to travel through the shunt into the esophagus. Fujimoto, Madison, and Larrigan (1991) looked at the effect of the valve on developing good voice as opposed to using finger closure of the stoma, finding that there were no real differences in quality of voice between the two methods. The patient who must use his or her hands in work might profit from wearing the stoma valve; otherwise, occluding the open stoma when one wants to speak might be best achieved by using one's finger to close off the stoma. It does appear, however, that recent research favors the low-pressure prosthesis (see Figure 6–2) over the duckbill prosthesis for developing the best speaking voice (Pauloski, Fisher, Kempster, & Blom, 1989).

The teaching steps below are designed for the patient with a tracheoesophageal shunt, using finger occlusion of the stoma to speak:

1. The speech-language pathologist should review the procedures the patient has had. The Shedd and Weinberg (1980) book is helpful here because it summarizes most of the surgical procedures available.

2. A review of how normal voice is produced is helpful for the patient who may never have realized, for example, that all speech is produced on pulmonary expiration.

3. Practice should be given to producing precise articulation. The patient should be encouraged to practice intraoral whispers so that the words are distinct and clearly understandable to listeners.

4. The patient is asked to take in a normal breath, occlude his or her stoma with a thumb or a finger, and say a monosyllabic word on expiration. It is important that the patient be counseled to use the thumb or finger only as a diverting body to the airstream. Sending the air through the shunt (or the appliance in the shunt) does not require heavy finger pressure. Only a very light touch is required to divert the air from the stoma on expiration. If voice is achieved on the single word, the patient can go to the next step. If not, the patient should practice the timing of inspiration (open stoma) and expiration (closed stoma) in synchrony with saying one word. Trial-and-error repetitions may be needed here. Most patients can produce an effortless esophageal voice

with very little difficulty. It has been our observation that patients who cannot successfully divert tracheal air through the shunt are pushing too hard with their fingers. Only light touch on the stoma opening is needed.

5. Go from single words to phrases as soon as the patient can do so. It is important to keep the inspiratory breath a normal one. The patient needs no more breathing effort than he or she ever did. It takes some practice to time the inspiratory-expiratory phonation to match the words or phrases one is attempting to say.

6. Once the patient can say phrases, it has been our observation that, by using natural articulation, he or she begins injecting air into the esophagus from above and using the pulmonary air passing out through the esophagus. Therefore, some patients can speak some words and phrases without occluding their stomas, obviously renewing the air reservoir within the esophagus by injection. Extended daily practice of several hours for a week or two is required before a patient with a tracheal-esophageal shunt is able to use his or her new esophageal voice conversationally.

7. Review with the patient that the best voice seems to be produced with the least amount of effort—that is, a normal speaking breath, light finger touch, and so on.

Helping the Patient with a Laryngectomy   The patient with a new laryngectomy is facing a number of social obstacles. Research by Blood, Luther, and Stemple (1992) has found that 73% of 41 laryngectomy patients showed good adjustment to their problem. Fear of cancer reoccurrence and some loss of self-esteem are among problems the patients report. The speech-language pathologist working with the laryngectomee must provide some counseling and social guidance for the patient (Salmon, 1986). The patient needs exposure to other laryngectomy patients, some participation in laryngectomy clubs, and encouragement to participate again in life activities experienced before the operation. Successful rehabilitation after laryngectomy is highly related to the patient's overall life adjustment, coping skills, and general well-being.

Paralytic Aphonia

Loss of voice due to vocal fold paralyses happens suddenly. In unilateral paralyses, the paralyzed vocal fold is fixed usually in the paramedian position and cannot adduct medially. Unilateral paralyses are generally the result of cutting of or trauma to the recurrent laryngeal nerve on one side of the neck. Bilateral paralyses are more often the result of a central brain lesion usually in the brain stem or medulla.

Unilateral Adductor Paralysis   With the paralyzed vocal fold in the paramedian position, the patient experiences aphonia or a severe dysphonia, depending on the amount of vocal fold approximation that is possible. Because many such unilateral paralyses spontaneously recover within the first 6 months, conservative intervention measures are used. The surgeon, for example, would hold off doing any kind of surgical reconstruction until it was evident that the paralyzed side of the larynx would not recover spontaneously. Likewise, the speech pathologist would offer the aphonic or dysphonic patient with unilateral paralysis voice therapy that might help to establish the best possible voice (until possible nerve regeneration takes place).

During the interim period from onset to possible nerve regeneration, some techniques are useful for establishing usable voice, particularly for aphonic patients. First of all, in most cases, the superior laryngeal nerve is still functional. The superior laryngeal nerve innervates the cricothyroid muscles, which help in vocal fold adduction and produce variation of pitch. If the patient can speak in a slightly higher voice pitch, he or she often experiences a firmer voice with less breathiness. Such a patient can then use the pushing approach (see Chapter 5). In unilateral adductor paralysis, the involved cord, despite its paralysis and lack of movement to the midline, still vibrates somewhat due to the force of the passing airstream. Under conditions of pushing, the airflow rate is accelerated and thus produces a greater vibration of the involved cord; the result is a louder voice.

Other helpful facilitating approaches (described in Chapter 5) include digital manipulation, half-swallow, boom, and head positioning. Patients are also encouraged to speak with increased glottal attack, coupling the pushing approach with deliberate attempts at sudden voicing onsets. Some attention is also given to increasing the efficiency of respiration by encouraging the patient to speak on a larger percentage of air volume, perhaps by saying few words per expiration and by renewing inspirations more often. Remember that these voice therapy techniques are designed to regain temporarily the best voice possible under conditions of a unilateral adductor paralysis. The continued hope is that nerve regeneration and restoration of normal vocal fold function will follow, at which time these techniques of increasing vocal effort for substitute normal voice can be abandoned.

If after 9 months (about 3 months longer than spontaneous regeneration could be expected) normal innervation of the larynx has not occurred, there are several treatment options open to the patient. It is important to wait, however, for possible reinnervation to occur. McFarlane et al. (1991) state that "*most* otolaryngologists still agree to wait 9–12 months or longer from the onset of paralysis, before attempting any surgical treatment" (p. 66).

The surgical options that are available for restoring normal vocal fold function are Teflon or gelfoam injection of the paralyzed fold (Schramm, May, & Lavorato, 1978), thyroplasty (surgical alteration of the glottis) (Crumley, 1990), and nerve transfer (Crumley, 1991). The patient who receives Teflon or gelfoam injections usually requires some voice therapy to develop the best postsurgical voice possible. While Crumley (1992) argues that the best voice results are obtained from thyroplasty or nerve grafting, McFarlane et al. (1991) argue that equal results can be obtained from voice therapy.

Bilateral Adductor Paralysis With both cords fixed in an open, abducted position, the patient will be aphonic. Bilateral adductor paralysis is more often than not the result of central brainstem impairment rather than bilateral destruction of the recurrent laryngeal nerves. The patient's primary problem—more important than the aphonia—is the inability to close the airway. The aphonia resulting from bilateral cord paralysis is frequently accompanied by other symptoms of cerebral dysfunction, such as weakness or paralysis of the tongue, pharynx, or palate. Medical therapy might well include a tracheostomy to improve the efficiency of the airway as a temporary measure because many cases of bilateral adductor paralysis eventually improve spontaneously.

A permanent bilateral adductor paralysis is sometimes treated surgically. The surgical approach may include rotation of the arytenoids to a fixed, more adducted position, taking care to still preserve the opening of the airway. The surgical reinnervation therapy of Crumley and Izdebski (1986) has been used with some success with patients with bilateral adductor paralysis. Unless some return of vocal fold function is evident, voice therapy for the patient with bilateral adductor paralysis is not too helpful. Rather than receive voice therapy, such patients are often instructed on using the artificial larynx or introduced to some form of electronic speech output system, such as the Vocaid or Phonic Ear Vois.

Abductor Paralyses Both unilateral and bilateral abductor paralyses are relatively rare events among patients with vocal fold paralyses (Tucker, 1980). In unilateral abductor paralysis the paralyzed fold remains fixed in the midline position. Phonation is rarely affected because the two folds approximate each other quite well. Quiet, at-rest breathing is usually normal. Only when the patient becomes physically active is he or she likely to experience some shortness of breath because of the narrowing of the airway. Half of the airway is occluded by the fixed midline cord, so that marked abduction of the normal cord is required to achieve an adequate glottal opening for normal breathing. The primary concern of the laryngologist is that the airway be open sufficiently to permit normal breathing; rarely is surgery necessary in cases of unilateral abductor paralysis.

Often, a patient with unilateral abductor paralysis will initially experience a midline paralysis (abductor) that begins to lessen over time, such that the paralyzed fold eventually becomes fixed in the open paramedian position. The injured or severed recurrent laryngeal nerve may also regenerate, returning function to the involved fold. Some patients experience voice symptoms with unilateral abductor paralysis, temporarily or permanently. For example, singers, actors, or professional users of voice may suffer from loss of pitch range, double voice (diplophonia), and problems in pitch register. Effective voice therapy for these patients would be probing with various facilitating approaches to find the one that works best. We have often found ear training, establishing a new pitch, relaxation, and respiration training to be the most effective approaches for developing the best voice possible with a unilateral abductor paralysis (see Chapter 5).

SPECIAL VOICE PROBLEMS USING A POOR MODE OF PHONATION

Diplophonia

The diplophonic voice is usually produced by two distinct voicing sources, each phonating simultaneously with the other. Occasionally, diplophonia is produced by the true folds—if one of the folds has a different mass and tension from the other one. For example, in persistent paralytic dysphonia, the patient's voice may sound diplophonic as the paralyzed fold vibrates faster because of its thinner mass (as a result of lower motor neuron atrophy). Laryngeal webs sometimes phonate in the airstream, producing a high-pitched squeal that joins the vocal fold vibration (altered because of the shorter segments posteriorly beyond the edge of the web) and thus a double voice. The epiglottis may also produce a sound that, when added to the true fold vibration, produces a diplophonic voice.

The first step in treating a diplophonia is to identify the double-voice source. Video nasoendoscopy has been an excellent tool for examining the vocal tract, attempting to identify an extra phonation source. Occasionally, vigorous aryepiglottic muscle activity produces a tight pursing of the superior larynx, which may prevent the viewer from looking underneath. The aryepiglottic muscles can be the second sound source with the true folds vibrating underneath. The ventricular folds sometimes occlude from view the true folds underneath; in fact, the most common diplophonic voice sources identified are the ventricular folds, vibrating above the true folds. Any additive lesion to the vocal folds, particularly a unilateral lesion, can change the vibratory characteristics of the folds and produce a diplophonia.

The first consideration in the treatment of diplophonia is whether or not the second sound source can be reduced or eliminated. Surgical eradication of a unilateral additive lesion, for example, might bring the two vocal folds into size compatibility so that their vibratory characteristics were basically the same, eliminating the double voice. Symptomatic voice therapy can often be effective in reducing diplophonia. For example, inhalation phonation (see Chapter 5) is produced by true fold vibration. The voice on inhalation is usually a high-pitched, single voice. Once the single voice is established on expiration, the clinician can usually expand the single phonation into other voicing tasks. The yawn-sigh approach (see Chapter 5) is an excellent way to develop an open, supraglottal airway. As the patient produces a phonated sigh, the supraglottal larynx and pharynx are maximally dilated, which might well eliminate any supraglottal structure, such as the aryepiglottic folds, from vibrating and producing the double voice. Other facilitating approaches from Chapter 5 that might be helpful in searching for a clear, single voice include ear training, glottal fry, half-swallow, boom, and place the voice. Use various approaches as probes to find one that might eliminate the second voice. If a particular technique is effective, then design practice materials incorporating it as the therapy practice mode.

Pitch Breaks

As we discussed in Chapter 3, there are two kinds of pitch breaks. First, the upward pitch break experienced by some adolescent boys must be considered as a temporary developmental vocal inconvenience and not a voice problem per se. During the last months of puberty some boys experience a one-octave pitch break (the voice breaks upward) as they are using conversational voice. There is no need for voice therapy, because this kind of pitch break is temporary. As the laryngeal mechanism reaches full development, the pitch breaks disappear as suddenly as they first appeared. An occasional boy (or his parents) may need brief counseling about the temporary nature of the problem. This counseling is about the only role required of the speech-language pathologist to deal with such adolescent pitch breaks.

The second kind of pitch break is related to continuous vocal hyperfunction, particularly prolonged speaking at an inappropriate pitch level (Boone, 1991). The voice breaks either one octave upward or one octave downward. Occasionally, patients experience two-octave breaks. The voice breaks in the direction (down or up) where it "would like to be." Although we have well established in previous chapters that there is no such thing as an absolute optimum voice pitch, speaking at the very bottom or top of one's range for extended periods of time may contribute to vocal strain. Pitch breaks are a symptom of that strain. The primary focus of voice therapy for pitch breaks is establishing a new pitch, raising or lowering the fundamental frequency one or two notes. Upward pitch breaks, the most common form of pitch break, is usually related to speaking at the very bottom of one's pitch range.

Elevating pitch one or two notes usually eliminates the problem. With the new pitch level, the patient might profit from developing a voice legato with chant talk, using a relaxed voice with chewing, practicing yawn-sigh, eliminating hard glottal attack, and attempting the open-mouth approach (see Chapter 5). A downward pitch break, observed more often in adult women, can usually be corrected by developing a lower voice pitch and using the other facilitating approaches recommended for lowering the pitch level. The final step in eliminating pitch breaks is developing an overall easy, open vocal style as the result of ear training, matching one's voice with target voice models previously tape recorded by the patient and the clinician.

Puberphonia

The high-pitched voice in a young man who has already completed puberty is known as *puberphonia.*The voice may be either at the end of the normal, chest register or in the falsetto register. It is thus sometimes called *mutational falsetto.*The fundamental frequency of the voice is often in excess of 260 Hz (or at middle C in the singing range). The social penalties for men who speak at such high-pitched levels are obvious; an individual who does so is often judged to be effeminate and perhaps inadequate. It is difficult to find the original physical or psychological factors that may have caused puberphonia. The large majority of young men with inappropriately high voices have excellent voice therapy prognosis; many achieve normal pitch levels and vocal quality after only brief exposure to voice therapy.

In previous editions of this book and in the writings of Aronson (1990) and Case (1991), the primary voice therapy for puberphonia begins with the speech-language pathologist asking the patient to cough. If the patient is past puberty, the cough will be the typical low-pitched, abrupt cough of the adult male. The clinician explains to the patient that the vocal folds are able to produce an adult male voice, and then demonstrates a cough, holding on to the phonation, indicating the desirability of the prolonged phonation. The patient is then asked to cough again.

Each time the patient coughs, emphasis should be given to prolonging the phonation, usually extending a prolonged "ah" sound. A series of "ahs" are then produced without the need of the "starter" cough. Once phonation is established, the patient is asked to say monosyllabic words beginning with vowels. The single words are then followed by phrases and then sentences. This highly symptomatic voice therapy approach is similar in many ways to our therapy approach with functional aphonia—that is, capturing a vegetative phonation from a cough, and then extending the cough sound into the voicing of vowels.

Other methods for eliciting and establishing a natural voice for the puberphonic patient may include digital pressure against the thyroid cartilage, using glottal fry and the half-swallow, boom, and auditory masking (which may reveal the patient's natural voice). Once symptomatic therapy has revealed the natural voice, most patients eagerly accept the new voice. These young men are extremely motivated to find and use the same voice as their age peers. For the rare patient who has the physical equipment to use a lower voice but prefers the high one, referral for counseling or psychological management is indicated. As Aronson (1990) indicates, for most puberphonic patients the initial diagnostic-therapy session is usually all that is needed, perhaps supplemented by two or three other therapy visits.

Spasmodic Dysphonia

There are two types of spasmodic dysphonia (sometimes called spastic dysphonia): adductor and abductor. The overwhelming number of spasmodic dysphonia patients are, however, of the adductor type. Because of severe vocal fold compression, often accompanied by ventricular and aryepiglottic closure, the patient attempts voicing against the closed laryngeal valve(s), resulting in a tight, strangled voice.

Davis et al. (1987), in studying 24 spasmodic dysphonics of the adductor type in Sydney, Australia, found on endoscopic examination that the tight voice was produced by firm approximation of the true folds that was often accompanied by false fold and aryepiglottic closure, which, in effect, produced a total laryngeal shutdown. Some patients with spasmodic dysphonia also exhibit additional symptoms of neurological origin, such as tremor, whereas other patients show no other physical symptoms. Aminoff et al. (1978) had 12 patients with spasmodic dysphonia examined by psychiatrists, neurologists, and otolaryngologists (the Davis study involved similar examinations and findings) and found no evidence of psychiatric or laryngological involvement sufficient enough to cause the severe voice symptoms. The causes of spasmodic dysphonia of the adductor type may be as varied as the treatments used for the disorder.

There is some controversy (Karnell, 1992; Watterson & McFarlane, 1992) over whether the abductor type should be classified as a true spasmodic dysphonia. Certainly, the symptom presentation of the abductor type contrasts with the adductor type. The voice therapy approaches for abductor spasmodic dysphonia are similar to the management and therapy used for abductor spasms.

At present, in our opinion, the patient with adductor spasmodic dysphonia has three possible treatment options: voice therapy alone, recurrent laryngeal nerve (RLN) cut followed by voice therapy, or botulinum toxin (botox) injections followed by voice therapy.

Specific to voice therapy for spasmodic dysphonia, most clinicians report only modest success in developing satisfactory voice. There are successful outcomes with spasmodic dysphonia patients, however, reported by Cooper (1990), who uses his "direct voice rehabilitation," and Shulman (1991), who uses more conventional voice therapy methods.

The voice therapy methods that seem to improve the voices of this patient group include developing easy, more efficient respiration relaxation methods with hierarchy analysis, inhalation phonation, the yawn-sigh, and developing a more anterior tongue position. It would appear that voice therapy should always be the first treatment tried with the spasmodic dysphonic patient. If such therapy does not produce the desired results, surgical-medical treatment is indicated.

The RLN section (Izdebski, Dedo, & Boles, 1984) was the first surgical procedure that was widely used. The procedure appears to get best results when the surgeon and speech pathologist work closely together.

A thorough diagnostic evaluation by both the surgeon and the speech pathologist is followed by injection of Xylocaine into the RLN, which produces a temporary unilateral adductor paralysis. The patient's airflow, relative ease of phonation, and change of voice quality are assessed. If there is marked improvement in airflow (greater flow rates with less glottal resistance) and in both ease and quality of phonation, the decision may be made to cut the RLN permanently. Postoperatively, then, the patient usually has an easily produced but breathy voice, similar in sound to the patient with unilateral adductor paralysis. Voice therapy focusing on a slight elevation of pitch, some ear training, increasing glottal attack, and pushing have all been effective in developing a better-sounding voice.

The long-term results of RLN resection have been mixed. Wilson, Oldring, and Mueller (1980) reported a woman who had received RLN cut 13 months previously who then experienced a regeneration of the severed RLN and a return of spasmodic dysphonia; a second RLN resection again produced immediate relief from her phonatory struggle. Over 3 years Aronson and DeSanto (1983) followed 33 patients with spasmodic dysphonia who had each received RLN cut. Although all experienced improved voice and ease of airflow immediately after surgery, 3 years later 21 of them, or 64%, had failed to maintain their gains and were considered failures. Much different results were reported by Dedo and Izdebski (1983) on over 306 patients who had received RLN cut for spasmodic dysphonia; they reported that 92% of the patients maintained voice improvement and required less effort to phonate. Those few patients who did not maintain "easier" voices after RLN cut were treated with laser surgery designed to thin the vocal folds, which produced greater lateralization of the folds and an immediate reduction in vocal tightness (Dedo & Behlau, 1991). It would appear for better long-term results after RLN section that the patient undergo some voice therapy with efforts given to establishing easier expiratory air patterns, developing greater neck relaxation, and promoting a lower carriage of the larynx through the yawn-sigh technique.

A more recent approach to improving the voices of spasmodic dysphonic patients is to inject the vocal folds (unilaterally or bilaterally) with botulinum toxin (Botox) (Blitzer & Brin, 1991). For many years, patients with eyelid spasms (blepharospasm) and severe neck muscle contractions (torticollis) have been treated successfully with direct injection of Botox directly into the affected muscles. Similarly with patients with spasmodic dysphonia, direct injection into the thyroarytenoid muscle appears to give dramatic relief from the tight, strangled voice. Blitzer (1992) reports that he has treated over 600 patients with spasmodic dysphonia by botox injection with most patients experiencing a 90% return of normal voice. Murry (1992) and other speech pathologists report that the best voice is achieved by following Botox injection with voice therapy aimed at reducing supraglottal constriction. Relaxation methods and the yawn-sigh approach are two methods that appear successful in reducing supraglottal constriction. In order to maintain a relaxed, near-normal voice, most spasmodic dysphonic patients need to be reinjected with botox about every 3 or 4 months.

Ventricular Phonation

Ventricular phonation, sometimes called *dysphonia plicae ventricularis*, occurs in its pure form when a patient uses the ventricular or false folds for phonation. Such substitute phonation is characterized by a low-pitched voice related to the relative thickness of the ventricular folds as compared to the true folds. Because of this relatively large tissue mass, there is little chance for subtle changes in mass and thickness (certainly as compared to the normal vocal folds); the result is a monotonous pitch level with minimal frequency variation. A patient who, on laryngoscopy, appears to have a structurally normal larynx and yet speaks with an inappropriately low-pitched, monotonous voice might well be using ventricular phonation.

Nasoendoscopy of patients with harsh functional dysphonia often shows the ventricular folds coming together as part of a total laryngeal shutdown; the overall laryngeal aditus is closed by sphincteral closure of the aryepiglottic folds, which pull the cuneiform prominences seemingly together (Pershall & Boone, 1986). As this total laryngeal closure begins, first the true folds adduct and then the false folds come together. The aryepiglottic folds then cover over the open larynx, and neither true nor false folds are visible. Ventricular phonation may be part of such a strained phonation, although it is difficult to single out a particular closure site.

The clinical management of such total laryngeal closure is facilitated by using the yawn-sigh approach (described in Chapter 5). Under conditions of the sigh, using a prolonged /i/ vowel, supraglottal structures open up, revealing on endoscopy the approximation of the true folds. From the sigh-produced /i/, the clinician can extend the number of sounds and words that the patient can say with the open larynx. Glottal fry and tongue protrusion, described in Chapter 5, are also helpful techniques for eliminating ventricular phonation.

An occasional patient will develop a ventricular voice as a substitute voice because of extensive disease or involvement of the true folds. Some patients have such hypertrophied ventricular folds, often as part of a disease process, that their ventricular folds approximate during attempts at normal phonation and produce either a ventricular or a diplophonic voice.

The best therapy approach is to have the patient practice making prolonged inhalations with an open mouth, followed by sustained exhalations, with no attempt at phonation (see inhalation phonation in Chapter 5). This is followed by having the patient make an effort to phonate on inhalation. With some practice, most patients can produce some inhalation phonation. Inhalation phonation is usually true cord phonation. After inhalation phonation is achieved by the patient, efforts can be made to produce a matching exhalation phonation, usually a high-pitched squeaky sound. This is the difficult part of the therapy. Patients will be able to make the inhalation voice with relative ease, but they will have a greater deal of difficulty in producing the matched exhalation. This seems to be easier, however, if the patient attempts inhalation-phonation/exhalation-phonation on the same breath cycle. Perseverance in this task is usually the key to eliminating the ventricular dysphonia; several of our therapy failures with ventricular dysphonia seem to have been related to our not sticking with the matched inhalation-exhalation phonations long enough.

SPECIAL VOICE PROBLEMS RELATED TO CERTAIN CONDITIONS

The Aging Voice

Are there typical voice characteristics that identify the aging voice? One of the problems that prevent answering this question easily is that there is great variability (chronological and physiological) among the aging population. Another difficulty in generalizing about the aging voice is related to the age of the listener or judge. Hollien (1987) found that different listeners at different ages view the aging voice with some bias.

In our 15-year studies of communication and aging at the University of Arizona, we have found differences in response to almost any task between the young aged (65–80) and the older aged (80 years plus). Grouping this large population together as "aged" masks the marked differences both physiologically and socially between the younger and older aged persons.

Kahane (1987) and Chodzko-Zajko, Ringel, and O'Connor (1985), among others, have made detailed descriptions of the changing larynx and respiratory system with age. As the human larynx ages, there is increased ossification of cartilages and decreased collagenous fibers within the intrinsic muscles of the larynx. Undoubtedly, these laryngeal changes contribute in part to the acoustic changes that can be heard in the aging voice. Also, as people get older there is a marked decrement in respiratory competence caused by an overall decrease in lung elasticity, resulting in the older person saying fewer words per breath. Recognizing the direct relationship of overall physiological fitness to the status of the older person's voice, Chodzko-Zajko and Ringel have developed the Index of Physiological Status (IPS). The better the older subjects' IPS rating, the better the overall voice.

There have been many research studies over the years that have looked at how well judges can determine someone's age by listening to his or her voice. Because most such studies have demonstrated a very positive relationship to listener judgment and the aged subject's actual age, efforts have been made (Linville, 1987; Shipp, Qi, Huntley, & Hollien, 1992) to identify those characteristics that contribute to successful listener identification. In summarizing many studies, these factors have been reported. With increasing age, the fundamental frequency (Fo) of both sexes seems to lower with each successive decade through age 50. The female voice continues to lower in Fo throughout life; the male Fo begins to rise slightly in the 60s and continues to rise slightly with each decade after that. There is also greater Fo variability among both aged female and male speakers. Elevated jitter and shimmer have been reported in some studies. A slower speaking rate related to renewing breath more often is another characteristic of the aged person (more severe in the older old than the younger old).

From a management point of view, efforts to improve the overall physiological fitness of the patient will often have a positive influence on voice. Counseling the patient specific to good vocal hygiene is helpful. Direct work on improving respiratory efficiency can lead the patient to develop better expiratory control. Direct work at increasing the speed of one's speech may have a "rejuvenating" effect on the sound of the older patient's voice. Among other facilitating techniques found useful for improving the aging voice are ear training, feedback, masking, and glottal fry.

Dysarthria

Dysarthria is a motor speech problem. Besides the dysarthric patient experiencing marked problems with articulation and speech prosody, voice symptoms occur from problems of respiration, pitch control, vocal quality, and resonance. Dysarthria is observed in patients with various kinds of central nervous system (CNS) and peripheral nervous system (PNS) disorders. The degree and type of dysarthric symptoms depend on where the particular nervous system disease or disorder is located. The most common cause of dysarthria comes from cerebral vascular accidents (CVAs), such as a patient's experiencing a stroke (thrombosis, embolus, or hemorrhage) that results in weakness or paralysis of muscles essential for normal speech. Other causes of dysarthria include trauma to the nervous system, tumors, and degenerative diseases, like muscular dystrophy (MD), amyotrophic lateral sclerosis (ALS), or myasthenia gravis (MG).

If we group all of the speech and voice symptoms under general headings, as Darley et al. (1969) did, we see that dysarthria can manifest itself in symptoms of pitch, loudness, vocal quality, respiration, prosody, articulation, and a general impression of intelligibility and bizarreness. We sometimes see patients for voice evaluation whose problems at the time of the evaluation are the beginning of a serious neurological disease. For example, several times a year in our large hospitals with many outpatients, we see a patient who comes in with a "functional voice problem" who is actually showing the early symptoms of a degenerative disease, such as MD or ALS. The man described in the following case represents a typical patient with the beginning of a serious CNS disease that was first masked as a functional voice disorder:

> John, a 46-year-old college biology professor, began to experience increased hoarseness after lecturing. At times, he would lose his voice completely after a busy, vocally demanding day. Indirect laryngoscopy found that John had "normal vocal folds with good motility, free of lesions." During the peripheral oral evaluation it was noted that John "seemed to have some tongue atrophy with surface fasciculations whenever the tongue was extended." He was subsequently referred for a neurological evaluation where testing, including muscle biopsy of thigh muscles, confirmed that the patient had "lower motor neuron disease or amyotrophic lateral sclerosis." Over a 24-month period, John experienced an increasingly severe dysarthria accompanied by marked involvement of all four extremities. Although the patient is still alive, his progressive disease continues.

The preceding case illustrates how some alteration of voice, either in phonation, resonance, or both, may be the early symptom of a neurological disease or disorder.

The symptoms of dysarthria are sometimes lessened by medical-surgical intervention. Some dysarthrias related to disease can be treated with medication. For example, many patients with Parkinson's disease experience a remarkable lessening of symptoms with the administration of L-dopa, which provides them with the dopamine they are lacking, and thus reduces the hypokinetic symptoms and improves the clarity of speech. Symptoms of spasticity that may seriously interfere with speech may also be lessened with muscle-relaxant medications. Patients whose dysarthrias are related to tumors are sometimes helped by neurosurgical intervention—by the removal of the tumor.

Many dysarthric patients experience severe hypernasality, which requires the combined therapies of the prosthodontist and the speech pathologist, who focus on improving velopharyngeal closure (see Chapter 7). The typical dysarthric with hypernasality has a weak or paralyzed soft palate, which may require a palatal-lift prosthesis to make contact with the pharyngeal wall. Those patients with degenerative diseases, even severe ones like ALS, can maintain function and life itself with help from such habilitative therapies as physical therapy and inhalation therapy (McGuirt & Blalock, 1980). Speech pathology services with heavy emphasis on voice therapy can often improve the intelligibility of dysarthric patients, both for those with static and fixed conditions (like CVA) and those with degenerative diseases (like ALS).

For some dysarthric patients, speech and voice can be markedly helped by determining whether either volitional or involitional behaviors are facilitative. Some dysarthrias are related to diseases that produce greater symptoms during nonintention or automatic function (like Parkinson's), whereas others are exacerbated by intention (like multiple sclerosis). We see the effects of nonintention and intention clearly when we ask the patient to count from 1 to 15 forward and then backward. The Parkinson's patient with nonintention symptoms counts forward with a light voice, rapidly, with poor articulation; however, when the patient counts backward (which requires greater intention), the dysarthric symptoms may be markedly less, with a louder voice, slower speech, and greater intelligibility. Also, speaking under conditions of masking and speaking with a metronome require greater intention and prove to be good therapy strategies for improving loudness of voice.

The opposite situation is seen in the multiple sclerosis patient with intention pathologies; the patient's count forward sounds clearer than the attempts to count backward. The voice clinician should probe with the patient to see if the type of verbal stimulus—nonintention (counting, days of week, and so on) or intention (speaking with an accent, or speaking inappropriately loud)—facilitates improvement in voice. If there is a difference between nonintention and intention, the voice clinician should use this information to help the patient minimize his or her dysarthria. The patient needs much practice using the best intention mode. If there is no improvement of speech function with one intention mode or the other, the clinician must work on the various parameters of voice, using, in many cases, the same voice facilitating approaches recommended for the various voice disorders described in this text.

Altering tongue position, particularly bringing the tongue forward, is often useful (see Chapter 5). We have found that rapid production and forward carriage of the tongue is often facilitated when the patient replaces voice with whisper. Some patients have better intelligibility with whisper or light voice than with full voice. Many feedback devices, such as the endoscope showing velopharyngeal closure on a television monitor or the Visi-Pitch showing fluctuations in vocal frequency, are useful with dysarthric patients. Sometimes modeling, providing the patient with the prosody or pitch inflection needed to sound "more normal," can produce change; the procedures outlined in Chapter 5 under ear training are useful to follow. Sometimes hierarchy analysis, coupled with relaxation and easy phonation, enables the dysarthric patient to minimize voice symptoms. Much of what we do in voice therapy with dysarthric patients is to teach them speaking tricks, ways of using the speech and vocal mechanism in an easy, efficient way. Examples of "tricks" to facilitate better speech include speaking with less intensity, making deliberate efforts to employ more nonintention or intention vocal responses, speaking with greater (or less) oral opening, and so forth. Besides focusing on voice and resonance, the speech pathologist gives obvious attention to improving the patient's articulation and developing a more normal rate of speech, which, in turn, improves overall speech-voice prosodic patterns.

Hard of Hearing and Deaf

If the hearing loss is severe enough, it will affect the voice. The greater the hearing loss, the greater the likelihood that some voice problems will arise, centered around elevated pitch, excessive pitch variability, and cul-de-sac and nasal resonance. However, it has been established (Ling, 1976; Andrews, 1986) that most voice problems among hearing-impaired children can be minimized if adequate amplification is provided as early as possible. In young children who are born with profound hearing loss that prevents them from ever hearing normal voice or vocal prosody, voice symptoms can be quite severe. It has been found (Ling, 1976; Wilson, 1987) that even in children born with profound losses that voice therapy can do much to normalize the sound of the child's speech and voice. Older children and adults who acquire a hearing loss greater than 70 dB in the speech range (500, 1K, 2K Hz) after normal voice-articulation-language has been established may gradually experience some deterioration of voice and articulation.

Pitch Elevated pitch and excessive pitch variability are two vocal symptoms often observed in the deaf (Boone, 1966a; Monsen, Engebretson, Vernula, 1979; Wilson, 1987). Wilson presents useful procedures for both changing pitch levels and for working on the changing pitch levels of intonation. Apparently, the lowering of voice pitch as one moves from childhood through adolescence and then to adulthood requires some acoustic monitoring to match one's normal peer group. The deaf child, or adult, who lacks this auditory feedback appears to need some external guidance to use the acceptable pitch levels of age peers. How can a teacher of the deaf or a voice clinician help a deaf child develop a normally pitched voice as he or she grows older?

Any attempt to change a deaf child's pitch level must begin with a discussion about the need for such a change. This discussion should focus on the child's tested fundamental frequency as compared to normative values for the child's age and sex. The inventive clinician might prepare a chart or graph demonstrating for the child where his or her pitch is and where it ought to be. Lacking an adequate auditory model for his or her pitch target, the deaf child must rely on various visual devices to signal whether his or her voice pitch is too high or too low. Instruments such as the PM 100 Pitch Analyzer, the Phonatory Function Analyzer, and the Visi-Pitch, which are capable of making real-time measurements of frequency as the deaf child or adult speaks, are excellent feedback instruments for therapy. Oscillographic display panels or displays on computer screens can isolate the fundamental frequency for the patient and provide a locked-in display pattern of a frequency he or she has just produced. Most such display units provide a "hold" pattern on the screen that can be used as a target model for subsequent therapy trials.

Innovative clinicians have found several effective ways of making the child or adult aware of pitch level and possible pitch variability. One useful device for altering a deaf person's pitch level is to provide "cue arrows" pointing in the desired direction of pitch change. For example, for a typical deaf child attempting to lower the voice pitch, cards should be printed with an arrow pointing down. These cards should be placed wherever possible in the child's environment—in the wallet, on the bureau or desk, and so on. Also, the classroom teacher and voice clinician can give the child finger cues by pointing toward the floor. Another method for developing an altered pitch level is to have the child place his or her fingers lightly on the larynx and feel the downward excursion of the larynx during lower pitch productions and the upward excursion during higher ones. The ideal or optimum pitch is produced by minimal vertical movement of the larynx. Any noticeable upward excursion of the larynx, except during swallowing, will immediately signal that the child may be speaking at an inappropriately high pitch level. Once an appropriate pitch level has been established, the child may read aloud for a specified time period, placing the fingers lightly on the thyroid cartilage to monitor any unnecessary vertical laryngeal movement.

Resonance The typical voice of a deaf child who has had no training in developing a good voice is characterized by alterations in nasal resonance, often accompanied by excessive pharyngeal resonance, which produce a cul-de-sac voice. The major contributing factor to these resonance alterations is the excessive posterior posturing of the tongue in the hypopharynx, which markedly lowers the second formant (Boone, 1966a; Monsen, 1976). The tongue is drawn back into the hypopharynx and creates the peculiar resonance heard in deaf speakers; this back resonance sounds similar to the resonance sometimes heard in speakers with athetoid cerebral palsy, or oral verbal apraxia. The cul-de-sac voice has a back focus to it. In addition, the hearing-impaired child or adult may demonstrate marked variations in nasal resonance—too much nasal focus (hypernasality) or insufficient nasal resonance (denasality); such nasal resonance variations may be due in part to the posterior carriage of the tongue, as well as to the inability to monitor acoustically the nasalization characteristic of the normal speaker.

Altering the tongue position to a more forward carriage and tongue protrusion (see Chapter 5) can contribute greatly to establishing more normal oral resonance in the voice of a deaf speaker. In addition to the procedures outlined in Chapter 5 for altering tongue position, more detailed procedures and therapy materials for both children and adults are available in *The Boone Voice Program for Children* (1993) and *The Boone Voice Program for Adults* (1982). Once the tongue has been placed in a more "neutral setting" (Laver, 1980), the deaf patient needs to practice

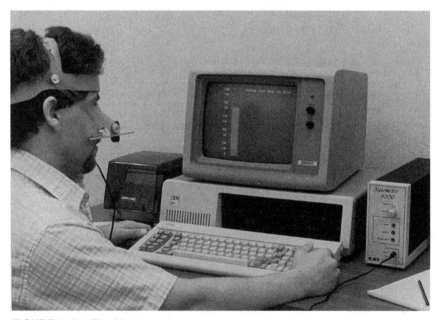

FIGURE 6–3   The Nasometer
The Nasometer produces visual feedback for the patient of his oral/nasal resonance ratio, thus providing a measurement of nasalence. The clinician can set a target level, and the patient's continuous performance can be monitored in relationship to that target level. The peak or highest level of nasal performance is also recorded.

making vocal contrasts between back-pharyngeal resonance and normal oral resonance. The deaf patient needs to develop an awareness of what it feels like to use the lips, the tongue against the alveolar processes, the tongue on the hard palate, and other front-of-the-mouth postures. Such front focus seems to develop only after intensive practice doing tasks that encourage anterior tongue carriage.

The deaf speaker must also work to eliminate hypernasality, if it is present. The patient first needs to become aware of excessive nasal resonance by reviewing feedback from various instruments that measure airflow in acoustic output simultaneously from both the oral and nasal cavities. How much of the perceived voice is oral and how much is nasal can be determined by the Nasometer. The Nasometer (see Figure 6–3) is a microcomputer-based system that can make an acoustic analysis of the relative amount of nasalence in a voice signal. The patient produces voice that is directed into two microphones that are separated by a nasal-oral separator. The computer screen provides real-time feedback about the relative acoustic output between the two channels. The Nasometer provides the same kind of nasal resonance feedback in therapy as the Tonar II (Fletcher & Daly, 1976); both instruments provide valuable visual feedback about vocal resonance for the deaf speaker.

Respiratory Problems Severely hearing-impaired children and adults have normal tidal breathing patterns, but may show marked deviations in expiratory flow while speaking (Forner & Hixon, 1977). They may begin phonation late on the expiratory cycle, taking breath refills at inappropriate times during connected speech. Loudness variations are frequently present (Boone, 1966a). Direct work on smoothing out the expiratory phase when speaking, such as learning to sustain both voiced and voiceless productions, is usually successful. Any kind of air-pressure/flow instrument can provide good feedback to the hearing-impaired speaker specific to appropriateness of breathing and voice loudness. Visual displays from oscillographs or instruments like the Visi-Pitch provide excellent feedback for training more appropriate breathing patterns.

SUMMARY

Each of the disorders of voice in this chapter requires that the voice clinician appreciate the uniqueness of the disorder. Therapy approaches for each of these conditions or disorders are often highly individualized. For example, the therapy approaches for functional aphonia might be markedly different from the approaches used in minimizing spasmodic dysphonia. Yet all of these voice disorders have some commonalities with one another. They can often be helped by combining individualized management steps customary for the particular disorder with some of the 25 facilitating approaches presented in Chapter 5.

Chapter 7

Therapy for Resonance Disorders

Hypernasality (excessive nasal resonance) is the most common resonance disorder. It can be an early sign of a neurological disease, or it can be the result of a congenital disorder such as cleft palate. It can also result from a surgical treatment. The cause of hypernasality must be determined as a prelude to successful treatment. Hyponasality, or denasality, can be caused by a number of obstructions, such as nasal polyps, allergies, or hypertrophied adenoids. Another nasalence problem, assimilative nasality, must be distinguished from either hypernasality or denasality. Speech-language pathologists play a primary role in the diagnosis and treatment of various nasality problems.

Resonance is selective amplification and filtering of the complex overtone structure by the cavities of the vocal tract after the tone has been produced by the vibration of the vocal folds. The vocal folds provide the source of vibration that gives rise to the complex sound waves. These periodic vibrations, characteristic of the normal voice, are *filtered* in the supraglottal space of the pharyngeal, oral, and nasal cavities, or the upper airway. Our discussion of resonance in Chapter 2 showed that the F-shaped upper airway amplifies and filters the sounds coming into it from the larynx, depending on the frequency of the sound waves and the shape and size of the particular cavity. The pharyngeal cavity constantly changes its horizontal and vertical dimensions by active movement of muscles, which in turn changes its overall configuration (Pershall & Boone, 1986; Watterson & McFarlane, 1990). An open coupling between the pharyngeal cavity and the oral cavity (particularly when the velopharyngeal mechanism is closed) enables the traveling sound wave to be further filtered by the continuous modifications of oral cavity size that occur during speech. What emerges as voice resonance is the fundamental frequency (laryngeal vibration) modified by the natural resonant frequencies occurring at the various *supraglottal* sites (above the vocal folds), within the pharynx, and through the oral cavity. When the velopharyngeal port is open, the pharyngeal-oral coupling with the nasal cavity is then possible so that sound waves are further absorbed and filtered as they pass through the chambers of the nasal cavity, as for the production of /m/, /n/, and /ng/ in English. Problems in pharyngeal-oral coupling, structural and functional, cause the most common resonance problems. We consider the evaluation, management, and therapy of nasal resonance problems.

NASAL RESONANCE PROBLEMS

Under the broad heading of nasal resonance fall three types of disorders: hypernasality, denasality, and assimilative nasality. Although individuals listening to speakers with these problems might only be able to say that the voices all sound nasal, distinct differences among the three types call for differential management and voice therapy approaches. As a prelude to our discussion of separate approaches, let us define the three terms:

Hypernasality is an excessively undesirable amount of perceived nasal cavity resonance during the phonation of vowels and voiced consonants. Voiced consonants and vowel production in the English language are primarily characterized by oral resonance with only slightly nasalized components. If the oral and nasal cavities are tightly coupled to each other by lack of velopharyngeal closure (for whatever reason), the periodic sound waves carrying laryngeal vibration will receive heavy resonance within the nasal cavity. Only three phonemes of the English language should receive the degree of nasal prominence produced by an open velopharyngeal port: /m/, /n/, and /ʒ/.

Denasality is the lack of nasal resonance for the three nasalized phonemes /m/, /n/, and /ng/. Therefore, denasality could be categorized as an articulatory substitution disorder. Generally, denasality also affects vowels, in that the normal speaker gives some nasal resonance to vowels. A voice with this inadequate nasal resonance sounds like the voice of a normal speaker suffering from a severe head cold and stuffed-up nose.

In *assimilative nasality*, the speaker's vowels appear nasal when adjacent to the three nasal consonants. The velopharyngeal port is opened too soon and remains open too long, so that vowel resonance preceding and following nasal consonant resonance is also nasalized.

Normal English consonants are produced with high intraoral pressures (3 to 8 cm H_2O) with essentially no nasal airflow except for the three nasal consonants that have low intraoral pressures (0.5 to 1.5 cm

H_2O) and high rates of nasal airflow (100 to 300 cc/sec), as reported by Mason and Warren (1980). Aerodynamic studies of cleft-palate speakers and problems of excessive nasality have provided some needed quantification to help differentiate patients with excessive nasal resonance from patients lacking sufficient nasal resonance (Warren, 1979). From his studies of air pressures and airflow patterns, Warren has estimated the size of the velopharyngeal port. Although most normal speakers demonstrate tight velopharyngeal closure with no air leakage (Thompson, 1978), speakers with openings as small as 5 mm or less may still have voice quality that is perceived by listeners as normal (Mason & Warren, 1980). Patients with nasal voices who produce high nasal airflow rates are perceived as having hypernasality, whereas denasality is accompanied by low nasal airflows. Probably no area of voice therapy is more neglected or more confusing than therapy for nasal resonance problems. Historically, the implication in the early literature was that most problems of nasality (usually hypernasality) could be successfully treated by voice therapy—that is, by ear training, by blowing exercises (Kantner, 1947), by the exercises for the velum suggested by Buller (1942), or by the treatment Williamson (1945) used for 72 cases of hypernasality, which put some emphasis on relaxing the entire vocal tract. Most of these early approaches were developed for functional hypernasality but were later applied by various clinicians to organically based problems of palatal insufficiency and cleft palate. For most of these structural problems, however, such approaches as blowing and relaxation were ineffective. If the velopharyngeal mechanisms were structurally unable to produce velopharyngeal closure, no amount of relaxation or exercise could have much effect in reducing excessive nasal resonance by closing an inadequate velopharyngeal port mechanism. Realistic management and therapy for any problem in nasal resonance, therefore, requires that the patient have a thorough differential evaluation, including detailed examination of the *velopharyngeal port* (VP) mechanism, aerodynamic studies, functional speech-voice testing, a detailed acoustical and perceptual analysis of voice, and videoendoscopic studies (McFarlane,1990; Watterson & McFarlane,1990; Watterson, 1991).

EVALUATION OF NASAL RESONANCE DISORDERS

There are more similarities than differences between patients with resonance disorders and those with phonation disorders. For this reason, the evaluation procedures outlined in Chapter 4 are equally relevant here. In addition to obtaining the necessary medical data (such as what treatment has already been provided), clinicians must pursue case-history information (description of the problem and its cause, description of daily voice use, variations of the problem, onset and duration of the problem, etc.). Clinicians must observe closely how well the patients seem to function in the clinic and during out-of-clinic situations. Considering how subjective our judgments of resonance disorders are, it is crucial that clinicians know how their patients perceive their own voices. A mild resonance problem, for example, can be perceived by a patient and/or others as a severe problem, but a severe resonance problem may be ignored.

Analysis of Voice in Speech

An obvious way to begin the evaluation of a person with a nasal resonance disorder is to listen carefully to his or her voice during spontaneous conversation. This can provide a gross indication of what the problem may be (assimilative nasality, hypernasality, etc.). The perceptual aspect of nasal resonance disorders is extremely important. It is, however, extremely difficult to make a clinical judgment about nasality by listening to someone as he or she speaks; in fact, such a judgment is likely to be wrong. For example, Bradford, Brooks, and Shelton (1964) found that neither a group of four experienced judges nor one of four inexperienced judges could reliably judge the recorded voice samples of children producing /a/ and /i/ with nares open and closed (by digital pressure). The judges were similarly unreliable when judging nasality from conversational speech samples. Although the casual judgment that "something is nasal about the speech" is usually correct, few examiners can quickly and reliably differentiate the type of nasality (hypernasality, assimilative nasality, denasality) on the basis of such a conversational sample. Voice quality judgments are more accurate if made on the basis of tape-recorded samples of a patient's conversational speech, his or her vowels in isolation, and his or her sentences (some with only oral phonemes and some loaded with nasal phonemes). The taped sample allows the clinician repeated playback. Focusing on a specific parameter (loudness, pitch, quality) on each playback may increase the clinician's objectivity. To counter the "halo" effect, the influence of a speaker's articulation on the judgment of his or her nasality, Sherman (1954) developed a procedure of playing the connected speech sample backward on the tape recorder, thus precluding the identification of any articulation errors. Reverse playback is most helpful in differentiating between hypernasality and denasality. Spriestersbach (1955) found that the reverse playback of speech samples of cleft-palate subjects reduced the correlations between articulation proficiency/pitch level and judgments of nasality. We have found that asking patients to repeat or read aloud passages that are totally free of nasal consonants, such as "Betty takes Bob to the show" (Boone, 1993), or passages that are loaded with nasal consonants, such as "many men in the moon" (Boone, 1993), helps us differentiate hypernasality, denasality, and assimilative nasality from one another.

We have also found that if we use the following simple screening procedures, we get a good, quick clinical classification of the type of resonance disorder present. These quick tests are simple and require no instruments to perform. First, we have the patient say these two sentences while holding the nose: "My name means money" and "Mary may make many messes." If these sound "plugged" when the nose is held and not plugged when the nose is released, the problem is hypernasality. If there is no difference between the nose-held and nose-released conditions, the problem is denasality. Next, we have the patient sustain a loud /s/ while the nose is held and quickly released. If a "snap" is heard on releasing the nose, the problem is probably hypernasality Next, we have the patient say, "This horse eats grass" and "I see the teacher at church." If we hear any "snorting" back in the pharynx, we can assume that it is probably due to inadequate closure of the velopharyngeal port and that the problem is hypernasality. We next ask the patient to say, "Maybe baby, maybe baby." If there is no difference between the two words (*maybe* and *baby*) and both sound like *maybe* the problem is hypernasality; however, if both words sound like *baby* the problem is denasality. Finally, we ask the patient to sustain the /i/ and the /u/ vowels, while we gently flutter the nose by occluding the nares with the thumb and forefinger. If we hear a pulsing change in the acoustic signal, the problem is hypernasality. Patients with hypernasality often have laryngeal abnormalities, as well. For example, children with velopharyngeal closure problems are reported to have a higher than normal incidence of vocal cord nodules and polyps (McWilliams, Lavorato, & Bluestone, 1973). Therefore, the clinician must not only make judgments about resonance abnormality, he or she must also listen closely to voice quality (for problems of hoarseness, breathiness, etc.). The voice sample should then be analyzed for resonance, vocal quality, and articulation. Besides listening to the voice, the clinician must employ stimulability testing (to assess the functional potential for improvement) and other testing techniques.

Stimulability Testing

Although stimulability testing was designed for use with problems of articulation, it is also effective with problems of voice. The basic purpose of stimulability testing, as first described by Milisen (1957), was to see how well the patient can produce an erred sound when he or she is repeatedly presented with the correct sound through both auditory and visual stimuli. One way of distinguishing between true problems of velopharyngeal structure (the mechanism is wholly incapable of adequate closure) and functional velopharyngeal inadequacy (the mechanism has the capability of closure) is to see if the patient can produce oral resonance under stimulability conditions (Morris & Smith, 1962). Obviously, the patient's success in producing oral resonance would be a strong indication that velopharyngeal closure is possible. Shelton,

Hahn, and Morris (1968) wrote:

> If repeated stimulation consistently results in consonant productions which are distorted by nasal emission and vowels which are unpleasantly nasal, the inference can be drawn, at least tentatively, that the individual is not able to change his speaking behavior because of velopharyngeal incompetence. (p. 236)

Success in producing oral resonance under conditions of stimulability would be a good indicator for voice therapy, and a good prognostic sign.

Another, simple stimulability test is to hold the patient's velum up with a tongue depressor while fluttering the nose during the patient's production of a sustained /i/ vowel. Next, remove the tongue depressor and repeat the process, listening for a difference in resonance. If the difference is dramatic, the patient will not likely be able to benefit from voice-speech therapy alone but will require a palatal lift, speech obturator, or surgical management. Watterson and McFarlane (1990) describe five classes of velopharyngeal function based on videoendoscopic observations during speech testing. The classes of VP function are I. Normal VP function; II. Consistent VPI (velopharyngeal incompetency); III. Task Specific VPI; IV. Irregular VPI; and V. Abnormal Resonance without VPI.

Articulation Testing

Articulatory proficiency can provide a good index of a patient's velopharyngeal closure. Nasal emission, the escape of air through the nose, is a most common articulation error on plosive and fricative phonemes among subjects with inadequate velopharyngeal closure. Even though a patient may have his or her articulators in the correct position, in relation to their lingual-alveolar-labial contacts, the error occurs because increased oral pressure escapes nasally through the incomplete posterior palatal closure. The presence or absence of nasal emission, therefore, is a most important diagnostic sign of velopharyngeal adequacy. It is important in articulation testing to distinguish between errors that result from faulty articulatory positioning and errors related to inadequacy of the velopharyngeal structure.

An excellent articulation test for assessing competency of velopharyngeal closure is found in the 43 special test items from the Templin–Darley Tests of Articulation (Templin & Darley, 1980), known as the Iowa Pressure Articulation Test. This test is particularly sensitive for identifying the presence of nasal emission during the production of certain consonants. However, any standardized articulation test is useful for determining those phonemes that are distorted because of inadequate velopharyngeal closure. The clinician must closely assess the identified errors to determine if lingual placements are accurate to make the target phoneme correctly. Many younger children with velopharyngeal problems exhibit sound substitutions and omission errors in addition to the nasal emission and nasal snort distortion they produce because of inadequate velar closure. Older children and adults with nasal emission problems may well have correct articulatory lingual placements, and their distortions are a product of posterior nasal escape of the airstream. Following successful pharyngeal flap surgery or the proper fitting of an appliance, nasal emission sometimes continues until it is modified through speech remediation. The past learning and the muscular "set" for making distorted nasal emission may continue even though the closure mechanism may now be considered normal. It is usually possible, however, to eliminate nasal emission through therapy, once structural adequacy has been achieved.

The 16 so-called pressure consonants provide the best test of the adequacy of the velopharyngeal mechanism. These pressure consonants should be included in any testing of the adequacy of the velopharyngeal port mechanism, since these sounds require the greatest degree of VP closure and greatest intraoral air pressure. Denasality in its purest and most overt form would be exhibited on an articulation test with these oral substitutions for the nasal phonemes. The sentence "My name means money" would be produced, for example, as "By dabe beads buddy."

Assimilative nasality would be observable only for vowels in words containing nasal phonemes. Nasal emission would be most common in patients with palatal insufficiency in affricates (such as t), fricatives (such as s), and plosives (such as p). Hypernasality per se would not be isolated on an articulation test. Clinicians should be alert to the relatively high number of articulation errors often present in the speech of patients with cleft palate or those with VPI unrelated to cleft palate. From a speech therapy point of view, there is often more merit in focusing on articulation errors in cases of cleft palate than on resonance per se; as speech intelligibility improves, the hypernasality of these patients interferes less with effective communication. The type of articulation test or tasks used to assess articulatory proficiency is a matter of clinical choice, but with the increasing availability of diagnostic aids for determining adequacy of velopharyngeal closure, clinicians must not abandon their articulation assessments, which may well be among the most valid tools for indirectly diagnosing velopharyngeal inadequacy during speech tasks. In addition to the obvious articulation errors in the speech of patients with velopharyngeal inadequacy, such as glottal stops and pharyngeal fricatives, errors may include tongue tip sounds made too far back in the mouth, posterior productions of other sounds, and weakened plosives, fricatives, and affricates.

The Oral Examination

By direct visual examination, the clinician can make a gross observation of the relationship of the velum to the pharynx, note the relative size of tongue, make a judgment of maxillary-mandibular occlusion, view the height of the palatal arch, survey the general condition of dentition, and determine if there are any clefts or open fistulas in the palate. Remember that direct visualization of palatal length and movement provides only a gross indication of velopharyngeal closure because the anatomic point of closure is superior by some distance to the lower border of the velum. That is, a lack of velar contact with the pharynx at the uvular-tip end of the velum is not an indication of lack of closure further up, where closure usually occurs. A markedly short palate or a palate with obvious pharyngeal contact can be noted on direct inspection of the oral cavity, and such a notation would be diagnostically important. The less obvious problems of borderline closure cannot be determined by direct inspection and probably require videoendoscopic or fluorographic confirmation, which we discuss in the next section.

The degree of velar movement can be determined with some validity by viewing the soft palate. It is important to know when crucial management decisions are being made—that is, when it is being decided whether a child should have a pharyngeal flap or an appliance, or speech therapy. Direct observation is only possible during vowel productions; however, the degree of closure of the velopharyngeal port is more critical on consonants and consonant clusters than on vowels. A degree of openness is acceptable on vowels and is not acceptable on consonants. Thus, instrumentation needs to be employed to make accurate observations during the critical production of consonants. Zwitman (1990) describes the use of oral endoscopy for observation of the VP mechanism during vowel production and plosive-vowel production. Watterson and McFarlane (1990) describe the use of nasal videoendoscopy for making valid observations of the VP mechanism during connected speech.

Velar movement is sometimes impaired in what might appear to be a normally symmetrical palate; here, the patient has a sluggish palate, sometimes as a symptom following a severe infectious disease (influenza, encephalitis, etc.). Adequacy of pharyngeal movement is almost impossible to determine by direct oral examination; it is best seen by lateral-view video fluorographic film or with endoscopy (nasal or oral).

In some problems of nasality, particularly those not associated with palatal insufficiency, the relative size and carriage of the tongue may have some diagnostic relevance. For example, some problems of "functional" nasality may be related to inappropriate size of the tongue for the size of the oral cavity, or to innervation problems of the tongue.

The clinician should make a thorough search for any openings of the hard or soft palate that might contribute to an articulation distortion or to some problem of nasal resonance. Some patients have small openings (*fistulas*) or lack of fusion around the border of the premaxilla, particularly in the area of the alveolar ridge. In some individuals such fistulas may produce airstream noises, creating articulatory distortion (by loss of intraoral air pressure), but almost never will such isolated openings this far forward on the maxilla produce nasal resonance. The absence or presence of soft-palate and hard-palate clefts should be noted; if such clefts have been previously corrected surgically, the degree of closure should be noted. In the case of a bony-palate defect, for example, sometimes the bony opening has been covered by a thin layer of mucosal tissue, not thick enough to prevent oral cavity sound waves from traveling into the nasal cavity. This same observation applies to the occasional submucosal cleft at the midline of the junction of the hard and soft palates. The major signs of a submucosal cleft are bifid or split uvula, inverted A-shape defect in the velum, lack of a palpable posterior nasal spine, or a thin soft palate (which may appear darker in color) in the midline portion. Any other structural deviations—of dentition, occlusion, labial competence, and so on—should be noted and considered with regard to their possible effects on speech production and nasal resonance.

Evaluation Measures

Many instruments can help the clinician evaluate various aspects of nasal resonance. These instruments can also be valuable in the process of deciding what to do for a patient with a nasalization problem. We consider separately instruments that provide aerodynamic data, acoustic information, radiographic visualization, and visual probe information.

Aerodynamic Instruments Pressure transducers and pneumotachometers are instruments of choice for measuring the relative air pressures and airflows emitting simultaneously from the nasal and oral cavities during speech (Warren, 1979). Pressure and flow data are measured from the two channels simultaneously, which permits relative comparisons. Normal speakers, except during the production of nasal consonants, exhibit relatively no nasal pressure or flow. Speakers with nasality problems show deviations in the relative amount of nasal and oral flows, as is well documented in the recent work of Mason and Warren (1980) and Warren (1979). The aerodynamic procedures basically provide the clinician information about possible leakage through the nose when the velopharyngeal mechanism should be closed. Manometers have also been useful for measuring relative nasal-oral airflows. Manometers measure the amount of pressure of the emitted airstream and do not measure resonance per se, since resonance is a perceptual event. Two types of manometers are used clinically, the water-filled U-tube and the mechanical pressure gauge. Both of these measure airflow pressure and not nasality; however, in comparing oral with nasal readings, some indication of velopharyngeal competence is given, which may, of course, have some relevance to the judgment of nasality. The water-filled U-tube works this way: A glass U-tube is partially filled with a colored liquid, and one end of the tube is fitted into a rubber hose. The free end of the hose is fitted with a nasal olive. The olive is emplaced nasally, and any utterance of the patient that is characterized by nasal emission will displace the liquid and thus provide the patient and clinician with some visual evidence of nasal emission. The second type of manometer, a mechanical pressure gauge, is available, but it has not proven to be an effective clinical tool for evaluating poor velopharyngeal function.

Acoustic Instruments The Tonar II was designed by Fletcher (1972) to provide relative data of the acoustic signal emitting from both the oral and nasal cavities: How much of the perceived voice signal is "coming" through the nose, how much from the mouth? The Tonar II provides for a running speech sample, a continuous feedback of the oral-nasal acoustic ratio, which is displayed on the instrument display panel. Because the oral-nasal acoustic ratio fluctuates with each utterance, a 1-second or 10-second averaging may be set on the instrument by the clinician. The patient is asked to read or repeat a continuous verbal passage, speaking directly into the two separate microphones, one receiving the oral signal and one the nasal signal. The oral signal value is divided into the nasal signal value to yield the actual oral-nasal acoustic ratio, a process that is done automatically at 1- or 10-second intervals (depending on the interval set by the clinician) by the Tonar II (Fletcher, 1972). The typical speaker with normal nasal resonance will experience a "top" oral-nasal ratio of under 10%. Speakers with severe hypernasality will experience ratios in excess of 80%. One advantage of using the Tonar II to analyze relative nasality is that it provides a continuous value specific to relative nasal and oral resonance in running speech.

Use of spectrographic and acoustic analysis has increased in the evaluation of patients with various voice disorders (Murry & Doherty, 1980; Takahashi & Koike, 1975) but has not been particularly useful in differentiating the types of nasal resonance deviations. It has been demonstrated spectrographically that speakers with increased nasalization demonstrate more prominent third formants with an increase in formant bandwidth, accompanied by a rise in fundamental frequency. In his acoustic study of nasality using the spectrograph, Dickson (1962) concluded there was no way to "differentiate nasality in cleft-palate and non-cleft palate individuals either in terms of their acoustic spectra or the variability of the nasality judgments" (p. 111). It is doubtful that the visual write out provided by the spectrograph can give the clinician any more information about the type of nasality he or she hears than does listening carefully to the same samples. The spectrograph can help to identify the aperiodic noise of nasal emission, but differentiating "blindly" between spectrograms of speakers with hypernasality and those with denasality or assimilative nasality is most difficult. As clinicians learn to use what spectral analyses the spectrograph can provide, however, the instrument may well become a most useful tool for studying various parameters of nasality. It has not however become a common clinical tool to date due to these stated shortcomings.

A newer instrument that we have used is the Nasometer, produced by Kay Elemetrics. This adaptation of the Tonar II is clinically very useful. It provides visual feedback on a computer screen for the patient. It also allows the clinician to set a predetermined level of acceptable nasal to oral ratio. The peak of nasal productions is also demonstrated on the screen. Watterson, McFarlane, and Wright (1993) discuss some of the problems with measurements of nasalence using the Nasometer. Hardin, Van DeMark, Morris, and Payne (1992) also discuss some of the cautions in using the Nasometer scores and its data measurements when compared to perceptual judgments.

Radiographic Instruments Radiographic studies of the velopharyngeal mechanism during speech provide ready information about structural and physiological limitations of the mechanism in those patients who demonstrate velopharyngeal incompetence. For example, through a lateral-view film we can determine the relative amount of velopharyngeal opening during speech, the length of the velum, relative movements of the velum and the posterior pharyngeal wall, and so on (Bowman & Shanks, 1978). However, there are limitations to the use of lateral views attempting to view closure because lateral wall movement of the pharynx, which may contribute heavily to velopharyngeal closure, cannot be visualized. Sometimes the patient is asked to swallow barium, and as the barium passes through the pharynx, measurements are made of the relative pharyngeal opening as it relates to the velopharyngeal closing mechanism (Skolnick, Glaser, & McWilliams, 1980). The most useful radiographic views of velopharyngeal closure require the patient to make some speech utterances, including phrases and sentences that include pressure consonants. The speech-language pathologist needs to work closely with the radiologist, presenting the speech tasks as the films are made and "reading" the films when they are completed. Sometimes a radiographic display can demonstrate a problem in velopharyngeal closure that cannot be detected by any other method except for nasovideoendoscopy.

Visual Probe Instruments Shelton and Trier (1976) have written that direct measures of velopharyngeal competence through the use of endoscopes, nasopharyngoscopes, and ultrasound apparatus offer some advantages in making treatment decisions. The oral endoscope (Zwitman et al., 1976) has been a useful instrument for determining the degree and type of velopharyngeal closure, as Figure 7–1 shows. The body of the oral endoscope is extended above the tongue within the oral cavity so that the lighted tip and viewing window lie just below the uvula and within the oropharyngeal opening. By turning the viewing window up toward the velopharyngeal area, the velum, the lateral pharyngeal walls, and the posterior pharynx may be visualized. Two views of varying degrees of velopharyngeal closure in the same subject are shown in Figure 7–2.

Shelton et al. (1975) have used the oral panendoscope to provide subjects visual feedback about their particular closure patterns; by watching their panendoscopically viewed closure patterns on a television monitor, subjects have been able to modify their closure patterns. Distinct variations in patterns of velopharyngeal closure have been demonstrated by Zwitman, Sonderman, and Ward (1974) and Zwitman (1990). Some subjects have only velar movement without associated pharyngeal wall movement, some subjects primarily have lateral and posterior pharyngeal wall constriction, and some subjects achieve closure by a combination of velar and pharyngeal movements. A nasal fiber-optic endoscope has been developed that places a small flexible scope through the nose and down into the pharynx, offering a view of velopharyngeal closure from above the closure site (Miyazaki, Matsuya, & Yamaoka, 1975; Watterson & McFarlane, 1990). The primary advantage of the nasoscope is that it is not invasive to the oral cavity and consequently does not impede tongue or lip movements during dynamic articulation (a limitation of the oral endoscope). The oral and nasal endoscopic probes are effective instruments for assessing velopharyngeal competence in patients with nasal resonance problems, because they offer direct observation of velar length and movement, degree of lateral and posterior pharyngeal wall movement, and the kind of velopharyngeal closure the patient is using. Perhaps, most importantly, this examination allows the clinician and the patient to see the various types and degrees of velopharyngeal closure during a variety of phonetic contexts. As mentioned earlier Watterson and McFarlane (1990) have described five useful classes of VP function and provide a basis for making recommendations for clinical treatment.

TREATMENT OF NASAL RESONANCE DISORDERS

Hypernasality

The presence of excessive nasal resonance (hypernasality) is relatively dependent on the judgment of the listener. That is, some languages and regional dialects require heavy nasal resonance and therefore consider pronounced nasalization of vowels to be normal. Others, however, such as general American English, tolerate little nasal resonance beyond the three nasal consonants. Thus, a native New Englander with a nasal "twang" exhibits normal voice resonance in Portland, Maine, but when he or she travels to New Knoxville, Ohio, the people there perceive his or her voice as excessively nasal. Variations do exist in the degree of nasality among the voices of the people in Ohio, of course, but a certain amount of

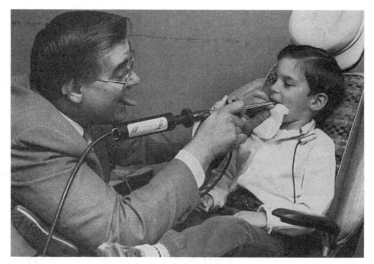

FIGURE 7–1   Oral Video Endoscopy
The velopharyngeal closure mechanism of a 4-year-old boy is examined by
oral video endoscopy. Children and adults are routinely evaluated in this
manner without the use of any topical anesthetic.

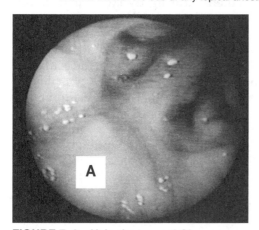
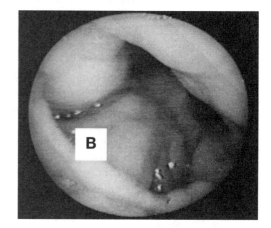

FIGURE 7–2   Velopharyngeal Closure
This oral video endoscopic view of velopharyngeal closure demonstrates two degrees of closure in a sequence
from (A) an open v-p mechanism, through (B) the bulging of Passavant's pad with posterior and lateral
pharyngeal wall movement and the velar movement.

resonance variability can exist among any particular population without
anyone's being bothered by it. If, however, a particular voice in Ohio (or
any other place) stands out as "excessively nasal," then that voice will be
considered to have a resonance disorder. The judgment of hypernasality,
then, is as dependent on the speech-language milieu of the speaker and
his or her listeners as it is on the actual performance of the speaker.

The speaker who is judged to be hypernasal increases the nasalization of his or her vowels by failing to close his or her velopharyngeal port. This failure to close the velopharyngeal opening may be related to structural-organic defects, or it may have a functional etiology. Hypernasality frequently accompanies unrepaired cleft palate or a short palate. Among other organic causes of the disorder are surgical trauma (e.g. postadenoidectomy), accidental injury to the soft palate, and impaired innervation of the soft palate as a result of poliomyelitis or some other form of bulbar disease. Sometimes temporary hypernasality may follow adenoid surgery and tonsillectomy as the patient attempts to minimize the pain by not moving his or her velopharyngeal mechanism. But when hypernasality persists for 2 to 3 months or more following an adenoidectomy, the adequacy or the velopharyngeal mechanism must be suspected and evaluated. Some people speak with hypernasal resonance for purely functional reasons, perhaps to maintain a lingering internal model of a previously acceptable form of resonance, or perhaps to imitate the voice of someone they consider particularly attractive (such as a famous political figure or performer). Although the majority of persons with hypernasal voices probably have some structural basis for their lack of velopharyngeal competence, the ease of imitating a hypernasal voice tells us that it could be relatively easy to become hypernasal with perfectly adequate and normal velopharyngeal equipment. Hypernasality is one voice problem in which the distinction must be made between organic and functional causes, as the treatment recommended is quite specific to the diagnosis.

If there are any indications of physical inadequacy of velopharyngeal closure, the primary role of the speech pathologist is to refer the patient to a specialist who can provide the needed physical correction—a plastic surgeon, say, or a prosthodontist. The postsurgical result must be evaluated by the speech pathologist after plastic surgery treatment is completed. If a prosthetic form of management is used, then the speech pathologist will be involved in the initial fabrication and fitting of the velar lift or obturator. Subsequent modifications of these devices will be directed by the speech pathologist, based upon the results of his or her speech testing and the patient's response to clinical speech stimulation. There is very little evidence that voice therapy to improve resonance has any positive effect in the presence of physical inadequacy. In fact, there is some indication that voice therapy to improve the oral resonance of patients with palatal insufficiency (those who lack the physical equipment to produce closure) will usually not only fail, but will also be interpreted by the patient as his or her own fault—as a defeat indicating low personal worth—and thus will take an obvious toll on the patient's self-image. An example of the uselessness of speech therapy in the presence of a severe inadequacy of velopharyngeal closure is provided by this case of a teen-aged girl who had received speech therapy for both articulation and resonance for a period of 7 years:

> Barbara, aged 14, had received 7 years of group and individual speech therapy in the public schools and in a community speech and hearing clinic for "a severe articulation defect characterized by sibilant distortion, and for a severely nasal voice." Barbara's mother was upset with Barbara's continued lack of progress and her tendency to withdraw from social contact with her peers, which the mother felt was due to her embarrassment over her poor speech. Barbara was evaluated by a comprehensive cleft-palate team, which, after reviewing her history, found that her nasality dated from a severe bout of influenza when she was 6 years old. The influenza had been followed immediately by a deterioration of speech. Subsequent speech therapy records were incomplete, although the mother reported that the therapy had included extensive blowing drills, tongue-palate exercises, and articulation work. Physical examination of the velar mechanism found that Barbara had good tongue and pharyngeal movements, but bilateral paralysis of the soft palate; even on gag reflex stimulation, only a "flicker" of palatal movement was observed. Lateral cinefluorographic films confirmed the relatively complete absence of velar movement. The examining speech pathologist found that Barbara had normal articulation placement of the tongue for all speech sounds, despite severe nasal emission of airflow for fricative and affricate phonemes. Low back vowels were relatively oral in resonance, whereas middle and high vowels became increasingly nasal. It was the consensus of the evaluation team that, with her structural inadequacy, Barbara was a poor candidate for speech therapy. It was recommended that she receive a pharyngeal flap and be evaluated again several weeks after the operation. The surgery was successful and had an amazingly positive effect on Barbara's speech. Although hypernasality disappeared, some slight nasal emission remained. Barbara was subsequently enrolled in individual speech therapy, where she experienced total success in developing normal fricative-affricate production.

Such a case shows the futility of continued speech therapy when real structural inadequacy exists. Without the operation, Barbara could have had speech therapy for the rest of her life, with no effect on her speech. If velopharyngeal insufficiency is found, there are two primary alternatives for treatment, surgical or dental. When structural adequacy is achieved, remediation services of the speech-language pathologist can produce further changes in the patient's speech and resonance.

Surgical Treatment for Hypernasality   The evaluation may reveal the existence of such structural inadequacies as open fistulas, open bony and soft tissue clefts, submucous clefts, and short or relatively immobile soft palates. The plastic surgeon is usually the medical specialist most experienced in making decisions about when and if surgical closure of palatal openings is required, based on the recommendation of the speech-language pathologist. The speech pathologist is best able to assess the adequacy of the velopharyngeal port mechanism during speech. Usually, the major reason (often the only reason) for surgical or prosthetic treatment in these patients is to improve speech.

A plastic surgeon wrote, "The surgeon requires the involvement of the speech pathologist in diagnosis as well as therapy" (Grace, 1984, p. 152). This includes preoperative testing, pressure and flow measurements, and mutual evaluation of cineradiographic studies. Paralleling the widespread use of direct endoscopic visual observation in medicine, the development of oral and nasoendoscopy has become an indispensable tool for diagnosing many speech disorders. Although nasoendoscopy is used by some plastic surgeons, it is often used by speech-language pathologists. It should be routinely available in centers managing organically based disorders (Grace, 1984).

When the diagnostic tests have been completed, the speech pathologist and surgeon must plan management. The speech pathologist should know available options for anatomic correction and participate in the decision for surgery. "The surgeon must know the alternative treatments and anticipated results of his operations. The timing of surgery can be a mutual decision" (Grace, 1984, p. 152). For patients who have cleft palate, the primary surgical procedure usually involves closing the cleft and still maintaining adequate palatal length. Most patients with cleft palate, however, require multiple secondary surgical procedures at later times, such as rebuilding structures or eliminating earlier surgical scars. Many patients with hypernasality have velums that are too short for closure or velums that do not move adequately for closure. Such patients often profit from a surgically constructed pharyngeal flap. Here, the surgeon takes a small piece of mucosal tissue from the pharynx and uses it to bridge the excessive velopharyneal opening, attaching the tissue to the soft palate. This tissue acts as a substitute structure for an inadequate velum by deflecting both airflow and sound waves into the oral cavity. Bzoch (1964), discussing the physiological and speech results for 40 patients who had received pharyngeal flap surgery, reported that the procedure was most effective in reducing both hypernasality and nasal emission (if present) in most of the subjects. Although pharyngeal flap surgery, or any other form of palatal surgery, must not be considered a panacea for all resonance problems, it often helps align oral-nasal structures in such a way that (allowing open or closed coupling of the nasal and oral cavity), for the first time, speech and voice therapy can be effective. Grace (1984), a plastic surgeon, stated:

> Postoperative speech testing is mandatory to objectively evaluate the results of surgery and reassess speech goals. The surgeon may profit from

observing a postoperative evaluation, much as the speech pathologist would profit from seeing surgery. All too often there is a tendency for the surgeon to divorce the patient when the surgery is completed, with the expectation that the battle will be won or lost by the speech pathologist. (p. 154)

When speaking of surgery in cleft palate patients, Grace further stated, "In truth, the success of surgery varies widely from patient to patient, and it can not be assumed that anatomy is restored to normal upon completion of the operation" (p. 154).

Dental Treatment of Hypernasality   Both orthodontists and prosthodontists may play important roles in treating individuals with hypernasality, particularly those with cleft palate. The orthodontist may have to expand the dental arches so that the patient can experience more normal palatal growth and normal dentition. The prosthodontist, by constructing various prosthetic speech appliances and obturators, may be able to help the patient preserve his or her facial contour and by filling in various maxillary defects with prostheses, may cover open palatal defects such as fistulas and clefts. The prosthodontist may also be able to build speech-training appliances to provide posterior velopharyngeal closure. In evaluating 21 adults with acquired or congenital palate problems, Arndt, Shelton, and Bradford (1965) found that both groups made significant "articulation and voice gains with obturation." Many cleft-palate subjects are fitted by prosthodontists with acrylic bulbs at the ends of their appliances; if the bulbs are well positioned near the posterior and lateral pharyngeal walls, often a noticeable reduction of both nasality and air escape results. Articulation, which depends upon adequate intraoral air pressure and normal resonance, may be achieved with speech-voice therapy in conjunction with a properly fit speech appliance such as an obturator or palatal lift device. Two lateral views of obturators are shown in Figure 7–3. Figure 7–4 shows a palatal lift device designed for an adult male with a paralyzed palate following traumatic brain injury in an accident.

When commenting on the role of the speech pathologist in the prosthodontic management of patients with velopharyngeal inadequacy, Ahlstrom (1984), a prosthodontist, stated, "One of the primary diagnostic services that a speech pathologist can offer is the determination of velopharyngeal competence in patients. This helps the prosthodontist to determine what type of appliance or procedure may be necessary" p. 150). Many patients with dysarthria, which may include a hypernasality component, have immobile velums and thus lack sufficient velar movement to achieve closure. Such patients, who experience weakened or paralyzed soft palates, might well profit from consulting a prosthodontist about being fitted with a lift appliance to hold the immobile palate in a

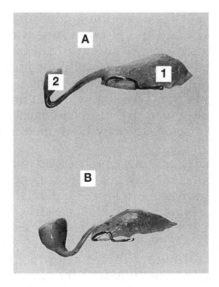

FIGURE 7–3 Two Views of Speech Appliances (Obturators)
(A) is from an adult with a neurogenic (dysarthria) problem of hypernasality; (B) is from a 5-year-old girl with structural (cleft palate) hypernasality with an extremely short velum following surgical repair. (1) is the palatal part, and (2) is the pharyngeal part. Note that the size of the pharyngeal part of the adult appliance is smaller than the corresponding part of the child's prosthesis.

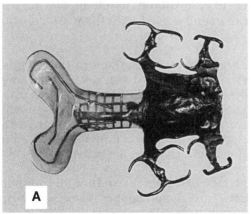

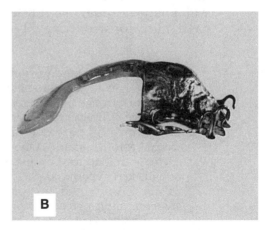

FIGURE 7–4 A Palatal Lift Device
(A) is a superior or top view; (B) is a lateral or side view.

higher position so that some pharyngeal contact will be possible (Mazaheri, 1979). The palatal lift in Figure 7–4 was made for just such a patient who now has normal resonance with the device. For nasality problems related to velopharyngeal inadequacy, speech pathologists should freely consult both orthodontists and prosthodontists for their ideas on how to achieve adequate functioning of the oral structures.

Voice Therapy for Hypernasality Any voice therapy for hypernasality should be deferred until both the evaluation of the problem and attempts at physical correction (surgical or prosthodontic) have been completed. The primary requirement for developing good oral voice quality is the structural adequacy of the velopharyngeal closing mechanism. Without adequate closure, voice therapy will be futile. However, for individuals who speak with hypernasality for functional reasons, voice therapy can help to develop more oral resonance. Added to this group are occasional patients who have had surgical or dental treatment that has left them with only a marginal velopharyngeal closing mechanism; in voice therapy, this mechanism may be trained to work more optimally.

The Nasometer is a less expensive and more practical adaptation or outgrowth of the Tonar. The computer display gives the patient instant feedback information about the peak nasalence level, the target level of oral-nasal ratio, and the moment to moment level of nasalence. If the patient is capable of developing greater oral resonance, he or she works incrementally using the Nasometer feedback system, toward goals of acceptable oral resonance. The following facilitating techniques (described in Chapter 5) may be used successfully with the Nasometer or with a tape recorder, nasal listening tube, U-tube manometer, See Scape, nasal mirror, or stethoscope. They can even be used with the unaided ear.

1. *Altering Tongue Position*. A high, forward carriage of the tongue sometimes contributes to nasal resonance. Efforts to develop a lower, more posterior carriage may decrease the perceived nasality.
2. *Change of Loudness*. A voice that has been perceived as hypernasal will sometimes be perceived as more normal if some other change in vocalization is made. One change that often accomplishes this is an increase in loudness; by speaking in a louder voice, the patient frequently sounds less hypernasal.
3. *Ear Training*. If the patient is motivated to reduce his or her hypernasality, a great deal of therapy time should be spent learning to hear the differences between his or her nasal and oral resonances.
4. *Establishing New Pitch*. Some patients with hypernasality speak at inappropriately high pitch levels, which contribute to the listener's perception of nasality. Speaking at the lower end of one's pitch range seems to contribute to greater oral resonance.
5. *Counseling*. No voice therapy should ever be started without first explaining to the patient what the problem seems to be and the general course of therapy that is being planned.
6. *Feedback*. Developing an aural awareness of hypernasality and some oral-pharyngeal awareness of what hypernasality "feels" like is a most helpful therapeutic device.
7. *Open Mouth*. Hypernasality is sometimes produced by an overall restriction of the oral opening. In such cases, efforts to develop greater oral openness may reduce the listener's perception of excessive nasality.
8. *Focus*. Although for some patients, focusing on the facial mask area seems to increase nasality, for other patients, particularly those whose

hypernasality is of functional origin, doing so noticeably improves resonance.

9. *Respiration Training*. Increased loudness is often achieved by respiration training.

These techniques get results by altering the speech production—for example, by pitch modification, increased or decreased airflow, reduced air pressure on the velopharyngeal port, or enhanced feedback to the patient by using mirror fogging, acoustic changes, or changes in the location of vibratory patterns. We find these methods very successful with patients who have resonance disorders or whose velopharyngeal ports are "borderline adequate" or better. When the velopharyngeal mechanism is less adequate, surgical or prosthetic management is in order prior to initiating voice therapy techniques. When the degree of velopharyngeal mechanism adequacy is seriously in question, a period of intensive trial voice and articulation therapy may determine the need for other management approaches. This trial therapy should be intensive (three sessions per week minimum) but of short duration (6 weeks), and it should be conducted with the understanding that it is a trial to determine if further therapy is indicated or if some other management approach is required. *Under no circumstances should voice therapy for resonance disorders be continued when success is not forthcoming.*

Denasality

Except for the nasal resonance required for /m/, /n/, and /ng/, vowels in American English require only slight nasal resonance. In severe cases lack of nasal resonance produces actual articulatory substitutions for the three nasal phonemes as well as slight alterations of vowels. Denasality (hyponasality) is characterized by the diversion of sound waves and airflow out through the oral cavity, which permits little or no nasal resonance. This problem is usually related to some kind of nasal or nasopharyngeal obstruction, such as excessive adenoidal growth, severe nasopharyngeal infection, or large polyps in the nasal cavity. Some patients who are hypernasal before surgical or dental treatment emerge from such treatment with complete or highly excessive velopharyngeal obstruction. Perhaps the pharyngeal flap is too broad and permits little or no ventilation of the nasopharynx, or an obturator bulb fits too tightly and results in no nasal airflow or nasal resonance. Such obstruction is the usual reason for a denasality problem, and the search for it must precede any voice therapy. We have seen cases, however, in which denasality was caused by psychological or other functional factors.

Nasal airflow competence can be tested as part of an overall resonance evaluation: Ask the patient to take a big breath, close the mouth, and exhale through the nose. Then test the airflow through each nostril separately, compressing the nares of one nostril at a time with finger. If there is any observable decrement in airflow, the nasal passage should be investigated medically. *Appropriate medical therapy should precede any voice therapy for denasality.* Only rarely do patients have markedly denasal voices for wholly functional reasons. Even though their denasal resonance may originally have had a physical cause, that cause is no longer present, and the denasality may remain as a habit, a "set." One television newsman with whom we worked had a denasal voice quality after many years of suffering from allergies. After moving to a new area of the country where the allergies were no longer a problem, he maintained his denasal voice by strength of habit until voice therapy produced a normal voice quality. Occasionally a patient has chosen a denasal voice as a model, for whatever reason, and has learned to match its denasality with some consistency. Voice therapy for increasing nasal resonance might include the following:

> 1. *Ear Training.* Considerable effort must be expended in contrasting for the patient the difference between the nasal and oral production of /m/, /n/, and /ng/. Oral and nasal resonance of vowels can also be presented for listening contrast.
> 2. *Counseling.* The resonance requirements for normal English must be explained to the patient, and his or her own lack of nasal resonance, particularly for /m/, /n/, and /ng/, pointed out. If the patient's problem is wholly functional, this explanation is of primary importance.
> 3. *Feedback.* Emphasis must be given to contrasting what it sounds like and "feels" like to produce oral and nasal resonance. The patient should be encouraged to make exaggerated humming sounds both orally and nasally, concentrating on the "feel" of the two types of productions.
> 4. *Nasal-Glide stimulation.* This technique is one of the most powerful for denasality treatment.
> 5. *Focus.* Direction of the tone into the facial mask is usually successful.

Assimilative Nasality

The nasalization of vowels immediately before and after nasal consonants is known as assimilative nasality. Performance on stimulability testing will provide a good clue whether such nasal resonance is related to poor velar functioning or is functionally induced. A few neurological disorders such as bulbar palsy or multiple sclerosis, prevent the patient from moving the velum quickly enough to facilitate the movements required for normal resonance. The velar openings begin too soon and are maintained too long, lagging behind the rapid requirements of normal speech and nasalizing vowels that occur next to nasal phonemes. *Any patient who has a sudden onset of hypernasality or assimilative nasality should be suspect for a neurological disorder or disease until proven otherwise.* Most cases of assimilative nasality, however, are of functional origin, and the patient shows good oral resonance under special conditions of stimulability. Remember that in connected speech, all sounds are *interdependent*; as one sound is being produced, articulators are positioning for the next sound. This phonemic interdependence allows for a certain amount of assimilation, even in normal speech. Assimilative nasality, therefore, is another perceptual problem—that is, whether the speaker's nasalization of vowels adjacent to nasal phonemes is excessive or not depends on the perception of the listener. The perception of assimilative nasality is related to the perception of excessive nasality; a normal, minor amount of nasality in the vowels following nasal phonemes would not be perceived, and increased amounts of nasal resonance would be judged quite differently by different listeners, according to their individual standards and experience. Therapy for assimilative nasality is likewise highly variable. It is largely related to the locale (in some areas such resonance is a normal voice pattern), the standards of the speaker or clinician, their motivations, and so on.

The Nasometer is a useful therapy instrument for the patient who wants to reduce his or her assimilative nasality. The clinician should be aware of the limitations of such instrumentation (Hardin et al., 1992; Watterson, McFarlane, & Wright, 1993). The clinician and the patient can set oral-nasal ratio goals that favor orality and then work incrementally toward eliminating the assimilative nasal resonance. Voice therapy for assimilative nasality is best attempted only by those patients who are strongly motivated to develop more oral resonance. Facilitating approaches (see Chapter 5) might include the following:

1. *Ear Training*. Ear training should help patients discriminate between their nasalized vowels and their oral vowels. Patients should listen to recordings of their own oral-consonant/vowel/oral consonant words as contrasted with their nasal consonant/vowel/nasal-consonant words, such as these pairs: bad-man, bed-men, bead-mean, bub-mum, and so on. Voice and diction books often contain word pairs matching mono syllabic words using /b/, /d/, and /g/ with those using /m/, /n/, and /ng/. Once the patient can hear the differences between oral and nasal cognates, see if he or she can produce them.

2. *Counseling*. Because nasal assimilations are difficult to explain verbally, any attempt at explanation should be accompanied by demonstration. The best demonstration is to present the contrast between oral and nasal resonance of vowels that follow or precede the three nasal phonemes.

3. *Feedback*. Although feedback can certainly be attempted with the problem of assimilative nasality, experience has found that few patients can monitor well what they are doing during conditions of ongoing feedback. Learning to listen to oneself critically with delayed feedback provided by some kind of auditory loop tape device has been helpful.

THERAPY FOR ORAL-PHARYNGEAL RESONANCE PROBLEMS

Although during speech both the oral and pharyngeal cavities are constantly changing in size and shape, the oral cavity is the most changeable resonance cavity. Speech is possible only because of the capability for variation of such oral structures as the lips, mandible, tongue, and velum. The most dramatic oral movements in speech are those of the tongue, which makes various constrictive-restrictive contacts at different sites within the oral cavity to produce consonant articulation. Vowel and diphthong production are possible only because of size-shape adjustments of the oral cavity that require a delicate blend of muscle adjustment of all oral muscle structures. Although many individuals display faulty positioning of oral structures for articulation, and thus articulate "badly," fewer individuals are recognized to have problems positioning their oral structures for resonance. Slight departures in articulatory proficiency are much more easily recognized than are minor problems in voice resonance. Even though an articulation error may be viewed consistently as a problem, faulty oral-pharyngeal resonance is usually accepted as "the way he or she talks," or a regional dialect. Nasality problems are more likely to be recognized by lay and professional listeners as requiring correction than are oral-pharyngeal resonance departures. Any judgment of resonance is heavily influenced by the appropriateness of pitch, the degree of glottal competence as heard in the periodic quality of phonation, and the degree of accuracy of articulation. Because quality of resonance, then, appears basically to be a subjective experience, the goal in resonance therapy must be to achieve whatever voice "sounds best."

Singing teachers have long been aware of the vital role the tongue plays in influencing the quality of the voice, and they devote considerable instructional and practice time to helping singing students develop optimum carriage of the tongue (Coffin, 1981). Although the postures needed to produce various phonemes will attract the tongue to different anatomic sites within the oral cavity, with noticeable changes of oral resonance, more objective evidence of the role of the tongue in oral resonance may be obtained through spectrographic and videofluorographic analysis. In the spectral analyses afforded by the spectrograph, we can study the effects of tongue positioning and the distribution of spectral formants. The second formant seems to "travel" the most, changing position up and down the spectrum for various vowel productions. Boone and McFarlane (1993) demonstrate this in their study of the yawn-sigh technique (Chapter 5). The primary oral shaper for production of vowels appears to be the tongue. Decisions about quality resonance (e.g., is the voice hypernasal or denasal) are, however, almost impossible to render from the visual inspection of spectrograms. It is most difficult to quantify formant variations and relate them to variations in voice quality. In describing the difficulty of spectrographic analysis, Moll (1968) has written that "this presumably more 'objective' measure involves overall judgments which probably are more difficult than those made in judging nasality from actual speech" (p. 99). Visual inspection of the spectrogram is a difficult task, particularly when one attempts to relate formant positioning to judgments of voice quality. As for the videofluorograph, its use for studying tongue, velar, mandibular, and pharyngeal movements, when such movements apply to voice quality, becomes far more effective when a voice track is added. The addition of the speaker's voice not only enables the viewer to match the sound of the voice with the analysis of the speaker's movements, but, more important, provides the viewer with the primary vehicle for determining whether a problem of quality exists; quality judgments cannot be made from the visual study of oral movements alone, but depend primarily on hearing the sound of the voice. By using both the pitch and intensity readings at the same time on the Visi-Pitch, we have found that the stored tracings on the Visi-Pitch scope give useful information specific to better resonance. Often the resonance that sounds better to the ear is represented on the scope as less aperiodic (the frequency write out has less scatter) and more intense (greater amplitude of the intensity curve). The "better-sounding" voice often comes quite unexpectedly as the clinician and the patient use various facilitating approaches in their search for good oral resonance. Once the "good" voice is achieved, the Visi-Pitch offers useful feedback for the patient, often confirming by improvement in the scope tracings the subjective judgments the clinician and patient have made.

Reducing the Strident Voice

One of the most annoying oral-pharyngeal resonance problems is the strident voice. We use the term *stridency*, which means the unpleasant, shrill, metallic-sounding voice that appears to be related to hypertonicity of the pharyngeal constrictors (walls of the pharynx). Fisher (1975) described the strident voice as having brilliance of high overtones sounding "brassy, tinny, blatant." Physiologically, stridency may be produced by the elevation of the larynx and hypertonicity of the pharyngeal constrictors, which decrease both the length and the width of the pharynx. The surface of the pharynx becomes taut because of the tight pharyngeal constriction. The smaller pharyngeal cavity, coupled with its tighter, reflective mucosal surface, produces the ideal resonating structure for accentuating high-frequency resonance. Stridency may be developed deliberately—for example, by a carnival barker or a dime-store demonstrator for its obvious attention-getting effects—or it may emerge when a person becomes overly tense and constricts the pharynx as part of his or her overall response to stress. A person who has this sort of strident voice—and who wants to correct it—can, in voice therapy, often develop some relaxed oral-pharyngeal behaviors that decrease pharyngeal constriction (increasing the size of the pharynx) and lessen the amount of stridency. Anything that an individual can do to lower the larynx, decrease pharyngeal constriction, and promote general throat relaxation will usually reduce stridency. The following facilitating techniques (described in Chapter 5) are most helpful in greatly reducing stridency:

1. *Inhalation Phonation.* This tends to increase the size of the pharynx, relax the walls of the pharynx and open the laryngeal aditus.

2. *Ear Training.* Explore various vocal productions with the patient, with the goal of producing a nonstrident voice. When the patient is able to produce good oral resonance, contrast this production with recorded strident vocalizations using loop tape feedback devices and following the various ear-training procedures.

3. *Establishing New Pitch.* The strident voice is frequently accompanied by an inappropriately high voice pitch. Efforts to lower the pitch level often produce a voice that sounds less strident.

4. *Counseling.* Although it is difficult to explain problems of resonance to someone else, sometimes such an explanation is essential if the patient is ever to develop any kind of self-awareness about the problem.

5. *Glottal Fry.* The glottal fry produces two beneficial effects. First, the fundamental frequency is somewhat lower following production of the glottal fry; and second, the resonating cavity of the laryngeal aditis is enlarged following the production of the glottal fry (especially an ingressive glottal fry). The relaxation of the folds and the opening of the laryngeal aditis effectively reduce strident vocal quality.

6. *Hierarchy Analysis.* For the individual whose voice becomes strident whenever he or she is tense, it is important to try to isolate those situations in which his or her nonstridency is maintained.

7. *Open Mouth.* Because stridency is generally the product of over-constriction, oral openness is an excellent way to counteract these tight, constrictive tendencies.

8. *Relaxation.* It is difficult to produce strident resonance under conditions of relaxation and freedom from tension. Either general relaxation or a more specific relaxation of the vocal tract is helpful in reducing oral-pharyngeal tightness.

9. *Yawn-Sigh.* Because the yawn-sigh approach produces an openness and relaxation that is completely the opposite of the tightness of pharyngeal constriction, it is perhaps the most effective approach in this list for reducing stridency.

10. *Tongue Protrusion.* This increases the length and width of the pharynx (the whole throat cavity).

Improving Oral Resonance

Two problems of oral resonance are related to faulty tongue position, a *thin* type of resonance produced by excessively anterior tongue carriage and a *cul-de-sac* type produced by backward retraction of the tongue. The thin voice lacks adequate oral resonance, and its user sounds immature and unsure of himself or herself. This problem, which is somewhat common among both men and women, is characterized by a generalized oral constriction with high, anterior carriage of the tongue and only minimal lip-mandibular opening. The user of such a voice appears to be holding back psychologically, either withdrawing from interpersonal contact by demonstrating all the symptoms of withdrawal, or retreating psychologically to a more infantile level of behavior by demonstrating a "babylike" vocal quality. The first type, the person who withdraws from interpersonal contact, employs his or her thin resonance situationally, particularly when he or she feels most insecure; the second type uses the thin voice, the "baby resonance," more intentionally, in situations in which he or she wants to appear cute, to "get his or her own way," and so on. The following facilitating approaches (described in Chapter 5) have been useful in promoting a more natural, adult oral resonance:

1. *Altering Tongue Position.* We discussed the problem of the thin voice in Chapter 5. Specific procedures are developed there to promote a more posterior tongue carriage.

2. *Change of Loudness.* When the resonance problem is part of a general picture of psychological withdrawal in particular situations, efforts to increase voice loudness are appropriate for overall improvement of resonance.

3. *Digital Manipulation.* This is especially helpful when the pitch of the voice is too high or the quality is breathy.

4. *Establishing New Pitch.* The thin voice is perceived by listeners to be drastically lacking in authority. Frequently, the pitch is too high. Efforts to lower the voice pitch often have a positive effect on resonance

5. *Feedback.* Those patients whose anterior resonance focus is related to situational tensions may use feedback apparatus to become aware of their varying states of tension. Feedback is best used with relaxation and hierarchy analysis.

6. *Hierarchy Analysis.* Symptomatic voice therapy is based on the premise that it is often possible to isolate particular situations in which we function poorly, with maladaptive behavior, and other situations in which we function comparatively well. By isolating the various situations and their modes of behavior, we can often introduce more effective behavior into "bad" situations to take the place of the maladaptive behavior. For individuals who use a thin voice in specific situations, particularly during moments of tension, hierarchy analysis may be a necessary preliminary step to eliminate the aberrant vocal quality.

7. *Open Mouth.* The restrictive oral tendencies of a thin-voiced speaker may be effectively reduced by developing greater oral openness.

8. *Relaxation.* If the thin vocal quality is highly situational and the obvious result of tension, relaxation approaches may be helpful, particularly when used in combination with hierarchy analysis.

9. *Respiration Training.* Sometimes direct work on increasing voice loudness requires some work increasing control of the airflow during expiration.

10. *Yawn-Sigh*. The yawn-sigh approach is an excellent way of developing a more relaxed, posterior tongue carriage.

11. *Glottal Fry*. The larger pharyngeal adjustment produced by glottal fry is generally helpful to produce improved resonance.

Patients with a thin voice are often judged by listeners to be immature, young, or lacking in authority. We have provided successful voice therapy to several attorneys, managers, and executives who suffered from thin voice quality that was ineffective for their work. We helped one attorney improve his voice and his performance in the courtroom and during client conferences by using the open-mouth and glottal fry technique.

The cul-de-sac voice is found in individuals from various etiologic groups: patients with oral apraxia; cerebral palsied children, particularly the athetoid type, who have a posterior focus to their resonance added to their dysarthria; some patients with bulbar or pseudobulbar-type lesions, who have a pharyngeal focus to their vocal resonance; and deaf children. The cul-de-sac voice, regardless of its initial physical cause, is produced by the deep retraction of the tongue into the oral cavity and hypopharynx, sometimes touching the pharyngeal wall and sometimes not. The body of the tongue literally obstructs the escaping airflow and the periodic sound waves generated from the larynx below. Although such a voice is often found in individuals with neural lesions who cannot control their muscles, and among deaf children and adults, it is also produced situationally by certain individuals for wholly functional reasons. Such posterior resonance is very difficult to correct in patients who have muscle disorders related to various problems of innervation, particularly dysarthric patients. Resonance deviations in the deaf may be changed somewhat in voice therapy, as described in Chapter 6. For individuals who produce cul-de-sac resonance for purely functional reasons (whatever they are), the following facilitating approaches from Chapter 5 are useful:

1. *Altering Tongue Position*. Speech tasks designed to promote front-of-the-mouth resonance are helpful here. Review the section on resonance changes in the deaf in Chapter 6. The approaches described there for altering tongue position in deaf children apply to anyone working for more forward resonance.

2. *Feedback*. Posterior focus of voice resonance may for some patients be situationally related to tension. Feedback is often useful for helping these patients monitor their varying tension states.

3. *Ear Training*. If, in the search for a better voice, the patient is able to produce a more forward, oral-sounding one, this should be contrasted with his or her cul-de-sac voice.

4. *Hierarchy Analysis*. If cul-de-sac resonance occurs only in particular situations, perhaps at those times when the individual is tense and under stress, the hierarchy approach may be useful. If the individual can produce

good oral resonance in low-stress situations, he or she should practice using the same resonance at levels of increasing stress, on up the hierarchy.

5. *Glottal Fry.* The production of the glottal fry opens the pharynx and the laryngeal aditis, thus enlarging the resonance cavity and adding to the openness of the whole vocal tract. The whole pharynx is relaxed, and thus the cul-de-sac resonance is eliminated.

6. *Focus.* The forward focus in resonance required to place the voice in the facial mask makes the approach a useful one for patients with a cul-de-sac focus. High front vowels and front-of-the-mouth consonants are particularly good practice sounds to use with the place-the-voice approach.

7. *Relaxation.* Posterior tongue retraction during moments of stress is often a learned response to tension. The patient who can learn a more relaxed positioning of the overall vocal tract may be able to reduce excessive tongue retraction.

8. *Tongue Protrusion /i/.* Because the tongue is extended outside of the mouth and the pitch is elevated, the base of the tongue is pulled forward and out of the oral pharynx and this is emphasized with the /i/ vowel. This eliminates the retracted tongue position that produces the back quality.

9. *Nasal-Glide Stimulation.* This helps to get a forward placement of the tongue and the sound and can be used in conjunction with focus.

SUMMARY

Resonance deviations of the voice are often produced by physical problems of structure or function at various sites within the upper airway. Primary efforts must be given to identifying any structural abnormalities and correcting these problems by dental, medical, or surgical intervention. Speech-language pathologists play an important role in the early evaluation and diagnosis of a resonance problem, as well as in providing needed voice therapy to correct the problem. For both organic and functional resonance problems, specific facilitating approaches were listed to help patients develop better nasal and oral resonance.

Chapter 8

Evaluation and Voice Therapy in Various Settings

The reader can be confused by the wide variety of clinical settings that are available today for voice evaluation and voice therapy. Within the various settings, there is great variability in the quality of treatment that is offered. In some clinical situations, because of having good instrumentation and a strong financial-time base, the well-trained voice clinician can reach out and offer an advanced, cutting-edge voice evaluation followed by all the voice therapy that a client may require. In other, less fortunate settings, lack of instrumentation and severe financial and time constraints may limit all clinical efforts, despite the qualifications of the clinician. In this chapter we take a close look at various clinical voice settings, with the hope that greater standardization and optimization of treatment will one day occur across different clinical settings.

Not only does the quality and extent of voice therapy vary in different settings, but there are extreme differences in the training and experience of the voice practitioner within particular settings. The director of voice research in the university clinic may have several years of postdoctoral training in contrast to a staff vocal coach who may have little academic preparation but extensive professional voice experience. In the typical clinical setting, such as in the public schools or in hospitals, the clinician will have a minimum of a Master's degree in speech-language pathology with several years of clinical experience. The amount of time, however, spent working with voice cases may not be as great as the speech-language pathologist's total clinical experience would indicate.

Presently, there are few speech-language pathologists who have had extensive academic preparation in normal voice, voice diagnosis-evaluation, and voice therapy. One might predict that the number of such voice specialists will be growing, as a natural outcome of a recently created national special interest group in voice disorders, formed by the national professional organization, the American Speech-Language-Hearing Association (*ASHA*, 1992). At the present time, ASHA does not offer specialty certification for any particular clinical area, including voice disorders. Therefore, the practice of voice therapy comes out of the generalized clinical preparation and experience by the speech-language pathologist, somewhat dependent on where he or she happened to go to school and the size of the community where the school was located. The formal academic training and available clinical practicum in voice disorders are still highly variable. ASHA's minimum required clinical practicum in voice evaluation and therapy is quite low in number of hours, requiring the clinician who wants to specialize in voice therapy to acquire this special skill after he or she has started professional employment.

There is a great variety of settings where the practice of voice therapy may take place: in the public schools, private practice, consultation for professional voice, university and/or research clinics, community clinics, and ENT and hospital clinics (McFarlane, 1989). The instrumentation available in each setting depends greatly on the wants of the clinician and the budget realities of the institution. Some clinicians, who often had little exposure to instrumentation in their training programs and little use of instrumentation in their clinical practicum settings, may be fearful of instrumentation and may not appreciate what it can do for them. Others may be frustrated that the instrumentation they had previously used is no longer available because of budgetary limitation or they may have been told that "the voice case load is too small to justify the expenditure of funds for voice equipment."

There is probably no factor that contributes more to the quality of voice service available to the patient than the cost-time factor. Evaluation time and voice therapy time cost money. Within the public schools the quantity of therapy offered is often adequate. A voice evaluation and therapy for school-age children is available within public school settings, provided by the school speech-language pathologist (SLP) as part of his or her overall case load. Voice disorders related to health problems are often adequately treated for the preschool child. A preschool child with a voice problem often has an airway problem that requires the medical intervention of the otolaryngologist and follow-up with the hospital SLP; these services are usually covered by medical insurance. On the other hand, voice therapy services for adults are often not covered by health insurance. An adult with a functional voice problem, such as functional dysphonia related to vocal nodules, may have a difficult time securing medical insurance coverage for nonsurgical treatment of the problem—that is, voice therapy. The voice evaluation and any subsequent voice therapy might require the patient to pay costs out of pocket; this can seriously limit the scope of treatment. Or the older adult female, for example, with a voice problem related to bowing of her vocal folds may be denied Medicare coverage and, therefore, be unable to pay for any costs beyond her voice evaluation. The private-practice voice clinician or the speech pathologist in the hospital or medical clinic may continually encounter resistance from third-party payers (such as Blue Cross/Blue Shield or Medicare) for badly needed diagnostic evaluations and voice therapy. There are few voice settings today where cost-time is not an overriding variable. One of the few such settings (and they are becoming increasingly rare) might be the university research clinic, which can study the voice patient in depth, both from a diagnostic-evaluation perspective and in following the patient in voice therapy over an extended period of time.

Let us now look at particular settings as listed in Table 8–1, which lists the settings and gives one negative and one positive factor for each setting. We will then look at each setting individually. For each setting, we will consider the typical personnel working there who may have some expertise in voice management. We will then discuss probable equipment availability for that particular setting. The typical kind of client or patient load will then be presented followed by a critical look at the cost-time factor. Negative and positive features for each treatment setting will then be summarized.

Table 8–1   Voice Evaluations and Therapy in Different Settings

Setting	Advantage	Disadvantage
Schools	Excellent cost-time factor	Poor instrument availability
Community Clinic	Specialty clinical services	Limited financial base
Private Practice	Preference of patient type	Poor cost-time factor
Professional Consultation	Excellent cost-time factor	Limited training and competence
University Clinic	Instrumentation availability	Clinician inexperience
ENT Office-Hospital	Excellent patient management	Deteriorating cost-time factor

VOICE EVALUATION AND VOICE THERAPY IN THE SCHOOLS

Our commentary is reserved for the typical *public* school. Also, the reader should be cautioned that these opinions apply only to a hypothetical public school setting. There are many school situations better than this and undoubtedly there are some that are worse.

Typical Personnel   In most of the public schools in the United States, the speech-language pathologist has a minimum academic entry requirement of a Master's degree. Special state credentialing is usually required, as well as the Certificate of Clinical Competence (CCC) in Speech-Language Pathology. Certified SLPs have had the training to work with children with functional voice disorders related to problems of voice abuse and misuse. In larger school districts there will be several SLPs, often with a consulting supervisor available for discussion of clinical problems. Some districts also provide an aide for the SLP to use to help in the provision of evaluation and therapy services to children. The school psychologist may also be of help with some children with voice problems. One observation commonly heard regarding personnel is that in the school setting, the SLP is often on his or her own and often must make management and treatment decisions with very little consultation.

Equipment Availability　There have been tremendous equipment advances for voice evaluation and therapy in the past few years. Unfortunately, much of this new equipment is not available in the schools. The typical school SLP has available an audiometer with masking capabilities (useful in voice therapy), an audiocassette recorder, a videocamera-recorder-playback unit, and a frequency-intensity analyzer (such as those shown in earlier chapters). There is a trend for larger school districts to set up a central voice clinic in which voice equipment (such as listed in Chapter 4) can be housed, rather than in each particular school. Children are evaluated in the central clinic, and findings (such as videoendoscopic recordings) are then sent to the referring SLP for use with children in therapy in their particular schools.

Typical Voice Problems　One only has to hear playground noises to realize that for many children yelling is a way of life. The primary voice problem in the schools is vocal hyperfunction, which can lead to a number of functional voice disorders, such as functional dysphonia, vocal nodules, and vocal polyps. Other voice problems seen by the SLP may be the result of papilloma, laryngeal web, granuloma, and velopharyngeal insufficiency. It is estimated that about 3% of the children in the primary grades may have phonation and resonance disorders; in the middle and high schools, only about 1% demonstrate voice problems (Hull et al., 1976).

Cost-Time Factors　Although SLPs in the public schools commonly complain that their case loads are too large, voice therapy is available for most schoolchildren who need it. There are few other population groups in the United States that have the opportunity of voice evaluation and therapy without struggling with the cost-time factor. With the federal mandates of PL 94-142, PL 95-561, and PL 99-457 (summarized in Boone & Plante, 1993), local school districts that receive federal monies must make available speech-language-hearing services for handicapped children. Children with voice disorders are listed as speech-handicapped children. Therefore, any child with a voice problem is eligible to receive diagnostic-habilitative services for this problem.

SPLs in the public schools develop their voice case loads from selective screening (certain grades are screened annually), from direct observation, and from referral (other professionals, parents, and teachers). Large case loads sometimes only permit group voice therapy where children of similar problems and ages are grouped together. Smaller and more selective case loads permit individualized voice therapy.

Negative and Positive Features   A negative feature of voice therapy in the public schools is the lack of adequate instrumentation. Such instrumentation, if it were available, permits quantification of various voice parameters and can provide excellent visual feedback for the child in therapy. Other negative features are large case loads, which may prevent individualization of treatment and may limit the amount of therapy that can be provided; also, the relative isolation of the SLP in the schools may limit consultation with other SLPs and other professionals.

An advantage in the schools is the availability of voice evaluation and therapy for children. The cost-time factor is perhaps more favorable in the schools than in any other setting. Other advantages are that the child does not have to leave the school setting to get voice treatment, carryover activities can be facilitated within the classroom and playground, and screening-referral procedures can offer early detection of a voice symptom that may be the first symptom of a serious laryngeal disorder.

VOICE EVALUATION AND VOICE THERAPY IN PRIVATE PRACTICE

The range of private practice in speech-language pathology varies from a part-time SLP who may work a few hours weekly to a practice that includes many full-time SLPs in one setting.

Typical Personnel   A private practitioner must have a graduate degree, be licensed in a state that has licensing, and have ASHA certification. The typical SLP in private practice sees children and adults across the array of clinical disorders. Few such practitioners limit their practice only to voice disorders, although their numbers are growing. For solo practitioners, cross-consultation with other SLPs is often lacking. Other professional consultation, such as with psychologists or laryngologists, may be more available in the private-practice setting.

Equipment Availability   Mobility of the private practice speech-language pathologist often limits the amount of equipment available for voice diagnosis and therapy. SLPs provide their services in many settings, such as in their office, the patient's home, a nursing care facility, or a hospital. Equipment availability in such varied settings is not as good as it may be for the practitioner who works primarily in the same office. Budget limitations for the purchase of equipment is often another reason for its lack of use in private practice. Most SLPs, however, in private practice working with voice patients have available an audiometer, an audiocassette, a VCR unit, a pitch analyzer of some type, an air volume/pressure measuring system, and some kind of acoustic analyzer (see Chapter 4) that permits measurement of frequency, intensity, and perturbation. More elaborate instrumentation, such as the glottograph or a video stroboscopic unit, may be found in selective private practice settings.

Typical Voice Problems   Although a few children are seen in private practice, such as preschoolers, most voice cases are adults. In review of our private-practice files for children with voice problems, we have seen a few preschoolers with moderate to severe resonance problems, vocal nodules, and vocal cord paralyses. A few school-age children with severe phonatory or resonance problems were seen for evaluation-consultation. The biggest private-practice voice case load is with adults with problems related to nodules, polyps, functional dysphonia, aphonia, resonance disorders, spasmodic dysphonia, dysphonia after microsurgery, and laryngectomy.

Cost-Time Factors   One learns quickly in private practice the need for marketing, letting the local area know of your private practice, the kind of patients you see, and the services that you offer. While the potential for earning good money is available in a voice private practice, there are many cost barriers that must be recognized. Many voice disorders are not considered as medical conditions that warrant diagnostic and therapeutic intervention by the SLP; this observation (which is frequently unwarranted) may make it difficult for a third-party payer to authorize payment for the services provided. Voice problems related to medical conditions such as surgical removal of a lesion, vocal cord paralysis, laryngeal web, or laryngectomy will usually result in reimbursement for SLP diagnosis-evaluation-therapy. Voice problems related to resonance defects, functional dysphonia, aphonia, or spasmodic dysphonia are often classified by insurance carriers as voice improvement endeavors and may not qualify for medical insurance payment.

The fiscal constraints in private practice are very real: professional dues and licensing fees, rent, support personnel, equipment costs, utilities, telephone, and so forth. The bills must be paid before the SLP can be reimbursed for his or her professional services. Accordingly, the SLP with a voice private practice has continuing financial pressures that require realistic billing for consultative services, for family conferences, for all diagnostic services, for both group and individual voice therapy. Attending professional meetings and even taking vacations are all activities the typical SLP takes for granted. In private practice with voice patients, such absences contribute no revenue to the practice.

Negative and Positive Features   The cost-time factors described above are perhaps the most negative features of private practice. There is pressure to make money. In working with voice patients, there are constant fiscal obstacles that seem to prevent good evaluation and management. Third-party payers often deny reimbursement for voice therapy; for example, the Medicare carrier in one state turned down voice therapy for a 69-year-old woman "with bowed vocal folds." Only after several calls by the SLP and after providing detailed treatment plans (following the criteria that Medicare wanted) could therapy be reimbursed. Working out "private pay" arrangements with some voice patients can be trying. Patient cancellation without much advance warning is a continuing negative in private practice. Other negatives for voice private practice is lack of needed equipment, the need for travel to various settings, and the overall lack of personnel benefits.

A great excitement for private practice in voice is seeing the kind of patients that one likes to see. When possible, the practice is limited to the age and kind of problem for which the SLP feels most competent and interested in treating. A successful practitioner may experience the thrill of providing the exact kind of voice therapy the patient requires, producing outstanding results. It should be mentioned that an SLP working with voice patients who gets poor results soon loses his or her referral base. A good private practitioner in voice develops a continuing referral source from other professionals (physicians, psychologists, singing teachers, theater directors) in the community. Occasionally, patients are referred from other communities for consultation and management, usually the sign of a successful practitioner.

CONSULTATION FOR THE PROFESSIONAL VOICE

The care of the performing voice is receiving much attention from professional users of voice. By professional voice user, we mean any person who makes his or her livelihood from using voice (singer, actor, teacher, politician, preacher, salesperson). While caring for and extending the voice is the focus of the intervention of vocal coaches and teachers, much attention is given to vocal artistry.

Typical Personnel   Some of the most innovative voice evaluations and voice therapy available are offered by the vocal coach, the voice teacher, and the singing teacher. There are also a few speech-language pathologists who limit their practice to caring primarily for the professional voice. The typical vocal coach or voice teacher may have had limited formal voice training but has had extensive performance experience. The range of formal education can range from almost no education to postdoctorate in performing arts. Professional experience in performing, directing, singing, and voice teaching is equally varied. Of all the settings in this chapter where voice intervention of some kind is offered, the heterogeneity of training and experience of clinicians or teachers is most marked. This lack of uniformity is primarily the result of the lack of a required credential and/or license for such personnel.

Equipment Availability   Most vocal coaches and voice and singing teachers work with very little equipment. Typically, they use a piano, a pitch pipe, and audio or video recorders. Some of the more elaborate voice studios have some respiratory measuring devices that can illustrate various volume and flow measures. Some studios may have some kind of spectral analyzing equipment that provides digital or oscillographic displays. Occasional laryngologists, who include care of the professional voice as part of their practice, have endoscopic or stroboscopic equipment available. Overall, in settings where work is done with the user of professional voice, very little equipment is used. There will no doubt be greater use of equipment in these settings in the future.

Typical Voice Problems   The speech-language pathologist working with professional users of voice is often confronted with a voice in trouble. Evaluation may reveal that the patient lacks sufficient air support, may be using the voice in a hyperfunctional manner, or is using a voice that lacks proper focus (see Chapter 5). The performer may or may not have a structural problem with the larynx (nodules, polyps, web, paralysis) but will generally demonstrate some physiologic abnormalities (he or she does not use the vocal mechanisms correctly). It should be remembered that the professional user of voice may experience some of the same vocal pathologies experienced by the population in general (infections, allergies, vocal fold irritation and swelling, nodules, etc.). Any such organic deviation for the professional voice user may have profound negative effects on performance and, therefore, may require some kind of immediate medical intervention (Sataloff, 1991).

The typical singing or voice teacher puts his or her emphasis on using the voice (respiration, pitch, quality, vocal attack, resonance, artistry interpretation) correctly. What to do about the disordered voice is often beyond the competence of coaches or teachers; it is sometimes observed that they might be unaware of their limitations and proceed anyway to work with disordered voices. Similarly, the SLP may extend beyond necessary training and experience when he or she begins to work on artistry and performance. In the area of professional voice training, it is very easy for the professional trainer (laryngologist, SLP, vocal coach, or teacher) to extend his or her "expertise" beyond one's actual knowledge-experience base. When possible, this should be avoided.

Cost-Time Factors   In general, the cost-time factors in providing care for the professional voice are very favorable. The professional voice user needs help in caring and extending the professional voice. As part of developing vocal skills, the actor or singer seeks professional training and expects to pay for it. There is usually direct payment without insurance. The teacher, preacher, or politician who is experiencing some kind of vocal limitation may seek professional help; direct payment is often the method of payment, although medical insurance may be available for some problems. Perhaps of all the settings described in this chapter, the cost-time factor is the most favorable for the provider of voice training for the professional user of voice.

Negative and Positive Features   The lack of uniform coaching and teaching is a primary negative factor. Without credentialing or licensing, the quality and type of treatment are highly variable. Lack of formal training or professional experience, as well as the relative lack of equipment, may limit the options for the client. The settings may be a noisy corner of a stage or a theater or the spare room of an apartment. The well-equipped clinic or studio is often lacking. There is a potential negative among the clientele seeking help for the professional voice; such clients may be temperamental, high-strung, manipulative, challenging to authority, any of which might make consultation and teaching more difficult. Or they may be exceedingly cooperative and grateful.

The biggest positive in providing care for the professional voice is experiencing the powerful improvement in performance of these professional voices. The capability of the trained speaking or singing voice is a remarkable experience to witness. To work with an actor or singer in a way that facilitates his or her performance is a thrilling experience for the clinician. The SLP who experiences successful intervention with professional voice users may receive far greater reward than financial. The financial aspects of such management and therapy are, however, very good and a strong positive. For the "frustrated performer" who ends up as a coach or SLP, working with performers may offer intangible awards—that is, it is "fun" to work with them.

VOICE EVALUATION AND VOICE THERAPY IN THE UNIVERSITY AND/OR RESEARCH CLINIC

Most training programs in the United States operate clinics in speech-language pathology. There are a few university clinics that offer extensive diagnostic-clinical services in voice disorders.Within the university clinic is a small clinical practicum in voice disorders, usually reserved for the advanced graduate student.

Typical Personnel   The typical graduate program in speech-language pathology has one faculty member who teaches the basic voice science courses and another faculty member who teaches clinical voice courses and supervises the clinical practicum. In small programs, the basic science and clinical voice faculty member may be the same person (usually possessing a doctorate). Many university clinics have in addition to several doctoral level faculty, several Master's-level clinical supervisors who supervise the voice practicum. All university clinical faculty generally have clinical certification. In large clinical research programs, different doctoral faculty members may have special skills, such as in endoscopy, glottography, or acoustic analyses. The typical speech-language pathology clinic in the university will also have a number of faculty available as consultants to the voice program, representing other areas like child language, neurogenics, stuttering, or articulation.

Equipment Availability   The latest in new voice equipment in the past 5 to 10 years is often used in university programs before it is found in applied clinical programs. Students and faculty who were fortunate to work in such departments with ample instrumentation were able to provide the voice client with "cutting-edge" evaluations and therapy. Certainly, the few voice programs in the United States with special funding (from foundation support or federal grants, such as those provided a few universities by institutes within the National Institutes of Health) are able to offer extensive clinical services as part of overall voice research.

The typical university program is always trying to find ways to fund the purchase of more equipment. The graduate student in clinical training may be able to get training in using an audiometer, videoendoscopy and stroboscopy, a glottograph, a spirometer, a pneumotachometer with pressure transducer (see Chapter 4), an acoustic analyzer (such as a Visi-Pitch), a spectrograph, and instruments for measuring velopharyngeal adequacy. The student needs special training in using such equipment rapidly (a reality in the clinical world) and selectively as it may be needed (and not subject every voice patient to a battery of tests).

Typical Voice Problems   Not too many university clinics attempt to meet the needs of the university's students. If they did, programs would be flooded with young adults with problems of phonation and resonance. Typically, these kinds of cases are hard to find in university clinics. In fact, in the typical training program, voice clients are "hard to come by." A few children—often with serious problems that require the university clinic instrumentation—are seen. Perhaps the most common child voice problem is related to the evaluation and management of problems related to velopharyngeal insufficiency. Other problems seen in children in university clinics are related to severe hearing loss, vocal nodules, web, papilloma, and functional dysphonia. There are relatively few middle-aged adults seen in such clinics; those that come in usually have problems of functional dysphonia, vocal nodules, and vocal fold paralyses. The older population patients usually have problems of spasmodic dysphonia, vocal fold paralyses, microsurgery, or laryngectomy.

Cost-Time Factors   There is no clinical setting more affordable than the university voice clinic. The time of evaluation and treatment may take a lot longer. Students are looking for voice hours and voice clients. Evaluation clinics may be set up that permit a full battery of tests (data gathering for some kind of research project) where the patient will come back for several diagnostic sessions. Unfortunately, in many university clinics the emphasis is given to diagnostic evaluations over the provision of voice therapy. In programs that combine laryngology, voice science, and clinical voice services, the diagnostic evaluations can be quite detailed, sometimes offering insights into the patient's problems that would be unavailable in the typical, more limited evaluation.

Therapy intervention can often be extended and perhaps more casual than what the patient might experience in a private practice or hospital setting. Time is a lot cheaper in the university setting than in other settings. The new graduate in his or her clinical fellowship year (CFY) often must learn painfully how to shorten the length of treatment time in clinical settings beyond the university clinic. Some university programs, however, are attempting to build better cost-time skills in new clinicians by making overall case management more similar to "real-world" clinical situations.

Negative and Positive Features   A student in training is not going to be able to offer the same quality of evaluation or therapy as the experienced clinician can. Supervision varies considerably in the university clinic; some clinics offer such poor supervision that the student clinician may be unguided in his or her treatment; in other clinics there may be so much supervision that students are asking for greater freedom. The typical university clinic focuses more on evaluation than on therapy. It appears that some faculty and students "hide" behind their equipment and their test scores, rather than use the equipment to facilitate diagnostic knowledge and improve the quality of treatment. Occasional university clinics may lack the quality of treatment space and sufficient equipment to do adequate voice evaluations and therapy. Other negatives might include the constant changeover of student clinicians, the excessive number of days spent on holidays and vacations, or the extended management of voice problems that should not take so long to fix.

Advanced instrumentation can often be found in university clinics. Many such clinics offer the best there is in instrumental evaluations and in using equipment as feedback devices in therapy. The relatively low financial cost to the patient and the family makes the university clinic attractive. The entire consulting faculty within the clinical department may be available for those patients needing such consultation. Other positives include working with caring young clinicians, having a leisurely clinic schedule, and having the opportunity for needed on-site consultation specific to the appropriateness of the treatment being offered. Another plus often not appreciated by the patient is the clinical data obtained in the university often add to the data base specific to the overall management of particular kinds of voice problems.

VOICE EVALUATION AND VOICE THERAPY IN COMMUNITY CLINICS

There are two kinds of community clinics that may offer voice evaluation and voice therapy. One is the nonprofit clinic for certain disorders or patient groups, like a cerebral palsy clinic or a crippled children's clinic, which offers habilitative services from many disciplines, including hearing and speech. The other kind of clinic is the hearing and speech center, usually nonprofit, which serves the community.

Typical Personnel   In the general community clinic, like a cerebral palsy center, there will be a number of personnel from various disciplines like physical therapy, occupational therapy, educational psychology, and speech-language pathology services. The key personnel in each of these disciplines will generally be certified and/or licensed within their profession. They will be assisted by therapy aides. The speech-language pathologist in the community clinics will usually have a Master's degree, clinical certification, and state licensing. In the community speech and hearing clinic, one may find an occasional doctoral-level SLP, but most are at the Master's level. The general thrust of the agency is in improving the communicative competencies of its clients or patients. In speech-language pathology, more emphasis is generally given to providing needed therapy than in providing extensive evaluations. In the typical community clinic, one does not usually find a SLP who specializes in voice disorders.

Equipment Availability The typical community clinic does not have a lot of instrumentation available for voice evaluation and voice therapy. A crippled children's agency, for example, may have an audiometer and a cassette tape recorder; there may be a computer available that can assist the clinician in word processing. The speech and hearing center has often set up a voice evaluation lab that might include some kind of respiratory pressure-flow measuring device, a good tape recorder, a VCR, some kind of acoustic-spectral measuring instrument, and perhaps an instrument that can assist in evaluation and therapy with resonance disorders (such as a Nasometer). The typical community agency is hard-pressed to find monies for the purchase of voice instrumentation, and it does not have the funds available for a disproportionately small number of voice patients as compared to the total number of patients in the agency.

Typical Voice Problems Among children seen in community agencies, voice problems can be quite severe. Many children with various neurogenic disorders may exhibit severe dysarthrias requiring help in respiration, pitch control, pitch inflection, quality, and resonance. Voice as the primary component in prosody of language may be markedly impaired. Some community clinics may specialize in certain problem areas that may impact heavily on voice, such as asthma, cerebral palsy, severe hearing loss, muscular dystrophy, or spinal injury.

In the community speech and hearing center, voice problems in preschool children are usually the result of severe hearing loss and respiratory limitations. Only a few school-age children are seen, usually for such problems as neuromuscular diseases or cleft palate. Young and middle-age adults are more likely to present voice problems related to vocal nodules and polyps, functional dysphonia, and aphonia. For the population over age 60, the SLP may see more serious voice problems, related to such problems as spasmodic dysphonia, dysarthria, vocal fold paralysis, laryngeal trauma, laryngeal microsurgery, and laryngectomy.

Cost-Time Factors The typical community agency is a nonprofit clinic with some budget dependency on foundation or community support, such as the United Way. Although professional personnel have relatively low salaries, total agency costs are high. Despite the need for more agency revenue, most community speech and hearing programs have sliding fee scales for their clientele. No one is turned down because of inability to pay. Each client pays what he or she can afford to pay. Community volunteers often provide clerical assistance or help the clinician as an aide in therapy.

For the voice patient, there is often a lack of third-party payment for evaluation and treatment. Consequently, evaluation time blocks for voice patients may be limited to an hour. More emphasis may be given to the therapy process than to a detailed diagnostic evaluation. The fiscal restraints of many community agencies result in lack of needed voice instrumentation, hiring personnel without extensive voice experience, and conducting evaluation and therapy with more emphasis on perceptual evaluation than on instrumental analysis and feedback. The overall cost-time factor for voice management in community agencies is not usually as good as it is in most of the other settings described in this chapter.

Negative and Positive Features   The poor cost-time factor is a prominent negative feature of voice evaluation and therapy in the community clinic. Financial limitations can be severe. Salaries for professional personnel may be lower than in other clinical settings. Accountability of cost and time of the SLP plays an important role and may influence decision making specific to voice management. Lack of needed voice instrumentation may be a problem in some agencies.

Some community agencies offer excellent services for problem populations, such as those with cerebral palsy or deafness. The entire agency may have a patient focus where the complete professional staff will interface with each patient, planning in detail the patient's total program. For patients who have a lack of financial resources, the community agency can offer the voice patient needed habilitative services. Some of the finest voice therapy available may be found in the community clinic.

VOICE EVALUATION AND VOICE THERAPY IN ENT AND HOSPITAL CLINICS

With the advent of new instrumentation and well-trained personnel in the past few years, there has been an impressive upgrade in the quality of voice diagnostic-therapy services offered in medical clinics. The practice of voice therapy in the ENT clinic may be located in a professional clinic outside the hospital or as part of an otolaryngology department within a hospital. Voice evaluation and therapy may also be offered within the hospital in free-standing audiology/speech-language pathology departments, as in veterans' medical centers, or within such hospital departments as physical medicine and rehabilitation, neurology, pediatrics, or plastic surgery.

Typical Personnel Perhaps the best-trained clinical voice clinicians are found in medical settings. Both doctoral-level and Master's-level SLPs may be found in the ENT practice or within a speech-language pathology service in the hospital. All have credentials and licensing (if available). Some voice scientists or SLPs with extensive voice training and experience may be housed in the medical voice clinic. The voice patient may access the SLP either directly or by referral from the laryngologist or other medical specialist. The opportunity for cross referral to other specialists within the hospital like the laryngologist, the neurologist, or plastic surgeon gives the SLP real advantages in patient management.

Equipment Availability The primary concern within the medical setting over preservation of the airway gives impetus to having equipment available that can closely examine the airway and, most importantly, its functions. Accordingly, most voice clinics in ENT offices or in hospital departments are well equipped. Typical instrumentation found in medical settings includes audiometric-audiological examining equipment, spirometers and pressure-flow measuring devices, videoendoscopes and stroboscopes, a glottograph, an advanced spectrograph, acoustic analyzers (frequency-intensity-perturbation), palatographs, and acoustic analyzers that can measure the relative ratio of nasal-oral acoustic signals. Such instrumentation is well utilized in diagnostic evaluations and can often play an important feedback display role in voice therapy. Instrumental data are not only important to the SLP in quantifying airway function, but can give the patient feedback on quantitative data specific to a particular voice function. For the occasional patient who has severe voicing limitations, the SLP may have some augmentative devices available (artificial larynx, speaker system, or computer-assisted communication board).

Typical Voice Problems Serious threats to the airway from such problems as traumatic injury or laryngeal carcinoma would have priority in the voice laboratory over more routine voice problems. In children, any kind of airway obstruction might have serious life-threatening implications and would be given medical-surgical priority. Since hospital patients spend less and less time as in-patients (more from funding limitations than from any other factor), most voice evaluations and therapy are provided to out-patients.

In the voice practice in an ENT clinic, typical voice problems are dysphonias related to nodules and polyps, functional and paralytic aphonia, spasmodic dysphonia, laryngeal trauma, and postsurgical problems related to web, cysts, papilloma, granuloma, and laryngeal cancer. Airway and voice evaluation is a primary requisite before any voice therapy would begin. The amount and kind of therapy offered is highly individualized, depending on the individual needs of the patient.

In the hospital, the kind of voice patient the SLP sees is highly related to the kind of service unit that houses the voice clinic. In a free-standing speech-language pathology department, any kind of voice patient can be seen. In children, more often the voice problems are related to airway obstruction; in adults, the problems are more related to changes in voice with airway obstruction still important but seen as a problem in fewer patients. In the typical hospital department (ENT, neurology, or physical medicine and rehabilitation), airway and voice problems may be seen as the result of head trauma, direct injury to the larynx, severe cerebral-brain stem disease, or directly after airway or laryngeal surgery. Besides working on respiration and voice, the SLP may also be working on dysphagia and cognitive deficits displayed by the patient (voice quality might be of secondary concern).

Cost-Time Factors   All voice patients seen by the SLP in medical settings must be referred by a physician. In recent years, there is much more procedure and paperwork required for physicians and other medical clinics to make direct referrals to speech-language pathologists. Emergency and primary care of patients with airway or voice problems is usually good in medical settings. However, anything elective, such as improving your voice, may not be possible in the medical setting. Costs and insurance payments often control and limit what can be done. The hospital SLP seems in recent years to spend increasing time arguing with third-party payment clerks and filling out extensive diagnosis and treatment forms, with less time available for voice therapy.

The cost-time factor for voice management in medical settings is a serious problem. Evaluation time is expensive. Needed evaluation procedures may be curtailed because of fiscal limitation. Various group health plans and medical insurance policies may not cover the provision of voice therapy for hospital out-patients. Or the amount of therapy may be limited to a prescribed number of visits, regardless of what the patient may need. Voice clinics in ENT offices and hospitals often have to absorb heavy dollar losses for voice habilitation services that sometimes have not qualified for insurance reimbursement.

Negative and Positive Features   The cost-time factor is the biggest negative feature in offering voice evaluation and therapy services in medical settings. Certain insurance carriers may deny payment to the SLP in the ENT office for certain services. For example, voice therapy may be viewed as an elective procedure that is not a health problem and will require the patient to pay out-of-pocket costs. Even though speech therapy is a covered Medicare service, it requires the filing of several forms, the physician's signature on a therapy plan, and some severe limitations on the number of visits possible. Even following these procedures, the SLP may end up receiving only a fraction of his or her normal billing. Another negative of voice practice in a medical setting is that the SLP in some situations is viewed as the "low person" on the professional hierarchy, with the physician viewed as the king or the queen (among experienced and older SLPs, this is less a problem). Another negative in medical settings is the long hours of work each day with a very high case load of patients.

Instrumentation availability in the medical clinic is the best of all the settings described in this chapter. The typical SLP in the ENT or hospital clinic knows how to use this equipment, often providing excellent voice evaluation and therapy. This quality professionalism results in excellent voice outcomes for many patients. Other positives in the medical setting include the stimulation of seeing many interesting voice patients, working side by side with other professionals, and enjoying excellent work benefits specific to health care, vacations, professional leave, and so forth.

SUMMARY

The voice patient may emerge in many different clinical environments. We looked at some of the specifics of providing voice evaluations and voice therapy for this patient in different settings. We reviewed the differences and similarities between voice practice in the schools, in private practice, in professional voice consultation, in university clinics, in community clinics, and in ENT or hospital clinics. Although the speech-language pathologist is trained to work with many kinds of clinical problems in diverse settings, the reality of practice seems to be that certain SLPs become more specialized in what they do, which is somewhat dictated by the settings in which they work.

References

Ahlstrom, R. H. (1984). Speech pathology: Views from medicine and dentistry. In S. C. McFarlane (Ed.), *Coping with communicative handicaps*. San Diego: College Hill Press.

Ainsworth, S. (1980). Disorders of voice. In G. M. English (Ed.), *Otolaryngology* (Vol. 4, Chap. 13). Philadelphia: Harper & Row.

American Cancer Society. (1980). *Cancer facts and figures, 1980*. New York: Author.

Aminoff, M. J., Dedo, H. H., & Izdebskil, L. (1978). Clinical aspects of spasmodic dysphonia. *Journal Neurology, Neurosurgery and Psychiatry, 41*, 361–365.

Andrews, M. (1986). *Voice therapy for children*. New York: Longman.

Arndt, W. B., Shelton, R. L., & Bradford, L. J. (1965). Articulation, voice, and obturation in persons with acquired and congenital palate defects. *Cleft Palate Journal, 2*, 377–383.

Aronson, A. E. (1985). *Clinical voice disorders* (2nd ed.). New York: Thieme-Stratton.

Aronson, A. E. (1990). *Clinical voice disorders, an interdisciplinary approach* (3rd ed.). New York: Thieme-Stratton.

Aronson, A. E., & DeSanto, L. W. (1983). Adductor spastic dysphonia: Three years after recurrent laryngeal nerve resection. *Annals of Otolaryngology, Rhinology, Laryngology, 93*, 1–8.

Aronson, A. E., Peterson, H. W., & Litin, E. M. (1966). Psychiatric symptomatology in hypernasality in cleft palate children. *Cleft Palate Journal, 1*, 329–335.

Asha (1992). ASHA's special interest divisions. *Asha, 34*, 17.

ASHA, (1992). Vocal tract visualization and imaging. *ASHA Supplement No. 7, 34*, 37–40.

Baken, R. J., & Orlikoff, R. F. (1988). Changes in vocal fundamental frequency at the segmental level. *Journal of Speech and Hearing Research, 31*, 207–211.

Batsakis, J. G. (1979). *Tumors of the head and neck*. Baltimore: Williams & Wilkins.

Bickley, C. A., & Stevens, K. N. (1987). Effects of vocal tract constriction of the glottal source: Data from voiced consonants. In T. Baer, C. Sasaki, & K. Harris (Eds.), *Laryngeal functioning phonation and respiration*. Boston: Little, Brown.

Blakeley, R.W. (1991). Voice assessment without instrumentation. *Seminars in Speech and Language, 12*, 142–53.

Bless, D. (1984). In V. L. Lawrence (Ed.), *Transcripts of the eleventh symposium: Care of the professional voice*. New York: Voice Foundation.

Bless, D., & Miller, J. (1972). *Influence of mechanical and linguistic factors on lung volume events during speech*. Paper presented at American Speech and Hearing Association Convention.

Bless, D., & Saxman, J. H. (1970). *Maximum phonation time, flow rate, and volume change during phonation: Normative information on third-grade children*. Paper presented at American Speech and Hearing Convention.

Blitzer, A. (1992). Efficacy of Botox treatment in adductor and abductor spasmodic dysphonia of dystonic etiology. *Neurogenic vs Psychogenic Dysphonias, Differential Diagnosis & Management*. San Francisco: Pacific Voice Conference.

Blitzer, A., & Brin, M. F. (1991). Laryngeal dystonia: A series with botulinum toxin therapy. *Annals of Otolaryngology, Rhinology, and Laryngology, 100*, 85–90.

Blitzer, A., & Brin, M. F., Fahn, S., & Lovelace, R. E. (1988). Localized injections of botulinum toxin for the treatment of vocal laryngeal dystonia (spastic dysphonia). *Laryngoscope, 98*, 193–197.

Blood, G. W., Luther, A. R., & Stemple, J. C. (1992). Coping and adjustment in alaryngeal speakers. *American Journal of Speech-Language Pathology, 1*, 63–69.

Boone, D. R. (1966a). Modification of the voices of deaf children. *Volta Review, 68,* 686–692.

Boone, D. R. (1966b). Treatment of functional aphonia in a child and an adult. *Journal of Speech and Hearing Disorders, 31,* 69–74.

Boone, D. R. (1973). Voice therapy for children. *Journal of Human Communication, 1,* 30–43.

Boone, D. R. (1974). Dismissal criteria in voice therapy. *Journal of Speech Hearing Disorders, 39,* 133–139.

Boone, D. R. (1977). Voice disorders: Communicative disorders. *An Audio Journal for Continuing Education.* New York: Grune & Stratton.

Boone, D. R. (1982). *The Boone Voice Program for Adults.* Austin, TX: PRO-ED.

Boone, D. R. (1983). *The voice and voice therapy* (3rd ed.). Englewood Cliffs, NJ: Prentice Hall.

Boone, D. R. (1991). *Is your voice telling on you?* San Diego, CA: Singular Publishing Group.

Boone, D. R. (1993). *The Boone Voice Program for Children* (2nd ed.). Austin, TX: PRO-ED.

Boone, D. R., & McFarlane, S. C. (1993). A critical study of the yawn-sigh technique. *Journal of Voice, 7,* 75–80.

Boone, D. R., & Plante, E. (1993). *Human communication and its disorders* (2nd ed.). Englewood Cliffs, NJ: Prentice Hall.

Bouhuys, A., Proctor, D. F., & Mead, T. (1966). Kinetic aspects of singing. *Applied Physiology, 21,* 483–496.

Bowman, S. A., & Shanks, J. C. (1978). Velopharyngeal relationships of /i/ and /s/ as seen cephalometrically. *Journal of Speech and Hearing Disorders, 43,* 185–191.

Bradford, L. J., Brooks, A. R., & Shelton, R. L. (1964). Clinical judgment of hypernasality in cleft palate children. *Cleft Palate Journal, 1,* 329–335.

Brodnitz, F. S. (1971). *Vocal rehabilitation.* Rochester, MN: Whiting Press.

Buchayer, M., & Cornut, G. (1988). Microsurgery for benign lesions of the vocal folds, *Ear Nose and Throat Journal, 67,* 446–466.

Buller, A. (1942). Nasality: Cause and remedy of our American blight. *Quarterly Journal of Speech, 28,* 83–84.

Case, J. L. (1991). *Clinical management of voice disorders* (2nd ed.). Rockville, MD: Aspen Systems Corporation.

Casper, J., Colton, R., & Brewer, D. (1986). Selected therapy techniques and laryngeal physiological changes in patients with vocal fold immobility. *Folia Phoniatricia, 38,* 288–289.

Cherry, J., & Margulies, S. (1968). Contact ulcer of the larynx. *Laryngoscope, 78,* 1937–1940.

Chodzko-Zajko, W. J., Ringel, R. L., & O'Connor, P. J. (1985). Cardiovascular and pulmonary performance and sensory deterioration in aging. *Gerontologist, 25,* 215.

Coffin, B. (1981). *Overtones of bel canto.* New Jersey: Scarecrow Press.

Colton, R. H., & Casper, J. K. (1990). *Understanding voice problems: A physiological perspective for diagnosis and treatment.* Baltimore: Williams & Wilkins.

Cooper, M. (1973). *Modern techniques of voice rehabilitation.* Springfield, Il: Charles C. Thomas.

Cooper, M. (1977). Direct vocal rehabilitation. In M. Cooper & M. H. Cooper (Eds.), *Approaches to vocal rehabilitation.* Springfield, IL: Charles C. Thomas.

Cooper, M. (1990). *Winning with your voice.* Hollywood, FL: Fell.

Coulthard, S. W. (1987). Personal communication. Tucson: University of Arizona College of Medicine.

Crumley, R. L. (1990). Teflon versus thyroplasty versus nerve transfer: A comparison. *Annals of Otology, Rhinology, and Laryngology, 99,* 759–763.

Crumley, R. L. (1991). Update: Ansa cervicalis to recurrent laryngeal nerve anastomosis for unilateral laryngeal paralysis. *Laryngoscope, 101,* 384–388.

Crumley, R. L. (1992). Response to McFarlane and co-authors. *American Journal of Speech-Language Pathology, 1,* 65–67.

Crumley, R. L., & Izdebski, K. (1986). Voice quality following laryngeal reinnervation by ansa hypoglossi transfer. *Laryngoscope, 96,* 611–616.

Curry, E. T. (1949). Hoarseness and voice change in male adolescents. *Journal of Speech Hearing Disorders, 16,* 23–24.

Daniloff, R. G. (1973). Normal articulation process. In F. D. Minifie, T. J. Hixon, & F. Williams (Eds.), *Normal aspects of speech, hearing, and language.* Englewood Cliffs, NJ: Prentice Hall.

Darley, F. L., Aronson, A. E., & Brown, J. R. (1969). Differential diagnostic patterns of dysarthria. *Journal of Speech and Hearing Research, 12,* 246–269.

Davis, D. S., & Boone, D. R. (1967). Pitch discrimination and tonal memory abilities in adult voice patients. *Journal of Speech and Hearing Research, 10,* 811–815.

Davis, P. J., Boone, D. R., Carroll, R. L., Darveniza, P., & Harrison, G. A. (1987). Adductor spastic dysphonia: Heterogeneity of physiological and phonatory characteristics. *Archives of Otolaryngology, 97,* 179–185.

Dedo, H. H. & Behlau, M. S. (1991). Recurrent laryngeal nerve section for spastic dysphonia: 5-to-14 year preliminary results in the first 300 patients. *Annals of Otolaryngology, Rhinology, and Laryngology, 100,* 274–279.

Dedo, H. H., & Izdebski, K. (1983). Intermediate results of 306 recurrent laryngeal nerve sections for spastic dysphonia. *Laryngoscope, 93,* 9–16.

Dedo, H. H., & Jackler, R. K. (1982). Laryngeal papilloma: Results of treatment with the CO2 laser and podophyllum. *Annals of Otolaryngology, Rhinology, and Laryngology, 91,* 425–430.

Delahunty, J., & Cherry, J. (1968). Experimentally produced vocal cord granulomas. *Laryngoscope, 78,* 1941–1947.

Dickson, D., & Maue-Dickson, W. (1982). *Anatomical and physiological bases of speech.* Boston: Little, Brown.

Dickson, D. R. (1962). Acoustic study of nasality. *Journal of Speech and Hearing Research, 5,* 103–111.

Dickson, S., & Jann, G. R. (1974). Diagnostic principles and procedures. In S. Dickson (Ed.), *Communication disorders, remedial principles, and practices.* Glenview, IL: Scott, Foresman.

Diedrich, W. M., & Youngstrom, K. A. (1966). *Alaryngeal speech.* Springfield, IL: Charles C. Thomas.

Eckel, F. C., & Boone, D. R. (1981). The s/z ratio as an indicator of laryngeal pathology. *Journal of Speech and Hearing Disorders, 46,* 147–150.

Ellis, P. D. M., & Bennett, J. (1977). Laryngeal trauma after prolonged endotracheal intubation. *Journal of Laryngology, 91,* 69–76.

Eysenck, H. (Ed.). (1961). *Handbook of abnormal psychology.* New York: Basic Books.

Fairbanks, G. (1960). *Voice and articulation drillbook.* New York: Harper Brothers.

Fant, G. (1960). *Acoustic theory of speech production.* The Hague: Mouton.

Filter, M. D., & Urioste, K. (1981). Pitch imitation abilities of college women with normal voices. *Journal of Speech Hearing Association, Virginia, 22,* 20–26.

Filter, M. D. (1982). *Phonatory voice disorders in children.* Springfield, IL: Charles C. Thomas.

Fisher, H. B. (1975). *Improving voice and articulation* (2nd ed.). New York: Houghton Mifflin.

Fletcher, S. G. (1972). Contingencies for bioelectronic modification of nasality. *Journal of Speech and Hearing Disorders, 37,* 329–346.

Fletcher, S. G., & Daly, D. A. (1976). Nasalance in utterances of hearing impaired speakers. *Journal of Communication Disorders, 9,* 63–73.

Forner, L., & Hixon, T. J. (1977). Respiratory kinematics in profoundly hearing-impaired speakers. *Journal of Speech and Hearing Research, 20,* 373–408.

Frable, M. S. (1972). Hoarseness, a symptom of pre-menstrual tension. *Archives of Otolaryngology, 75,* 66–67.

Froeschels, E. (1952). Chewing method as therapy. *Archives of Otolaryngology, 56,* 427–434.

Fujimoto, P. A., Madison, C. L., & Larrigan, L. B. (1991). The effects of a tracheostoma valve on the intelligibility and quality of tracheoesophageal speech. *Journal of Speech and Hearing Research, 34,* 33–36.

Glenn, E. C., Glenn, P. J., & Forman, S. H. (1989). *Your voice and articulation.* Englewood Cliffs, NJ: Prentice Hall.

Gordon, MT. T., Morton, F. M., & Simpson, I. C. (1978). Airflow measurements in diagnosis assessment and treatment of mechanical dysphonia. *Folia Phoniatrica, 30,* 372–379.

Gould, W. J. (1975). Quantitative assessment of voice function in microlaryngology. *Folia Phoniatrica, 27,* 190–200.

Grace, S. G. (1984). Speech pathology: Views from medicine and dentistry. In S. C. McFarlane (Ed.), *Coping with communicative handicaps.* San Diego: College-Hill Press.

Gray, B. B., England, G., & Mahoney, J. L. (1965). Treatment of benign vocal nodules by reciprocal inhibition. *Journal of Behavioral Research Therapy, 3,* 187–193.

Green, G. (1989). Psycho-behavioral characteristics of children with vocal nodules: WPBIC ratings. *Journal of Speech and Hearing Disorders, 54,* 306–312.

Greene, M. C. L. & Mathieson, L. (1980). *The voice and its disorders* (5th ed.). London: Whorr Publishers.

Hardin M. A., Van DeMark, D. R., Morris, H. L., & Payne, M. M. (1992). Correspondence between nasalance scores and listener judgments of hypernasality and hyponasality. *Cleft Palate-Craniofacial Journal, 29,* 346–351.

Hirano, M., (1981). *Clinical examination of the voice.* New York: Springer-Verlag.

Hixon, T. J., & Abss, J. H. (1980). Normal speech production. In T. J. Hixon, L. D. Shriberg, & J. H. Saxman (Eds.), *Introduction to communication disorders.* Englewood Cliffs, NJ: Prentice Hall.

Hixon, T. J., Goldman, M. D., & Mead, J. (1973). Kinematics of the chest wall during speech production: Volume displacements of the rib cage, abdomen, and lung. *Journal of Speech and Hearing Research, 19,* 297–356.

Hixon, T. J., Saxman, J. H., & McQueen, H. D. (1967). The respirometric technique for evaluating velopharyngeal competence during speech. *Folia Phoniatrica, 19,* 203–219.

Hixon, T. J., Watson, P. J., & Maher, M. Z. (1987). Respiratory kinematics in classical (Shakespearean) actors. In T. J. Hixon (Ed.), *Respiratory function in speakers and singers.* Boston: College Hill Division, Little Brown.

Hollien, H. (1962). Vocal fold thickness and fundamental frequency of phonation. *Journal of Speech and Hearing Research, 5,* 237–243.

Hollien, H. (1987). Old voices: What do we really know about them? *Journal of Voice, 1,* 2–17.

Hoshiko, M. S. (1962). Electromyographic investigation of the intercostal muscles during speech. *Archives Physical Medicine & Rehabilitation, 43,* 115–119.

Hull, F. M., Mielke, P. W., Willeford, J. A., & Timmons, R. J. (1976). *National Speech Hearing Survey,* Final Report, Project 50978, Bureau of Education for the Handicapped, U.S. Office of Education, Washington D. C.

Isshiki, N. (1989). Medical displacement of the vocal cord. In *Phonosurgery: Theory and practice* (pp. 77–129). Tokyo: Springer-Verlag.

Isshiki, N., & von Leden, H. (1964). Hoarseness: Aerodynamic studies. *Archives of Otolaryngology, 80,* 206–213.

Izdebski, K., Dedo, H. H., & Boles, L. (1984). Spastic dysphonia: A patient profile of 200 cases. *American Journal of Otolaryngology, 5,* 7–14.

Izdebski, K., Ross, J. C., & Klein, J. C. (1990). Transoral rigid laryngovideostroboscopy (phonoscopy). *Seminars in Speech and Language, 11,* 16–26.

Jacobson, E. (1957). *You must relax.* New York: McGraw-Hill.

Judson, L. S., & Weaver, A. T. (1965). *Voice science.* New York: Appleton-Century-Crofts.

Kahane, J. C. (1983). Postnatal development and aging of the human larynx. *Seminars in Speech and Language, 4,* 189–204.

Kahane, J. C. (1987). Connective tissue changes in the larynx and their effects on voice. *Journal of Voice, 1,* 27–30.

Kantner, C. E. (1947). The rationale of blowing exercises for patients with repaired cleft palates. *Journal of Speech Disorders, 12,* 281–286.

Karnell, M. P. (1992). Adductor and abductor spasmodic dysphonia: Related until proven otherwise. *American Journal of Speech-Language Pathology, 1,* 17–18.

Kleinsasser, O. (1979). *Microlaryngoscopy and endolaryngeal microsurgery: Technique and typical findings.* Baltimore: University Park Press.

Koufman, J. A. (1986). Laryngoplasty for vocal cord medialization: An alternative to Teflon. *Laryngoscope, 96,* 726–731.

Koufman, J. A. (1991). The otolaryngologic manifestations of gastroesophageal reflux disease (GERD), *Laryngoscope, 101,* 1–78.

Laver, J. (1980). *The phonetic description of voice quality.* Cambridge, Eng.: Cambridge University Press.

Lavorato, A.S. (1991). Evaluation and treatment of the professional voice with minimal instrumentation, *Seminars in speech and language, 12,* 154–67.

Lavorato, A. S., & McFarlane, S. C., (1983). Treatment of the professional voice. In W. H. Perkins (Eds.), *Current therapy of communication disorders: Voice disorders.* New York: Thieme-Stratton.

Lavorato, A. S., & McFarlane, S. C. (1988). Counseling clients with voice disorders. *Seminars in Speech and Language, 9,* 237–255.

Lehmann, Q. H. (1965). Reverse phonation: A new maneuver for examining the larynx. *Radiology, 84,* 215–222.

Leeper, H. A. (1976). Voice initiation characteristics of normal children and children with vocal nodules: A preliminary investigation. *Journal of Communication Disorders, 9,* 83–94.

Lim, R. Y. (1985). Laser arytenoidectomy. *Archives of Otolaryngology, 111,* 262–263.

Ling, D. (1976). *Speech and hearing impaired child: Theory and practice.* Washington, DC: Alexander Graham Bell Association for the Deaf.

Linville, S. E. (1987). Acoustic-perceptual studies of aging voice in women. *Journal of Voice, 1,* 44–48.

Luchsinger, R., & Arnold, G. E. (1965). *Voice-speech-language clinical communicology: Its physiology and pathology.* Belmont, CA: Wadsworth.

Ludlow, C. L., Naunton, R. F., Fujita, M., & Sedory, S. E. (1990). Spasmodic dysphonia: Botulinum toxin injection after recurrent nerve surgery. *Otolaryngology Head and Neck Surgery, 102*, 122–131.

Lundquist, P. G., Haglund, S., Carlson, B., Strander, H., & Lundgren, E. (1984). Interferon therapy in juvenile laryngeal papillomatosis. *Otolaryngology Head Neck Surgery, 92*, 386–391.

Martensson, A. (1968). The functional organization of the intrinsic laryngeal muscles. In M. Krauss (Ed.), *Sound production in man* (pp. 91–97). New York: New York Academy of Sciences.

Mason, R. M., & Warren, D. W. (1980). Adenoid involution and developing hypernasality in cleft palate. *Journal of Speech and Hearing Disorders, 45*, 469–480.

Mazaheri, M. (1979). Prosthodontic care. In H. K. Cooper, R. L. Harding, M. M. Krogman, M. Mazaheri, & R. T. Millard (Eds.), *Cleft palate and cleft lip: A team approach.* Philadelphia: Saunders.

McFarlane, S. C. (1988). Treatment of benign laryngeal disorders with traditional methods and techniques of voice therapy. *Ear Nose and Throat I, 67*, 425–435.

McFarlane, S. C. (1989). Combining clinic, teaching, research, and administration. *Seminars in Speech and Language, 10*, 138–144.

McFarlane, S. C. (1990). Videolaryngoendoscopy and voice disorders. *Seminars in Speech and Language, 11*, 162–171.

McFarlane, S. C., & Brophy, J. W. (1992). Effects of drugs on voice. *ASHA Special Interest Division 2: Voice, 2*, 9–10.

McFarlane, S. C., Fujiki, M., & Brinton, B. (1984). *Coping with communicative handicaps: Resources for the practicing clinician.* San Diego, CA: College Hill.

McFarlane, S. C., Holt, T. L., & Lavorato, A. S. (1985). Unilateral cord paralysis: Vocal characteristics following three methods of treatment. *Asha, 27*, 114.

McFarlane, S. C., Holt-Romeo, T. L., Lavorato, A. S., & Warner, L. (1991). Unilateral vocal fold paralysis: Perceived vocal quality following three methods of treatment. *American Journal of Speech-Language Pathology, 1*, 45–48.

McFarlane, S.C. & Lavorato, A.S. (1983). Treatment of psychogenic hyperfunctional voice disorders, in W.H. Perkins (Ed.), *Current therapy of communication disorders: Voice disorders.* New York: Thiene-Stratton, Inc.

McFarlane, S. C., & Lavorato, A. S. (1984). The use of video endoscopy in the evaluation and treatment of dysphonia. *Communicative Disorders, 9*, 117–126.

McFarlane, S. C., & Shipley, K. G. (1979). Spastic dysphonia: Laryngeal stuttering? *Asha, 21*, 710.

McFarlane, S. C., & Watterson, T. L. (1990). Vocal nodules: Endoscopic study of their variations and treatment. *Seminars in Speech and Language, 11*, 47–59.

McFarlane, S. C., & Watterson, T. L. (1991). Clinical use of laryngograph and the electroglottogram (EGG) with voice disordered patients. *Seminars in Speech and Language, 12*, 108–114.

McFarlane, S. C., Watterson, T. L., & Brophy, J. (1990). Transnasal videoendoscopy of the laryngeal mechanisms. *Seminars in Speech and Language, 11*, 8–16.

McGuirt, W. F., & Blalock, D. (1980). The otolaryngologist's role in the diagnosis and treatment of amyotrophic lateral sclerosis. *Laryngoscope, 90*, 1496–1501.

McWilliams, B. J., Lavorato, A. S., & Bluestone, C. D. (1973). Vocal cord abnormalities in children with velopharyngeal valving problems. *Laryngoscope, 83*, 1745–1753.

Michel, J. F., & Wendahl, R. (1971). Correlatives of voice production. In L. E. Travis (Ed.), *Handbook of speech pathology and audiology.* Englewood Cliffs, NJ: Prentice Hall.

Milisen, R. (1957). Methods of evaluation and diagnosis of speech disorders. In L. E. Travis (Ed.), *Handbook of speech pathology.* New York: Appleton-Century-Crofts.

Minifie, F. D. (1973). Speech acoustics. In F. D. Minifie, T. J. Hixon, & F. Williams (Eds.), *Normal aspects of speech, hearing, and language.* Englewood Cliffs, NJ: Prentice Hall.

Minifie, F. D. (1984). In V. L. Lawrence (Ed.), *Transcripts of the eleventh symposium: Care of the professional voice.* New York: Voice Foundation.

Miyazaki, T., Matsuya, T., & Yamaoka, M. (1975). Fiberscopic methods for assessment of velopharyngeal closure during various activities. *Cleft Palate Journal, 12*, 107–114.

Modisett, N. F., & Luter, J. G. (1984). *Speaking clearly: The basics of voice and articulation* (2nd ed.). Minneapolis: Burgess.

Moll, K. L. (1968). Speech characteristics of individuals with cleft lip and palate. In D. C. Spriestersbach & D. Sherman (Eds.), *Cleft palate and communication.* New York: Harper & Row.

Moncur, J. P., & Brackett, I. P. (1974). *Modifying vocal behavior.* New York: Harper & Row.

Monsen, R. B. (1976). Second formant transitions in the speech of deaf and normal-hearing children. *Journal of Speech and Hearing Research, 19*, 279–289.

Monsen, R. B., Engebretson, A. M., & Vernula, N. R. (1979). Some effects of degrees on the generation of voice. *Journal of Acoust. Soc. Amer., 66*, 1680–1690.

Moolenaar-Bijl, A. (1953). The importance of certain consonants in esophageal voice after laryngectomy. *Annals of Otolaryngology, Rhinology, and Laryngology, 62*, 979–989.

Moore, G. P., & von Leden, H. (1958). Dynamic variations of the vibratory pattern in the normal larynx. *Folia Phoniatrica, 10*, 205–238.

Morris, H. L., & Smith, J. K. (1962). A multiple approach for evaluating velopharyngeal competency. *Journal of Speech and Hearing Disorders, 27*, 218–226.

Moses, P. J. (1954). *Voice of neurosis.* New York: Grune & Stratton.

Murphy, A. T. (1964). *Functional voice disorders.* Englewood Cliffs, NJ: Prentice Hall.

Murry, T. (1992). Prolongation of Botox results by voice therapy. *Neurogenic vs. Psychogenic Dysphonias: Differential Diagnosis & Management.* San Francisco: Pacific Voice Conference.

Murry, T. & Doherty, E. T. (1980). Selected acoustic characteristics of pathologic and normal speakers. *Journal of Speech and Hearing Research, 23*, 361–369.

Myers, E. N., & Suen, J. Y. (Eds.). (1989). *Cancer of the head and neck.* New York: Churchill Livingstone.

Nation, J. E., & Aram, D. M. (1977). *Diagnosis of speech and language disorders.* St. Louis: Mosby.

Negus, V. E. (1957). The mechanism of the larynx. *Laryngoscope, 67*, 961–986.

Netsell, R. (1973). Speech physiology. In F. D. Minifie, T. J. Hixon, & F. Williams (Eds.), *Normal aspects of speech, hearing, and language.* Englewood Cliffs, NJ: Prentice Hall.

Netsell, R., & Hixon, T. J. (1978). A noninvasive method for clinically estimating subglottal air pressure. *Journal of Speech and Hearing Disorders, 43*, 326–330.

Newby, H. A. (1972). *Audiology.* New York: Appleton-Century-Crofts.

Newcombe, P. J. (1986). *Voice and diction.* Raleigh, NC: Contemporary.

Offer, D. (1980). Normal adolescent development. In H. I. Kaplan, A. M. Freedman, & B. J. Sadock (Eds.), *Comprehensive textbook of psychiatry* (3rd ed.). Baltimore: Williams & Wilkins.

Otis, A. B., & Clark, R. G. (1968). Ventilatory implications of phonation and phonatory implications of ventilation. In M. Krauss (Ed.), *Sound production in man* (pp. 122–238). New York: New York Academy of Sciences.

Pauloski, B. R., Fisher, H. B., Kempster, G. B., & Bloom, E. D. (1989). Statistical differentiation of tracheoesophageal speech produced under four prosthetic/occlusion speaking conditions. *Journal of Speech and Hearing Research, 32,* 591–599.

Paynter, E. T. (1991). Phonatory function analyzer. *Seminars in Speech and Language, 12,* 98–107.

Pearl, N. B., & McCall, G. N. (1986). *Laryngeal function during two types of whisper: A fiberoptic study.* Paper presented at ASHA convention, Detroit.

Perkins, W. H. (1971). Vocal function: Assessment and therapy. In L. E. Travis (Ed.), *Handbook of speech pathology and audiology* (pp. 122–238). Englewood Cliffs, NJ: Prentice Hall.

Perkins, W. H. (1977). *Speech pathology, an applied behavioral science* (2nd ed.). St. Louis: Mosby.

Perkins, W. H. (1983). Optimal use of voice: Prevention of chronic vocal abuse. *Seminars in Speech and Language, 4,* 273–286.

Pershall, K. E., & Boone, D. R. (1986). A video-endoscopic and computerized tomographic study of hypopharyngeal and supraglottic activity during assorted vocal tasks. In V. Lawrence (Ed.), *Transcripts of the Fourteenth Symposium: Care of the Professional Voice.* New York: Voice Foundation.

Peterson, G. E., & Barney, H. L. (1952). Control methods used in a study of the vowels. *Journal of Acoustical Society, 24,* 175–184.

Prasad, U. (1985). CO2 surgical laser in the management of bilateral vocal cord paralysis. *Journal of Laryngology and Otology, 99,* 891–894.

Ptacek, P. H., & Sander, E. K. (1963). Maximum duration of phonation. *Journal of Speech and Hearing Disorders, 28,* 171–182.

Rubin, H. J., & Hirt, C. C. (1960). The falsetto, a high speed cinematographic study. *Laryngoscope, 70,* 1305–1324.

Salmon, S. (1986). Adjusting to laryngectomy. *Seminars in Speech and Language, 7,* 67–93.

Sansone, F. E., & Emanuel, F. W. (1970). Spectral noise levels and roughness severity ratings for normal and simulated rough vowels produced by adult males. *Journal of Speech and Hearing Research, 13,* 489–502.

Sataloff, R. T. (1981). Professional singers: The science and art of clinical care. *American Journal of Otolaryngology, 2,* 251–266.

Schramm, V. L., May, M., & Lavorato, A. S. (1978). Gelfoam paste injection for vocal cord paralysis: Temporary rehabilitation of glottic incompetence. *Laryngoscope, 88,* 1268–1273.

Seashore, C. E., Lewis, E., & Saetvuit, J. G. (1980). *Manual of instruction and interpretations for the Seashore Measures of Musical Talent.* New York: Psychological Corp.

Sever, J. C. (1982). An introduction to objective acoustic analyses of the voice. In M. D. Filter, (Ed.), *Phonatory voice disorders in children.* Springfield, IL: Charles C. Thomas.

Shanks, J. C. (1986). Evoking esophageal voice. In J. C. Shanks (Ed.), *strategies of rehabilitation of the laryngectomized patient.* New York: Thieme.

Shedd, D. P., & Weinberg, B. (1960). *Surgical and prosthetic approaches to speech rehabilitation.* Boston: Hall.

Shelton, R. L., Hahn, E., & Morris, H. L. (1968). Diagnosis and therapy. In D. C. Spriestersbach & D. Sherman (Eds.), *Cleft palate and communication.* New York: Academic Press.

Shelton, R. L., Paesani, A., McClelland, K. D., & Bradfield, S. S. (1975). Panendoscopic feedback in the study of voluntary velopharyngeal movements. *Journal of Speech and Hearing Disorders, 40,* 232–243.

Shelton, R. L., & Trier, W. C. (1976). Issues involved in the evaluation of velopharyngeal closure. *Cleft Palate Journal, 13,* 127–137.

Sherman, D. (1954). The merits of backward playing of connected speech in the scaling of voice quality disorders. *Journal of Speech and Hearing Disorders, 19,* 312–321.

Shipp, T., Mueller, P., & Zwitman, D. (1980). Letter: Intermittent abductory dysphonia. *Journal of Speech Hearing Disorders, 45,* 283.

Shipp, T., QI, Y., Huntley, R., & Hollien, H. (1992). Acoustic and temporal correlates of perceived age. *Journal of Voice, 6,* 211–216.

Shulman, S. (1991) Voice therapy for spasmodic dysphonia. *Proceedings of the Fourth Annual Pacific Voice Conference.* San Francisco.

Singer, M. I., & Blom, E. D. (1980). An endoscopic technique for restoring voice after laryngectomy. *Annals of Otolaryngology, Rhinology, and Laryngology, 89,* 529–533.

Skolnick, M. L., Glaser, E. R., & McWilliams, B. J. (1980). The use and limitations of the barium pharyngogram in the detection of velopharyngeal insufficiency. *Radiology, 135,* 301–304.

Sloane, H. N., & MacAulay, B. D. (1968). *Operant procedures in remedial speech and language training.* Boston: Houghton Mifflin.

Spriestersbach, D. C. (1955). Assessing nasal quality in cleft palate speech of children. *Journal Speech and Hearing Disorders, 20,* 266–270.

Staats, A. (1968). *Learning, language, and cognition.* New York: Holt, Rinehart, & Winston.

Stetson, R. H. (1937). Can all laryngectomized patients be taught esophageal speech? *Transactions of American Laryngological Association, 59,* 59–71.

Stone, R. E. (1982). Management of childhood dysphonias of organic bases. In M. D. Filter (Ed.), *Phonatory voice disorders in children.* Springfield, IL: Charles C. Thomas.

Stroebel, C. (1983). *Quieting reflex training for adults.* New York: BMA Audio Cassettes.

Strome, M. (1982). Common laryngeal disorders in children. In M. D. Filter (Ed.), *Phonatory voice disorders in children.* Springfield, IL: Charles C. Thomas.

Tait, N. A., Michel, J. F., & Carpenter, M. A. (1980). Maximum duration of sustained /s/ and /z/ in children. *Journal of Speech and Hearing Disorders, 45,* 239–246.

Takahashi, H., & Koike, Y. (1975). Some perceptual dimensions and acoustical correlates of pathologic voices. *Acta Oto-Laryngologica, 338,* 1–24.

Templin, M. C., & Darley, F. L. (1980). *The Templin-Darley Tests of Articulation.* Iowa City: Bureau of Educational Research and Service.

Thompson, A. E. (1978). *Nasal air flow during normal speech production.* Unpublished Master's Thesis, University of Arizona, Tucson.

Thurman, W. L. (1958). Intensity relationships and optimum pitch level. *Journal of Speech and Hearing Research 1,* 117–123.

Toohill, R. J. (1975). The psychosomatic aspects of children with vocal nodules. *Archives of Otolaryngology 101,* 591–595.

Tucker, H. M. (1980). Vocal cord paralysis—1979: Etiology and management. *Laryngoscope, 90,* 585–590.

Tucker, H. M., Wood, B. G., Levine, H., & Katz, R. (1979). Glottic reconstruction after near total laryngectomy. *Laryngoscope, 89,* 609–618.

Tyler, A. A., & Watterson, T. L. (1991). VOT as an indirect measure of laryngeal function. *Seminars in Speech and Language, 12,* 131–141.

Van den Berg, J. W. (1968). Register problems. In M. Krauss (Ed.), *Sound production in man.* New York: New York Academy of Sciences.

Warren, D. W. (1979). PERCI: A method for rating palatal efficiency. *Cleft Palate Journal, 16,* 279–285.

Watterson, T., Hansen-Magorian, H., & McFarlane, S. C. (1990). A demographic description of laryngeal contact ulcer patients. *Journal of Voice, 4,* 71–75.

Watterson, T., & McFarlane, S. C. (1992). Adductor and abductor spasmodic dysphonia: Different disorders. *American Journal of Speech-Language Pathology, 1,* 19–20.

Watterson, T., McFarlane, S. C., & Diamond, K. L. (1993). Phoneme effects on vocal effort and vocal quality, *American Journal of Speech-Language Pathology, 2,* 74–78.

Watterson, T., McFarlane, S. C., & Menicucci, A. (1990). Vibratory characteristics of Teflon-injected and noninjected paralyzed vocal folds. *Journal of Speech and Hearing Disorders, 55,* 61–66.

Watterson, T., McFarlane, S. C., & Wright, D. (1993). Nasalance (nasometer), nasality and speech intelligibility. *Journal of Communication Disorders, 26,* 13–28.

Watterson, T. L., & McFarlane, S. C. (1991). Transoral and transnasal laryngeal endoscopy, *Seminars in Speech and Language, 12,* 77–87.

Watterson, T. L., McFarlane, S. C., & Brophy, J. W. (1990). Some issues and ethics in oral and nasal videoendoscopy. *Seminars in Speech and Language, 11,* 1–7.

Watterson, T. L. (1991). Current trends in voice evaluation. *Seminars in Speech and Language, 12,* 57–64.

Watterson, T. L., & McFarlane, S. C. (1990). Transnasal videoendoscopy of the velopharyngeal port mechanism. *Seminars in Speech and Language, 11,* 27–37.

Watson, P. J., & Hixon, T. J. (1985). Respiratory kinematics in classical (opera) singers. *Journal of Speech and Hearing Research, 28,* 104–122.

Weber, R. S., Neumayer, L., Alford, B. R, & Weber, S. C. (1984). Clinical restoration of voice function after loss of the vagus nerve. *Head and Neck Surgery, 7,* 448–457.

Wetmore, S. J., Key, J. M., & Suen, J. Y. (1985). Complications of laser surgery for laryngeal papillomatosis. *Laryngoscope, 95,* 798–801.

Whited, R. E. (1979). Laryngeal dysfunction following prolonged intubation. *Annals of Otolaryngology, Rhinology, and Laryngology, 89,* 474–478.

Williams, T. T., Farquarson, I. M., & Anthony, J. (1975). Fiberoptic laryngoscopy in the assessment of laryngeal disorder. *Journal of Laryngology, 89,* 299–306.

Williamson, A. B. (1945). Diagnosis and treatment of seventy-two cases of hoarse voice. *Quarterly Journal of Speech, 31,* 189–202.

Wilson, D. K. (1987). *Voice problems of children* (3rd ed.). Baltimore: Williams & Wilkins.

Wilson, F. B., Oldring, D. J., & Mueller, J. (1980). Recurrent laryngeal nerve dissection: A case report involving return of spastic dysphonia after initial surgery. *Journal of Speech and Hearing Disorders, 45,* 112–118.

Wilson, F. B., & Rice, M. (1977). *A programmed approach to voice therapy.* Austin, TX: Learning Concepts.

Wolpe, J. (1987). *Essential principles and practices of behavior therapy.* Phoenix: Milton H. Erickson Foundation.

Yamaguchi, H., Yotsukura, Y., Kondo, R., Hanyuu, Y., Horiguchi, S., Imaizumi, S., & Hirose, H. (1986). Nonsurgical therapy for vocal nodules. *Folia Phoniatrica, 38,* 372–373.

Yanagihara, N. Y., & von Leden, H. (1967). Respiration and phonation. *Folia Phoniatrica, 19,* 153–166.

Yates, A., & Dedo, H. H. (1984). Carbon dioxide laser enucleation of polypoid vocal cords. *Laryngoscope, 94,* 731–736.

Zemlin, W. R. (1988). *Speech and hearing science* (3rd ed.). Englewood Cliffs, NJ: Prentice Hall.

Zwitman, D. H. (1990). Utilization of transoral endoscopy to assess velopharyngeal closure. *Seminars in speech and language, 11,* 38–46.

Zwitman, D. H., Gyepes, M. T., & Ward, P. H. (1976). Assessment of velar and lateral wall movement by oral telescope and radiographic examination in patients with velopharyngeal inadequacy and in normal subjects. *Journal of Speech and Hearing Disorders, 41,* 381–389.

Zwitman, D. H., Sonderman, J. C., & Ward, P. H. (1974). Variations in velopharyngeal closure assessed by endoscopy. *Journal of Speech and Hearing Disorders, 39,* 366–372.

VOICE INSTRUMENTATION

Artic Arion Products, 1022 Nicollet Avenue, Minneapolis, MN 55043.

B & K Real-Time Frequency Analyzer, Bruel & Kjaer, Naerum, Denmark.

Echorder and Echordette, RIL Electronics, Inc., Street Road and Second Street Pike, Southhampton, PA 18966.

Language Master, Bell and Howell, Co., 7100 N. McCormick Road, Chicago, IL.

Nasometer, Kay Elemetrics Corp., Pinebrook, NJ 07058.

Phonatory Function Analyzer, PS-77, Nagashima Medical Instruments, Richmond VA. Kelleher Medical Instruments.

Phonic Ear Vois, H.C. Electronics, Inc., 250 Camino Alto, Mill Valley, CA 94941.

PM 100 Pitch Analyzer, Kay Elemetrics Corp., Pinebrook, NJ.

Tonar II. This instrument, developed by S.G. Fletcher in 1970, is no longer commercially available.

Tunemaster III, Berkshire Instruments, Inc., 170 Chestnut Street, Ridgewood, NJ 07450.

Visi-Pitch, Model 6087, Kay Elemetrics Corp., Pinebrook, NJ 07058.

Vocaid, Texas Instruments, Communication Builders, PO Box 42030, Tucson, AZ 85733.

Vocal Loudness Indicator, LinguiSystems, Suite 806, 1630 Fifth Avenue, Moline, IL 61265.

Voice Monitor, Communication Research Unit, Hollins College, Hollins, VA.

Index

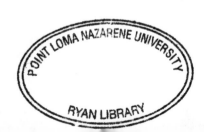